D0782281

THE ESTROGEN ERRORS

THE ESTROGEN ERRORS

Why Progesterone Is Better for Women's Health

Susan Baxter, PhD, and Jerilynn C. Prior, MD

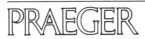

Westport, Connecticut
London

Library of Congress Cataloging-in-Publication Data

Baxter, Susan, 1954–
    The estrogen errors : why progesterone is better for women's health / Susan Baxter and
Jerilynn C. Prior.
        p.   cm.
    Includes bibliographical references and index.
    ISBN 978–0–313–35398–7 (alk. paper)
    1. Menopause—Hormone therapy–United States.   2. Progesterone—Therapeutic use—United
States.   3. Perimenopause—Hormone therapy—United States.   I. Prior, Jerilynn C., 1943–   II. Title.
    RG186.B39   2009
    618.1′75061—dc22   2008046772

British Library Cataloguing in Publication Data is available.

Library of Congress Catalog Card Number: 2008046772
ISBN: 978–0–313–35398–7

First published in 2009

Praeger Publishers, 88 Post Road West, Westport, CT 06881
An imprint of Greenwood Publishing Group, Inc.
www.praeger.com

Printed in the United States of America

The paper used in this book complies with the
Permanent Paper Standard issued by the National
Information Standards Organization (Z39.48–1984).

10 9 8 7 6 5 4 3 2 1

Contents

FOREWORD

Susan Baxter, PhD

The overarching theme . . . is authority—the authority of medicine. This authority is not the same as that of your physician. Rather, the authority of which I speak belongs to the institution of medicine, the organizational structure to which your physician must conform. To paraphrase Robespierre, institutions are born to die; it is the people who are born to live. The twentieth century has witnessed the birth of two institutions of medicine: the first elevated medicine to be the arbiter of normalcy; the second superimposed the trappings of enterprise and created the "health care delivery system."

—N. M. Hadler[1]

Since the turn of the twentieth century, gynecologists (the de facto authorities on women's health) and other experts on women's reproductive health have been convinced that without estrogen a woman just isn't a woman. Menopause, therefore, was a disease, an "estrogen-deficiency disease," for which the cure was obviously estrogen. Unfortunately, estrogen "replacement" therapy, or ERT, was discovered to cause endometrial cancer in women going through a natural menopause, first clinically and later with the PEPI trial.[2] So a dash of progestin (a synthetic form of progesterone) was added to the popular, best-selling estrogen pill (Premarin, made from the urine of pregnant mares) in the lowest dose possible, and the term became hormone replacement therapy or HRT.

The problem was that even though hundreds of thousands of women were being prescribed hormones, nobody had actually *tested* them. So, in the mid-1990s, the Women's Health Initiative (WHI) was set up under the auspices of the National Institutes of Health (at a time when its director was a woman, for some reason) to confirm what everyone knew in their heart of hearts[3] to be true, namely, that HRT would ward off all the evils of old age, from heart disease to dementia, and keep women youthful, healthy, taut, and unwrinkled. Nearly seventeen thousand women, therefore, were followed through the years, half of whom were given the standard hormone regimen and the other half, a placebo.

Then the unthinkable happened. It had always been known that hormones could increase a woman's risk of breast cancer, but what the WHI began to show was the risk was a lot higher than anyone had thought. Plus, *hormones didn't work.* It was the women taking the placebo who were healthier and not suffering from heart attacks and strokes, blood clots and cancer. The trial was stopped early, in 2002,[4] and the WHI made international headlines.

FIRST ENCOUNTERS OF A SURREAL KIND

I first encountered the idea of HRT in 1995, when the editor of a woman's magazine I wrote for asked me to write an article on the subject.[5] The editor and I were both in our thirties, and we figured it would be a quick job. I would research the basics, interview a few doctors, a few women, write up the plusses and minuses (maybe in a box)—the piece would practically write itself.

My first interview was with a gynecologist, a very pleasant man, who patiently explained to me that when a woman took hormones at menopause, all she was doing was "replacing" the hormones her body no longer made. The same way a diabetic had to take insulin or someone with an underactive thyroid took thyroxine. It just made sense.

Except it doesn't.

As the next doctor I spoke to, Vancouver endocrinologist Jerilynn C. Prior, explained, unless your menopause is prematurely early or you've had a hysterectomy, it is perfectly *normal* for the ovaries to reduce the level of hormones at midlife. Jerilynn further blew my uninformed mind by asking me how it was possible to consider hormone therapy a "replacement" when every single woman's hormones *naturally* waned as she got older. "You and I have no choice in the matter," she pointed out. Well, no, we didn't. Plus, women naturally have *two* hormones that balance each other out during each menstrual cycle: estrogen and progesterone. Yet somehow, the only hormone we seemed to care about was estrogen—and even when we added progesterone (as progestin, a synthetic variant), the amount was only about a quarter of what it should have been.

Yet as every first-year physiology student knows, our hormones ebb and flow during each normal menstrual cycle: during the first half of the cycle, leading up to ovulation, estrogen increases. Then, once the egg is released midcycle, progesterone rises, clearing the thickened endometrial lining that estrogen has made (in preparation for a possible pregnancy) and sets the scene for the new cycle to begin. Moreover, although both hormones start low and move up, when progesterone reaches its peak, it is nearly fifteen hundred times *more* than estrogen—so if we were intent on elevating one hormone over another, shouldn't that be progesterone?

How did progesterone get lost in all this?

NATURAL BALANCE

It was when I wrote a book on the immune system that I first realized just how warped and Western our concepts and heuristics in physiology and medicine are.[6] The same metaphors that we use for politics, economics, commerce, war, and everything else permeate our concepts of health and disease—except we don't know that; we just tell ourselves this is how things are, the way of the world, truth. Of course we've used that line to justify pretty much everything, from colonialism to slavery.

We valorize strength, size, and heft, so we spend untold amounts of money on arcane nutrients to strengthen our immune systems or enhance functioning. We are particularly fond of anything that will strengthen our body's defenses, never mind that an immune system that's too powerful can also cause damage. Autoimmune diseases such as lupus or rheumatoid arthritis are the result of an immune system spiraling out of control, like a boxer unaware of his own strength. These illnesses create excess scar tissue, fibrosis, and inflammation, which in turn can lead to crippling symptoms, or even death, if they strike a vital organ. What our military metaphors ignore is that having the capacity to destroy does not necessarily make something *good*, or an ally.

In fact, if our expressions and concepts actually reflected how the immune system really works, we would aim for something that would calm the immune system, because even a cold is the result of an overreactive immune system—probably fatigued by life stressors—overresponding to one of the many viruses always present. It is the immune *reaction* that results in the sore throat and sneezing, not the virus. But we think of our bodies as mini armies fighting the invader, as though a virus or bacterium is an enemy versus an ever-present (and often useful) aspect of all physiologic systems.* We are also fond of quantity: if something is good, then more has to be better—which means we use antibiotics and other drugs in higher amounts and potencies than anybody else in the world. (This explains why antibiotic-resistant bacteria run rampant in all our hospitals.) Common dosages for even an aspirin are almost twice as high in North America as they are in Europe.[7]

---

*So we take antibiotics, which kill all the bacteria—and attempt to put them back with probiotic yogurt.

Nowhere is this idea of nuance and balance more important than our reproductive hormones. Our monthly cycle is a subtle dance between estrogen and progesterone, one descending as the other rises—and nowhere is this idea of equilibrium more thoroughly ignored than in our fascination with estrogen. What is particularly odd is that during *perimenopause*, the transition into menopause still erroneously referred to as the "menopausal transition," a time when some 20 percent of women are highly symptomatic with night sweats, migraines, and depression, estrogen levels are actually often sky-high, and it is progesterone levels that are low. Yet since the early years of the twentieth century, any symptoms during this time are blamed on low estrogen.

Of course, part of our love affair with estrogen probably also had something to do with the fact that estrogen was conceptualized sooner and was more easily synthesized (from those pregnant mares' urine) and used commercially before natural progesterone.

UNCERTAINTY, AMBIGUITY, AND DOUBT

Much as we would like to believe that medicine and medical science deal in facts and truth—and that all those marvelous therapeutic interventions, such as quadruple bypass surgery, CT scans, and high-tech drugs, are the result of painstaking science (done by saintly scientists eager to do good)—the reality is that expedience, economics, serendipity, accidents of fate, turf wars, and a host of very human activities go into what we call scientific medicine, and hormones are no exception. Since the nineteenth century, when it was first discovered that these potent glandular secretions existed within the body, the endocrinology of women's hormones has been influenced by factors encompassing everything from the (often nonexistent) status of women within society to war, commerce, culture, politics, and social norms, in particular what it meant to be a woman (fertile).

As you will read in the Afterword, for Jerilynn Prior our preoccupation with estrogen is virtually a conspiracy, focused, pointed, pernicious, and, in all fairness, had I spent my entire career as she did, within this blatant hormone bias, I might agree. But my area of expertise is completely different: I deal in the critical, interdisciplinary analysis of medicine and clinical practice, concepts based in social science, clinical epidemiology, health economics, communications science, and history.

From my perspective, the estrogen debacle is part of a pattern. Over the years, there have been hundreds, if not thousands, of instances where medicine has lumbered on in spite of mounting evidence that various practices were not only not useful, but downright dangerous. When polio was common, Kenny packs were routinely used in hospitals to prevent paralysis. Nobody knew why some children ended up crippled, and those hot packs, pioneered by an Australian nurse (played by Rosalind Russell in the movie) were thought to help, which, as it turned out, they did not.[8] They even made the condition worse—and although doctors and nurses had suspected this for years, nobody said anything because they weren't sure, and it just didn't seem right to *deprive* children of something that could be beneficial. Or take radical mastectomies, which were the standard of care in treating breast cancer for years, long after many clinicians (and patients) had realized that this mutilating surgery did not save lives. One physician in particular, Oliver Cope, tried for years to publish his observations; no medical journal would touch his work. Finally, he ended up writing a piece in a women's magazine. Gradually, word did get out, women began demanding lumpectomies, and the practice died out. But it goes on. Even as we speak, opioids are being used to treat nerve pain, even though it has been known for years that the excruciating pain of shingles or an amputation requires a drug that affects the nerves, like gabapentin. A reaction to antibiotics or morphine ten days after surgery is persistently called "postoperative" delirium even though neither the timing nor symptoms fit. Drugs, tests, stents, and other technologies are used even though there is no evidence that they work. The list goes on.

SHIFTING MEDICAL DOGMA (OR AN OIL TANKER)

In medicine and science, knowledge is always changing, but every generation believes they have it right. Beliefs become entrenched and dogmatic; expert knowledge becomes insistent and resistant to change—even though true science is supposed to be characterized by doubt, new paths forged from the old, never rigid or static.[9] Newtonian physics made way for Einstein and quantum physics, even as other explanations of the universe fell by the wayside.

Medicine is enormous, however, like an oil tanker carried along by its own momentum, route, and rationale. Change requires time and effort. It's a tanker, remember: massive, propelled by forces like money and power as well as years of practice, and people. People repeating what they were taught, what was done before. Women, furthermore, have not had much of a voice, and anything outside of reproduction has only recently been included in women's health issues. With this book, I hope that we can at least radio that tanker, let it know that it might be heading in the wrong direction. As with radical mastectomies and AIDS and other things where people made a difference, I am hoping that the women who read this, along with their primary care physicians, will weigh the evidence and shift women's health in the right direction.

We are inundated with health information these days, on the Internet, on TV, on radio, and in newspapers and magazines. Everywhere you look, someone is telling you what to check for and how to stay proactive. It's a full-time job, really. We are told to get our blood pressure and lipid levels checked to prevent cardiovascular disease; then we need to do all that screening: mammograms and bone density scans and colonoscopies. Then there's glucose and type 2 diabetes, which shrill headlines tell us is now an epidemic. What they omit to mention is that we have no idea whether any of these biomarkers, numbers like the ones used to determine cholesterol or glucose levels, are actually connected to any disease, because any evidence comes from large-scale, population-based epidemiological studies, and all those can show are correlations, not cause. What we are also not told is just how much such advice is driven by commerce.[10] Those expert panels that tell us what our ideal blood pressure or glucose should be meet up at posh hotels that are paid for by the same drug companies whose products we are told to take if our numbers don't measure up. Given how little we actually know about physiology, my overwhelming sense is one of caution.

Don't get me wrong: I'm no medical nihilist. If I fall off a ladder and hear something go crunch, or if a friend is doubled over with abdominal pain, I'm heading to the ER. Western medicine does very well much of the time, with acute care, trauma, and so on. But it doesn't have the best track record when it comes to figuring out *why* we get sick. The sad truth is that good health often has nothing to do with medicine; it is related to socioeconomic factors and whether we have enough money and are happy with our jobs and our lives.[11] In any event, it is one thing to suggest that people wear seatbelts or use bicycle helmets, what is called *passive prevention*; it is quite another to tell people to take drugs or have surgery—like a quadruple coronary bypass—"just in case." As the guru of evidence-based medicine, Dr. David Sackett, once wrote, such advice is not only arrogant, but presumptuous and overbearing: chasing people who feel perfectly well and telling them what to do to stay healthy.[12]

A case in point is estrogen.

For years we were authoritatively told to take estrogen because we became es- trogen "deficient" at menopause. Ironically, during perimenopause, the transition into menopause during which some of us have symptoms, it is not estrogen levels that are low, but *progesterone*. Although precisely what causes the hot flushes and night sweats and migraines and insomnia—all of which both Jerilynn Prior and I understand because we both went through it (much to our own astonishment)— remains a mystery.

A DIFFICULT PERIMENOPAUSE

Somewhere in my early forties, years before I had even considered peri- menopause, I began to have problems with my cycle: excess bleeding, night sweats, constant migraines, PMS (which I had never had, to the point where

I was one of those nauseating people who actually wasn't sure it existed), even mood and concentration.

As a writer, my ability to concentrate is key, and suddenly I couldn't focus. It felt as though I was coming down with something or as if there was a transparent film between me and the world. I had always disliked hot weather, but now it seemed as though heat was following me, like that Pig Pen character in *Peanuts* with the cloud of dirt. My sleep became fitful and disturbed. Never a good sleeper at the best of times, now I not only had trouble falling asleep, but would wake up umpteen times a night—feeling almost claustrophobic as well as hot. Almost without conscious thought, I would find myself up and moving, usually toward an open window. I recalled that my mother had also had similar symptoms, although later, in her fifties. She hadn't taken anything, but then, she hates taking pills.

For me, the solution was to take 300 mg of Prometrium (a bioidentical proges-terone) at bedtime. This, incidentally, is not some alternative product you send away for on the Internet; you get a prescription from your doctor. These little round capsules allowed me to get on with my life—balanced out what clearly were high levels of estrogen (the daily migraines were a clue: estrogen causes mi-graines). The bonus was that they also helped with deep sleep; in fact, the main side effect of progesterone is drowsiness, which is why you take it at night.[13]

I dug up the article I had written years before—the one where I had interviewed Jerilynn Prior—and reread my own advice. I also attended a lecture Jerilynn gave (one of my students at the university told me about it). She had handouts— updated, similar ones are reproduced at the end of the book in the appendices— and I eagerly took a few. Over the next few months, I faxed, photocopied, or e-mailed these handouts to countless women, from friends to casual acquaintances to virtual strangers, like the woman who came to measure my windows for blinds. All of these women were going through something similar, and none of them knew what to do, particularly because being told that low estrogen was the problem simply *felt* wrong. Women know what high estrogen feels like—with birth control pills, for instance. It's sore breasts and headaches, anxiety and bloating. It made intuitive and physiologic sense to all of us that during perimenopause estrogen was high and we needed progesterone. Various women asked me what to tell their doctors because most of them had gone to medical school at a time when it was all about estrogen, and it became patently clear that women needed a book on perimenopause and progesterone. It took me a few years, but here it is.

A GUIDE FOR WOMEN AND DOCTORS

When I convinced Debbie Carvalko, my editor at Praeger, that this would make a terrific book, it made sense to invite Jerilynn Prior to come on board. What

Jerilynn doesn't know about the endocrinology of women's hormones clinically isn't worth knowing, particularly on progesterone (and perimenopause). She is also a tireless researcher whose work has been published in prestigious journals like *The New England Journal of Medicine* and the *Annals of Internal Medicine*. She is a full professor at the Faculty of Medicine at the University of British Columbia and has long been an advocate and voice for women's health. She created the "Daily Menopause Diary" (which I convinced the editor to run in 1995) and has spent years trying to include women's experiences of perimenopause and menopause in the narrative. She has been a pioneer and a maverick and that's not an easy role. Questioning current medical dogma is difficult.

It seemed, moreover, that our combined expertise would make for a better book. Jerilynn knows hormones inside and out, and I understand medicine, at a time when most of medicine (and medical writing) is reductionist and piecemeal. As Bruno Latour, the philosopher of science, has said, we tend not to examine complicated subjects too closely today; we "black box" them.[14] Much as we do with a computer, where we focus on input and output, and everything else is just a black box where mysterious things happen that normal people don't understand. Except with medicine it is vital that normal people *do* understand, because nobody has the same vested interest in your health as you do. As they used to say, the doctor may be the expert on the illness, but you are the expert on the patient.

In my career as a medical writer, I spoke to hundreds, if not thousands, of doctors, nurses, patients, policymakers, and others; wrote detailed stories on every disease and condition you can think of and one thing I realized early on was that the one thing we all need in our dealings with medicine is *caution.* Medical advice is flung at us from all sides—a lot of it in bullet form, and most of it emphasizing the so-called magic of medicine. But magic, as the late media critic Neil Postman said, evokes wonder, not understanding,[15] and that is not useful when it comes to making medical decisions. People are confused about medicine, and with good reason. One minute, coffee gives you cancer; the next, it prevents heart disease. "Ideal" blood pressure changes from one day to the next. There is a great deal of information—unfortunately, most of it is wrong.

I have enormous respect for the ability of the lay public to understand complex medical subjects. Throughout my career I have spent many years describing complicated subjects—from the possible neural basis for clinical depression to the intricate workings of the immune system or CD4 cells in AIDS—to all kinds of people. I have always found that if I explain things well (if I understand it myself, in other words), nobody has any trouble. Unfortunately, we only get half the story much of the time, and what we are told is tainted by vested interests—from drug companies trying to promote their drugs to research labs touting their work (and trying to raise funds). So we overfocus on the "miraculous" and sensational,[16] whether it is genes or transplants, and underexplain the basics such as hormones or cardiac function. The hapless reader or patient is inundated with jargon and inappropriately complicated language even as the authority of medicine, as the quote at the start of this chapter explained, moves away from individuals and toward rules, guidelines, and impersonal advice.[17]

In this book, I hope to provide women (and their physicians) with the intellectual framework to comprehend their hormones. I am hoping to give women the confidence to ask more questions and, most important, to say no. Finally, this book is an attempt to explode the estrogen myth and explain how daft it is to discuss hormones so one-sidedly—because too many women just don't know, even if the WHI did make headlines (for five minutes).

THE MYTHS CARRY ON

A few months ago, I was at a meeting in California. I chatted with a few women during the break and casually mentioned that I was writing this book. These three attractive, bright, clearly capable women converged on me with questions. Should they take "HRT?" Wasn't it good for the heart or something? More important, they had heard that taking hormones kept you young—and living in Los Angeles, this meant a lot (well, if it was true).

The myth that estrogen keeps you young was promulgated in the 1960s with a book called *Feminine Forever*. In fact, a lot of the nonsense about estrogen that is still around came from this one book. Written by a gynecologist, supported by a drug company (the same company that makes Premarin), it started an estrogen narrative that just refuses to die.[18]

Alas, there is no elixir of youth; time touches us all. (As the poet W. H. Auden once said, "Time will say nothing but I told you so.") We all change with time. We were once little girls, then it was puberty, and then the menstrual years, followed by perimenopause, menopause, and beyond, when hormones settle back down to the same level as when we were girls. Each of these stages has its own character and hormone profile; each is natural at its time. What is important is not the hormones per se, but our progression as individuals, educationally, socially, personally, and even economically, because the single biggest predictor of health is socioeconomic status: having enough money and a job we like[19]—something women are still not always able to have.

This book combines the joint expertise of two very different slants on medicine: Jerilynn is a physician, an endocrinologist, a sub-subspecialist. Her knowledge has depth, whereas my strength is breadth, notably with respect to health and medicine. So this book is not just about hormones but how we got here and how the discourse developed. It is a guide to perimenopause and progesterone, but it is also a narrative about modern medicine and how we fit into that story. I have tried to make it easy to read, but serious in intent and content.

Part 1 is about the basics of women and hormones: menstruation, peri-menopause, and menopause (and how these were medicalized). Part 2 is on hormones and health; those areas where estrogen was said to play a part in keeping us well and reducing our risk for disease. This was not only wrong but a complete fabrication. Not only did hormones not protect women from disease, but they put women's health at risk. In this section we are hoping to bring women the intellectual and medical tools they need to question more of the medical advice they are given and understand the reasoning and history for much of what they are told.

Preventive medicine today has moved from the abstract and passive to the dangerously aggressive. We rarely realize, for instance, that the main drugs used to lower cholesterol can cause a horrible muscle-wasting disease (and the more people who take them, the more side effects there will be). We seldom are told about the risks of screening technologies: that CT scans contain four times as much radiation as an X-ray or that those colonoscopies Katie Couric wants us to have can nick the bowel and cause internal bleeding. (If you must, at least have a sigmoidoscopy; it's more flexible, shorter, and safer.) When you give your informed consent, make sure it is exactly that.

Finally, so much nonsense has been written (and repeated) over the last century about menopause that it was time: time for a book that was endocrinologically accurate and accessible, covering not only the science, but its sociocultural and political underpinnings. We have glossed over the importance of hormones to our health for too long, ignored our inherent nature, and manipulated pieces of a whole we did not understand. It is time to reclaim that understanding and realize our individual slant on this collective midlife experience we share with all women.

ACRONYMS

AAE—anovulatory androgen excess

ACTH—adrenocorticotropic hormone

BMD—bone mineral density

BMJ—British Medical Journal

CAD—coronary artery disease

CDC—Centers for Disease Control and Prevention

CT—computed tomography

DCIS—ductal carcinoma in situ

D&C—dilation and curettage

DES—diethylstilbestrol

DSM-IV—Diagnostic and Statistical Manual of Mental Disorders, fourth edition

ER—emergency room

ERT—estrogen "replacement" therapy (refers to the erroneous, reflexive therapy with estrogen in menopausal women)

FDA—U.S. Food and Drug Administration

FSH—follicle-stimulating hormone (estrogen)

HMO—health maintenance organization

HRT—hormone "replacement" therapy (refers to the erroneous, reflexive therapy with estrogen and a synthetic progesterone in menopausal women)

JAMA—Journal of the American Medical Association
LH—luteinizing hormone (progesterone)
NEJM—The New England Journal of Medicine
NIH—National Institutes of Health
PMS—premenstrual syndrome
PMT—premenstrual tension
RCT—randomized clinical trial
SES—socioeconomic status
WHI—Women's Health Initiative
WHO—World Health Organization

Part 1

WOMEN AND HORMONES

You're sure, Doctor?...
I mean, I'm getting divorced. My mother's getting divorced.
I'm raising twin boys. I have a lot of job pressure—I've got to find one....
Not long ago I lost a very dear friend, and...and my husband is involved...not just involved, but in love, I'm afraid...with this woman...who's quite a bit younger than I am.
And you think it's my [hormones] and not *my life?*

—*Lily Tomlin*[1]

1

INTRODUCTION AND OVERVIEW

The great enemy of the truth is very often not the lie—deliberate, contrived and dishonest—but the myth—persistent, persuasive and unrealistic.

—John F. Kennedy

Beginning in the seventeenth century, European and North American modernization fostered an "engineering mentality"—one manifestation of which was a concerted effort to establish increased control over the vagaries of the natural world through the application of science. As a result, by the eighteenth century, health came to be understood . . . as a commodity and the physical body as something that could be improved upon.

—anthropologist Margaret Lock[1]

Women and *hormones*. The terms are so inexorably linked in our collective imagination—conceptually, behaviorally, socially, medically, linguistically, and in every other way possible—that we take the connection for granted. We routinely describe ourselves as "hormonal" or refer to behaviors as resulting from "raging" hormones. *Pre-period, premenstrual PMSing, menopausal*: nobody thinks twice about these adjectives; they are ordinary, commonplace. Yet try switching genders, and suddenly it sounds ridiculous, comic, even surreal. We seem to forget that all of us, men and women alike, are a blend of hormones, from insulin (the hormone people with diabetes lack); to adrenaline and noradrenaline (sometimes referred to as the fight–flight hormones); thyroid hormone and more. At times, any one of these could "rage" (if we were to insist on anthropomorphizing hormones) given that these potent, albeit subtle, glandular secretions are involved in every part of our physiology, from regulating body temperature and metabolism to energy and sleep. So, clearly, more is going here when we talk about women and hormones than mere endocrinology, and the phrases are more a reflection of social mores and a culture that devalues women than of physiology.

By "ascribing causality to uncontrollable biological forces" such as hormones, furthermore, such concepts and phrases not only minimize personal responsibility (by implying that these factors are unchangeable and beyond our control),[2] but refer to some ideal of how women *should* behave. Rather than questioning the link, however, women also fall into this habit: blaming our hormones for ups and downs with mood and concentration; for anxiety, stress, fatigue, pain; and even problem skin or an itchy scalp.

Even more perplexing is that that the hormone in question is inevitably estrogen. Estrogen is considered the quintessential female hormone, fundamental to being a woman; nobody even blinks if a restroom door or a newspaper headline uses the term as shorthand for *women* (just as *testosterone* refers to men). So how did a single hormone, one of many, achieve such iconic status? Particularly because physiologic balance in women requires both estrogen and progesterone? (And all of us, men and women, have estrogen, progesterone, and testosterone; it is simply the proportions and amounts that differ.)

So what happened? How did progesterone just fade out of the medical and cultural lexicon in favor of estrogen?

PROGESTERONE: THE FORGOTTEN HORMONE

This book is an answer to that question, delving back in time to cover not only the history of hormones—and the late-nineteenth-century scientists and researchers who first identified these active and mysterious substances—but also analyzing a host of other influences that converged during the twentieth century, particularly after World War II, to make estrogen and estrogen "therapy" the fulcrum for women's biology, identity, and destiny. Based in medicine and endocrinology, shaded in with concepts from social science, this book is also an examination of the diverse elements—war, money, culture, science, medicine, the status of women, language, and the laboratory itself—that came into play in the discourse on women's hormones and their role in health. A counterbalance to the frequently inaccurate, contradictory, and prejudicial advice women are too often given with respect to hormones (from birth control pills to hormone "replacement" therapy, or "HRT," as it is routinely and erroneously called), this book clarifies what is usually referred to as the "menopausal transition" and provides women, especially at midlife, with a solid intellectual and medical framework for understanding how hormones function within their lives and health. Those earlier terms, incidentally, are in quotes because it makes no sense to call hormones a "replacement" at a time when *all* women's hormones naturally wane—this is not like a person with diabetes injecting insulin or someone taking thyroxine to replace that of a sluggish thyroid.

Furthermore, calling this time in a woman's life the "menopausal transition" ignores the difficult years of high estrogen and heavy flow within regular cycles, implying that any and all problems will halt abruptly at that "final" menstrual period (which is how menopause is officially defined), as though anyone at that point could even know it was really the last menstrual flow. Rather, the time leading up to menopause (before and for one year after that last flow), during which some 15 to 20 percent of women have troubling symptoms, is more accurately called *perimenopause.*

An enormous amount of nonsense has been said and written about women's ostensible lack of estrogen as they age. For years, even women not experiencing any problems at all were told to take estrogen for their heart, their bones, or to keep their hair and skin youthful. Yet estrogen has been repeatedly demonstrated to increase heart disease, breast cancer, blood clots, and so on (most recently in 2002, when the Women's Health Initiative [WHI] was stopped early due to the adverse effects of hormones). Nonetheless, it would appear that women's roles throughout Western history have been so inextricably linked to their fertility, their ability to conceive, that anything outside of those middle menstrual years was expeditiously labeled aberrant, even diseased. Women, unfortunately, believed the experts who told them menopause was an "estrogen deficiency disease" for which "replacement" hormones were necessary. This book is also, therefore, an analysis of the many myths about estrogen (and menopause) and a guide to help women understand their own hormones at various stages of life. Although we have tried to make this book accessible, it is not a lightweight work or a book on alternative medicine (not that there is anything necessarily wrong with that); we have provided extensive sources and notes. Readers can confidently use this book as a reference or when talking to their family doctors.

For those women for whom perimenopause is difficult (like the authors of this book), we explain why it is not estrogen that is low during this time, but progesterone. In fact, during perimenopause, estrogen levels often skyrocket, fluctuating wildly, which is what causes those vasomotor symptoms such as hot flushes and night sweats.[3] With this book, we hope to bring progesterone out of the shadows and back into the discussion because it has been forgotten for far too long. Yet without progesterone, there would be no menstrual cycle, no pregnancy, and no natural maturation. For reasons that elude us, however, whenever women's hormones are spoken of, it is inevitably estrogen that holds pride of place—even though the two hormones, estrogen and progesterone, work in tandem and complement each other physiologically. Estrogen and progesterone balance each other out.

During each menstrual cycle, estrogen is released through a single, pinhead-sized group of cells—called a follicle—that encircle one egg. At this time, estrogen levels increase; then, about midcycle, estrogen reaches its peak whereupon the levels decline, after triggering a spike in a pituitary hormone leading to ovulation (the release of an egg). At this point, progesterone takes over. At their maximum, progesterone levels far exceed the levels of the earlier estrogen peak, reaching levels more than one thousand times higher. Then, both hormones wane with the menstrual period, and the cycle starts all over again. Yet, for mysterious reasons, progesterone never seems to enter the popular (or medical) narrative; estrogen always seems to be the hormone that gynecologists and other experts turn to whenever there is a problem—such as menopause or perimenopause, both of which are conceptualized as a hormone "deficiency."

Logically, physiologically, estrogen without progesterone makes no sense, and could potentially be dangerous, because during that first half of the menstrual cycle, as estrogen levels rise, they also cause the uterine lining (the endometrium) to overgrow and thicken. This is to start preparing the uterus in case there is a pregnancy.[4] When there is no pregnancy, ovulation and the production of large amounts of progesterone transform the lining and then help it to fall away with the menstrual flow. Progesterone's role is essential because this endometrial thickening or hyperplasia could become pathological, even cancerous. Progesterone is like a cleansing rain, if we want to be fanciful, washing away accumulated dust; without progesterone, that earlier estrogen-based activity could clog (for want of a better word) the healthy menstrual cycle.* So clearly, there is an essential balance of these two hormones necessary to optimal health.

THE SOCIAL ROOTS OF MEDICINE

Explained in stark physiologic terms, it might strike the reader as bizarre that this essential balance of hormones has not seemed important. And it would be, were what we think of as purely scientific or medical explanations not so fundamentally rooted in sociocultural norms and beliefs. But, like everything else, science is the product of the society that creates it; it is neither objective nor somehow above the fray, as most of us believe. As Stephen Jay Gould once said, science is not something foreign but an integral part of our culture; medicine, similarly, is steeped in our prejudices and buffeted about by all manner of influences, from the political and commercial to the fashionable and expedient.

Most of us have a vague sense that the reason our grandmothers did not benefit from the drugs, surgeries, and other therapies we take for granted is that the science, the technology, simply had not been discovered; we feel lucky to live in a time of such stunning advances, when genetics, pharmacology, microsurgery, and so on could soon make disease obsolete. Television shows like *House* or *Nova* show us the "miracles" that modern medical science has wrought, and on the

---

*The menstrual cycle is described in length in the following chapter.

Internet and in newspapers and magazines we read that (any minute now) it will be possible for us to intervene therapeutically in ways that would have seemed like pure science fiction a few short years ago—we will cure cancer, grow new organs, use our genome to predict and prevent illness, even stop aging and push back death.

Unfortunately, attention-grabbing headlines and sensational health news are precisely that: sensational, attention-grabbing headlines. They are designed to sell things, not reflect reality. We rarely, if ever, hear of the true complexities of physiology or how difficult it is to predict, or even know, how the subtle interplay of our genes, our environment, and everything else about us might translate into disease (or health). We barely understand what even a single hormone might do, never mind DNA. (In any event, how much can we know about the latter when the largest piece of gene remains unidentified and is unhelpfully called "junk" DNA?) There continue to be more questions than answers. Plus, we rarely realize how much the media exaggerate, under- or overreport medical news, emphasizing the inaccurate, experimental, or merely hopeful. At the turn of twenty-first century, for instance, with the huge expenditures of The Genome Project, we were told that genetic therapies were on the horizon, and in five years we would reap the benefits. (It is always five years down the road for some reason.) Well, it is closer to ten years, and we still have nothing. Even old drugs and techniques, such as cardiopulmonary resuscitation, are presented on television as being far more effective than they really are.[5] We rarely (if ever) hear of the disasters, the side effects, the downside of those ostensible miracle drugs and procedures. The bulk of what we hear about health and medicine, moreover, is *disease*-oriented, and women's health, in particular, tends to highlight bad news—most commonly in terms of reproduction and reproductive hormones.[6]

These social, media, and other cultural narratives have a profound impact on how we think about medicine, ourselves, and our symbiotic link to our hormones. Since we were children, everything from advertisements and television shows to the books we read or the conversations we overheard contained the subtext that estrogen equaled being a woman (just as testosterone meant being a man), and that being female implied that we just did not measure up. We lacked, well, the *testosterone* for those powerful, male-dominated careers: president, prime minister, director, CEO, the "man" in charge.

Overtly and covertly, that belief continues to be reinforced, whether in some (highly fictional) movies featuring a woman as president of the United States, where her reluctance to blow up some small country (as her male entourage advises her to) is attributed to her maternal (i.e., hormonal) shortcomings, or an article in the business section on women executives suggesting that women are not competitive enough to cut it in the cutthroat global marketplace. From the time we are in school, both boys and girls (as well as adults, both real and fictional) easily dismiss female irritation or anger as PMS, and much of the time anything misaligned with social definitions of how a proper woman is supposed to behave is attributed to hormones. So if a woman is just not caring or communicative enough; if she is not sociable, or speaks her mind or gets angry; if a woman is not *nice,* then it must be "that time of the month." Would it even be conceivable to suggest that a man in a bad mood is hormonal—outside of a *Saturday Night Live* sketch?

As women, it is our ability to bear children—our status as incubators—that has subtly defined our role in the world. For a long time, in fact, the woman was not thought to contribute anything to procreation; it was the mighty sperm that carried the blueprint for life. (Not dissimilar to the way we currently perceive the genome.) So convinced of this were philosophers and scientists in the past that the seventeenth-century Dutch scientist Antonie van Leeuwenhoek, one of the first people to use a microscope, was positive he had seen a tiny man, complete with miniscule arms, legs, and head (a homunculus), when he observed sperm through his lens.[7] (Well, in vitro veritas, so to speak.)

HISTORY AND HORMONES

The endocrine secretions we now call hormones were first noticed in the late 1800s, although it was not until 1905 that these dynamic chemical messengers circulating in the blood were dubbed "hormones" (by the British scientist Ernest Starling). Hormones quickly led to a whole new kind of biologic determinism, particularly for women. It was soon realized that these potent glandular substances could exert powerful physiologic effects and were instrumental in regulating various physical processes. This in turn created a new slant on old views of existing gender roles.

As Nelly Oudshoorn, a lecturer at the University of Amsterdam and an expert in the history of hormones and social dynamics, writes in *On the Making of Sex Hormones,* sex hormones soon became linked with health, stamina, even eternal youth. Wild claims were made for the vitalizing effects of these hormones—and an early physiologist and neurologist, Charles-Edouard Brown-Sequard, a professor at the College de France, reported in 1889 that by taking "aqueous extracts of animal testes," he had totally rejuvenated himself, enhancing his strength and sexual potency. This early Viagra made Brown-Sequard an international star (although his exotic background may have helped; his father was a sea captain from Philadelphia and his mother was French).[8] Of course, the effects of surgically castrating men and women were also understood in considerable detail, for example, castrati in Italian opera. These endocrinological explanations, however, were a new and exciting way to describe physiology—and psychology.

By 1916, the burgeoning field of endocrinology was on its way, and the therapeutic use of hormones (then called *organotherapy*) had led to nearly ten thousand papers and some genuine therapeutic advances. An English physician, George Redmayne, treated a form of hypothyroidism (underactive thyroid) with an extract from the thyroid gland; Jokichi Takamine, a Japanese-American chemist working in the United States, isolated adrenaline, and in Canada, Frederick Banting and Charles Best isolated insulin—the lack of which was known to cause diabetes. By 1923, the knowledge claims for sex hormones had also expanded, thanks in part to gynecologists whose area of expertise—reproduction—coupled with their access to women patients, provided them with professional legitimacy in the new field. Endocrinology attracted huge numbers of researchers jockeying for position, and almost immediately estrogen became the focus for so-called women's diseases and reproduction. (Men, by this point, unlike Brown-Sequard, were no longer quite so keen on ingesting or injecting the testes of small animals.) "'Hormone treatment' of climacteric [menstrual and menopausal] complaints must be as old as 'hormone' preparations themselves," wrote P. van Keep of the International Menopause Society in 1990, even though it seems unlikely that these early preparations, such as "dried sheep's ovaries," had any "demonstrable" hormonal effects.[9]

A great plus was that this hormone research dovetailed nicely with the prevalent social, medical, and cultural beliefs—so now it could be said that it was women's *glands* that were responsible for their inability to excel (the way men so easily could). As Oudshoorn writes,

> The chemical substances believed to originate in the sex glands were designated sex hormones: the male sex hormone secreted by the testes, the female sex hormone secreted by the ovaries. This terminology constructed a sexual *duality*: sex hormones were conceptualized as the chemical agents of masculinity and femininity, thus emphasizing the ancient folk-wisdom that femininity and masculinity resided in the gonads. Although, in the 1920's and 1930's, scientists had to reconsider the conceptualization of sex hormones as strictly sexually specific both in origin and function, *the terminology was never revised* [italics added].[10]

This meant that the basic idea of men and women being opposites (and estrogen and testosterone being the physiologic expression of that opposition) could be said to have a scientific basis.

This ideology and terminology persists to this day: women are said to be fragile, weak, whereas men are strong. This is why men drive SUVs and hybrids are "chick" cars. (Although precisely how hormones determine mechanical choice is unclear, particularly because the significance of the car transcends gender, reflecting freedom and power, at least in North America.) But, we are assured, this is because men are hunters, which explains their penchant for cooking outdoors on a barbecue (even if it is gas). As for the exceptions, like men who are chefs—well, that is being in charge of a kitchen. These contradictory messages and narratives are so common that we barely notice them; so much so that we forget they are not facts at all but reflections of how we have constructed our social world. And being part of that world ourselves, it is impossible for us to put ourselves *outside* of it. So we forget it's just a way of explaining the world—not the world itself.

"We cannot dispense with metaphors in thinking about nature," geneticist Richard Lewontin dryly explains, so we start to believe the metaphors are real and not mere descriptors. Or, as Lewontin puts it, "We cease to see the world *as if* it were *like* a machine and take it to *be* a machine."[11] Women, then, as we are continually told (in stories, films, ads, and song) are domestic creatures, who prefer to stay close to home and hearth, cleaning and tidying after everybody else. This was, after all, their role through time immemorial: picking roots and berries, while man-the-hunter was out looking for something to kill. Never mind that archeological evidence suggests that the entire tribe, men, women, and children, had to help in catching large prey—probably making noise to scare it down a cliff onto a net of some kind. Our cultural narrative—and Hollywood—have given us the brave hunter, out alone with his teeny prehistoric knife (that could barely kill a mouse, never mind some large creature with sharp teeth), and so the gender stereotyping merry-go-round circles along, molding the questions we ask, shaping our science and our medicine, and defining what we make of, and how we describe, the natural world.

SCIENCE AND GENDER

Fundamentally, we believe the universe has an order similar to that of our own lives, reflecting our own hierarchical culture and society, wrote the late physician and neurobiologist Ruth Bleier in *Science and Gender*. A central premise in our "biological explanations of the asymmetrical positions of women and men" in current culture is therefore that women's subordinate position is "universal" and holds true "across all time and all cultures." We ignore any contradictions, gloss over obvious errors, and stick to our guns that this is what nature intended.[12] Paradoxes slide by. When ancient art is found in caves, at Lascaux, for instance, experts opine that it is simply not possible to know anything about the minds of the people who created that art. But gender roles? Those we have no trouble decoding—even though the end result seems to bear an uncanny resemblance to *Barbarella*. Which brings us full circle to our belief that there are intrinsic gender roles that our hormones embody.

These "universalistic assumptions" invite biological explanations and find them in women's capacity to bear children, which therefore must be rooted in her nature, or rather, her hormones[13]—specifically, estrogen—perhaps because it was the first hormone understood well enough to be synthesized. Progesterone was identified early on but proved more difficult to make in the lab and was not used therapeutically until much later.

Estrogen, on the other hand, was plentiful and easily available in pregnant mares' urine (since pregnancy increases estrogen in mares and humans). As Oudshoorn describes, in the Netherlands, the home of the first pharmaceutical company devoted entirely to hormone preparations, Organon, laboratory scientists and pharmaceutical industrialists were soon boasting that they had found "gold in the urine of pregnant mares." Estrogen became the treatment of choice for alleviating the symptoms of menopause or anything else menstrual.

By mid-century, estrogen was being touted, particularly in the United States, not merely as a cure for any midlife symptoms (actually, perimenopause), but as a magical substance that could keep women young, taut, healthy, and vital—and on a continent where anything that even vaguely promises to maintain youth and vigor is valorized, estrogen soon became one of the most frequently prescribed drugs in the country. As recently as 2001, 15 million midlife women were filling prescriptions for estrogen (with a smidgeon of a synthetic progesterone, progestin, added to prevent the endometrial cancer that estrogen alone could cause).[14] Premarin, the estrogen pill derived from the urine of those pregnant mares[15] (the derivation is obvious from the name: pregnant, mare, urine), had indeed become a gold mine for the pharmaceutical industry, all those years after those early Dutch scientists had predicted it would.*

How could this happen? How could so many women be in need of a cure for a natural progression that occurs in all women? Quite simply, it came about by making the template for "normal" in hormone levels that of a woman of about twenty-three, a standard that continues to this day. Older or midlife women (and their hormone levels, bones, and everything else) would be compared to younger versions of themselves and, not surprisingly, found wanting.

Conspicuously absent was the realization that all living organisms change with age, imperceptibly at first, then gradually more obviously. Women and men alike find that over time, their hair becomes gray, their bones become less dense, and their skin loses elasticity, and, depending on the person and the life he or she has led, internal organs also change. Arteries, like joints and muscles, become stiff and gradually harden.[16] No matter. For women, menopause was defined as a "lack" of estrogen since, after menopause, ovaries no longer create the same levels of hormone. This became the ostensible cause of menopause and its corollary, aging, and estrogen was the solution, the therapy, the *cure* for this "deficiency disease" that time had created. (If we applied the same logic elsewhere, incidentally, a headache would be an aspirin-deficiency disease.) Hundreds of thousands of menopausal women were authoritatively told that they had to take estrogen because menopause (and its dire consequences, like heart disease and osteoporosis)

---

*Apparently, slightly wetting a Premarin pill makes its origin obvious—all one has to do is smell it, at least according to the physician and author Christiane Northrup in her book *Women's Bodies, Women's Wisdom.*

was a sure sign that hormone levels literally needed topping up. The term *estrogen-deficiency disease* became the common medical description for menopause, and it is still around, even in medical journals.

Throughout their lives, women are said to somehow be victims of their hormones, and menopause is said to herald the start of heart disease, cancer, osteoporosis, dementia, and untold other problems (all of which often contain the prefix "postmenopausal"). From the outer body, where skin becomes dry and wrinkled; to the vaginal walls, which become itchy and irritated; inward to our organs and bones, we are literally and metaphorically told that menopause makes us brittle, dry, and breakable: old hags, if we don't mince words. Of course, it is usually phrased more politely than that—today, the language reflects our current obsession with risk and risk reduction, but the upshot is the same, as is the solution: taking hormones (estrogen). These are obligingly provided in pretty pink boxes when we are younger to pills, patches and injections, as vaginal inserts, creams, and all kinds of preparations, when we are older.

PERIMENOPAUSE AND THE ESTROGEN FALLACY

Throughout much of the twentieth century, but especially from the 1970s on, women whose menstrual cycles began to change (usually) as they hit their forties were not told that this was *perimenopause*, a natural transition between menstruation and menopause. Perimenopause was not even a word. Instead, women were told that lack of estrogen was the culprit—even though during this time, estrogen levels are actually high, and it is progesterone that declines; it is this imbalance that causes the tumult some women experience during those years.[17] Ironic—given estrogen's iconic status and the gynecologic insistence that estrogen makes women feel good—that it is during these years, when estrogen levels are flying out of control, surging unpredictably, that women have their worst symptoms. During perimenopause, estrogen levels are high and chaotic—one could even liken them to a hurricane.[18] These high levels of estrogen, furthermore, without sufficient progesterone to balance them out, cause menstrual flooding, instead of flow,[19] and three-week, rather than four-week, cycles. High estrogen leads to tender, swollen breasts for weeks rather than merely a day or two (as one is used to), at erratic times and for durations far longer than anything we have experienced before.

For up to 20 percent of us (the authors included), perimenopause is a miserable time—totally different from menopause, soothingly defined as a year without flow. It begins with typical changes in women whose periods are still regular (see Table 1.1).[20] These physiologic changes, which resemble PMS in their intensity, include sore breasts, new or increased migraines, shorter cycles, heavy flow, cyclic flow-related night sweats, sudden wakening in the middle of the night, and weight

Table 1.1
Experience Changes Characteristic of Perimenopause Onset in Regularly Cycling Women

Any three of the following can be used to define perimenopause:

- New heavy and/or longer menstrual flow
- Shorter menstrual cycle length (≤25 days)
- New sore, swollen, and/or lumpy breasts
- New or increased menstrual cramps
- New mid-sleep wakenings
- Onset of night sweats, especially around flow
- New or markedly increased migraine headaches
- New or increased premenstrual mood swings
- Notable weight gain without changes in exercise or food intake

gain (without any change in exercise habits) and are all attributable to dramatically changing estrogen levels—not downward changing, but upward. Contrary to what we have been led to believe with terms like *estrogen deficiency* and qualifiers for estrogen such as *low* and *diminishing*, the reality is that estrogen levels are often sky-high in the years leading up to menopause. So, for those women in whom hormone fluctuations during this time cause troublesome symptoms (why this happens in some women and not others we do not know), it stands to reason that hormone therapy with *progesterone* might help, not the estrogen women have traditionally been prescribed. (Although how many women were actually helped is a mystery because all we can track are the number of prescriptions, not how many women actually took it. What is called *adherence* to hormone therapy, furthermore, has always been low.[21]) The real question remains why we, why medicine, have focused on estrogen deficiency in perimenopause, when it is estrogen that is high and requires progesterone for balancing out.[22]

Going back to first principles, *menopause*—also known as "the change" or the change of life—is a term referring to the pause of the menses (both from the Greek, the latter from *meno*, meaning "month"). For many women, it is fraught not only with hot flushes (also known as hot flashes) and poor sleep, punctuated by night sweats, but also with unpleasant reminders of the passage of time and their aging bodies. As one of the authors of this book wrote in a 1995 text (a time when "HRT" was at its peak and menopause was defined as a deficiency disease), in a plea for sanity,

Menopause is defined in retrospect, after a year has elapsed without menstruation. The healthy woman will experience about four years of varying reproductive hormones and their symptomatic effects before her last period. . . . Effective therapy for the perimenopausal or menopausal woman cannot begin until she understands and begins to deal with the *social and emotional context* [italics added] of menopause.

> Goals of therapy [are] to help women deal with menopause as a sociocultural transi-
> tion, to educate women during perimenopause to the climacteric as a normal phase of
> life for all women, rather than an estrogen deficiency disease, to make patients aware
> of accessible community and support resources [and] to treat Menorrhagia (heavy
> bleeding), severe VMS [vasomotor symptoms] and endometrial cancer risk during
> the perimenopause; and severe VMS and low bone density during menopause.[23]

Not a fixed point in time, in other words, but a nebulous period often difficult
to pinpoint exactly—which is how physiology always works, along a continuum.

The ephemeral, non-fixed-in-time character of menopause is readily compre-
hensible to women, who know that their menstrual cycle does not begin at
precisely the same time each month and may vary by as much as weeks, or even
months. There are a variety of reasons for this variation, the most important
of which is individual physiology, and today our Western diet and environment
probably exacerbate this. Most of us are exposed to estrogen-mimicking synthetics
and other compounds in everything from plastic water bottles to treated fabrics.
Estrogen is also present in body fat and in our food (factory-raised animals are
treated with hormones so they will gain weight more quickly). But it is not this
ersatz estrogen we are exposed to that tends to worry us, any more than the actual
physiology of what is happening. What occurs is a kind of magical thinking, one
where estrogen is the solution for anything time throws our way.

In fact, so strong is the belief in the efficacy of estrogen, suggests Harvard
hematologist Jerome Groopman in his best-selling book *How Doctors Think*, that
it transcends reason. He quotes a female physician, a professor of obstetrics and
gynecology at Yale, who, in her "heart of hearts," as she told *The New York Times*,
believes in the benefits of estrogen, even though the evidence is vanishingly small.
She took estrogen herself and recommended it to her patients. But, as Groopman
writes, when a respected professor and doctor speaks out this passionately, she is
"speaking not objectively but from faith"[24]—faith that estrogen is the de facto
female hormone, the bedrock on which all that is female rests. (And this belief was
so widespread that for many years, women were prescribed "estrogen replacement
therapy" or "ERT.") Of course, to "replace" hormones that wane naturally in all
women already requires a leap of faith, which, by definition, requires no proof.

EMPOWERMENT?

Calling us hormonally deficient does not, we are assured, intend to make
victims of women, but to empower us—make us better, more complete, and
better able to make informed choices about our health. After all, what could be
more terrific than that, since we are *all* aspiring to be better (prettier, thinner,
more fit, etc.)? Why not move closer to the ideal of youth, vigor, and strength, if

all we have to do is take a pill? (It is, of course, rather depressing to think that age, experience, and learning can be so easily dismissed in favor of a youthful image that looks good on television, but that is not something we can change with one book.) The decision of whether or not to take hormones is thus presented as a choice, a medical option that we can decide to accept or not, much as we might have elective surgery to lift our eyelids or take analgesics (painkillers) for a painful knee.[25]

Taking hormones is, in fact, nothing of the kind. It is part and parcel of deeply felt attitudes steeped in long-held social norms and history dictating that a woman's value and her fertility are one and the same. As anthropologist Margaret Lock writes, too often what we think of as our own free, independent, individual will and pragmatic self-interest are really the result of having internalized, over time, various rules, systems, and roles that have been pushed on us, to the point that we think they are ours:

> In contemporary writing it is common to assert that . . . to cast women in a passive role is to perpetuate the very kinds of assumptions that feminists have been trying to challenge. Although active resistance to medicalization has contributed to the rise of the home birth movement and to widespread use of alternative therapies and remedies of various kinds, empirical research makes it clear that the responses of individuals to the availability of biomedical interventions are pragmatic, and based upon what are perceived to be in the best interests, not only of women themselves, but often of their families and at times their communities. This is particularly evident in connection with reproduction when, for example, women who believe themselves to be infertile make extensive use of new reproductive technologies despite the high failure rate and the expense and emotional upheaval that is involved.[26]

She adds that, as women, we internalize the norm that our primary task—our purpose in life—is to produce a family "of the ideal size and composition" because not doing so makes us failures. Whether it is a woman in India or China aghast at having given birth to a girl or a childless woman in North America feeling pressured to explain her choice to a random stranger in a restroom (as happened to one of the authors, S.B.), women are subliminally prodded to fulfill the roles and (often unspoken) assumptions and expectations our social world ordains—which, we are now told, is backed by science. But as the late Stephen Jay Gould once remarked, theories are most successful when they let us believe that "our social prejudices are scientific facts after all."[27]

Believing that estrogen deficiency led to a pathological state called menopause was a comfortable belief, one that everyone wanted to believe. And in any event, who needs proof when all that was really called for was a *super* book explaining the importance of estrogen? Particularly if the author was a kindly, well-spoken, gray-haired doctor with a British accent (supported by his wife, a nurse), who happily went on tour to preach the gospel according to estrogen.

FEMININE FOREVER

The book *Feminine Forever* appeared on the scene in 1966.[28] Written by a gynecologist named Robert Wilson, it proclaimed that menopause was not only preventable (with the exception of being able to have a child, naturally), but *curable* with estrogen. Later, much later, the book was revealed to be the result of a corrupt collaboration between the gynecologist and various drug companies, as surgeon Susan Love explains:

> In 1964—two years before Wilson's book was published—the Wilsons' trust [the Wilson Foundation], established to promote the use of estrogen, had received $17,000 from Searle, $8,700* from Wyeth-Ayerst Laboratories, and $5,600 from the Upjohn Company, all of which made hormones that Wilson promoted for the treatment of menopause.[29]

As Wilson proselytized to menopausal women, the drug companies turned their attention to convincing doctors—and, through a confluence of factors, *Feminine Forever* managed to alter medical practice for the rest of the century. Some would argue that the marketing of the idea of estrogen deficiency was the biggest international success since the development of the printing press. The book did have a general impact throughout the Western world, but the nation that fell for it hook, line, and sinker was the one whose founding philosophy and cultural basis relied totally on self-amelioration and the pursuit of happiness: the United States.

The elimination of menopause was, according to Wilson, "perhaps the most important technical advance by which women may equip themselves for an enduringly feminine role in modern life" (p. 30). In fact, he suggested, keeping estrogen from women could well be considered a fiendish sexist plot, given that the "lack of medical sympathy for menopausal women might simply be due to the fact that most doctors, being male, are themselves immune to this 'disease,'" namely, the "genital atrophy" and "castration" that estrogen deficiency caused as women got older (p. 35). This led to the tissues drying out, muscles weakening, skin sagging, and bones becoming brittle. Menopause, in other words, would result in everything women feared. During an era when American women had no power, no money, and very little status other than through their ability to "catch" a husband, have children, and (ideally) move to the suburbs, this was powerful imagery—rife with symbolism reflecting the desiccation, akin to dry crumbling leaves, of the menopausal woman.

True, a few feminist books had begun to make waves in the late 1960s, and a handful of feminists like Germaine Greer were prominent, but for the vast majority of women, already older and with few or no choices in life, especially were

---

*Bear in mind that this was serious money in the 1960s.

they to lose their husbands and their roles as housewife and mother, menopause was the final indignity. During World War II, some twenty years earlier, their mothers might have been employed in factories or government offices while the men were off fighting, but once the war was over, so were their working lives. Then came the real cultural backlash, along with the corsets and other trappings of American modernity: advertising, antibiotics, and all the other accoutrements that advances in science and technology had led to. As the series *Mad Men* cleverly depicts, women were not only constrained physically, mentally, and economically, but now medically as well. It was probably no accident that the roles and careers most suited to a lady at the time were those in which she was helpmeet and handmaiden: secretary, nurse, teacher. Without wishing to belittle the value of these professions, it is nonetheless obvious the attraction the estrogen-deficiency myth could have held at such a time and how it could flourish within this social, cultural, linguistic, and even sartorial landscape because medical science, like everything else, is part and parcel of society and the culture in which it exists.

Neither Wilson nor the drug company Ayerst (later Wyeth-Ayerst, and now Wyeth) ever admitted to the fraud they had perpetrated, and it was only after Wilson's death, when his son Robert Jr., who perhaps felt somewhat guilty that he had provided the "illustrations and dynamism" needed for the book according to the acknowledgments, came clean and admitted that his father had indeed (as many had suspected) been supported by the makers of Premarin, the most widely used form of estrogen available (who never admitted their involvement, up to and including the present).

Unfortunately, even once the truth about *Feminine Forever* was out, its ramifications continued, and estrogen remained central to gynecologists' prescribing pads. Medical practice, after all, is primarily based on teaching and mentoring; doctors repeat what they have been taught and perpetuate the same patterns, right or wrong, of their role models. Upholding medical orthodoxy is drummed into young doctors, who are primarily taught via retrospective case studies.[30]

Progesterone never captured anyone's imagination; even women often disliked it, blaming the synthetic form of progesterone, medroxyprogesterone—added to Premarin in the form of Provera, to prevent the endometrial cancer unopposed estrogen could cause—for every symptom the combination hormone "therapy" caused. Yet one of the authors of this book (J.C.P.) conducted a randomized, double-blind, one-year comparative study, giving forty-one menstruating women who had just had their uteruses and ovaries removed either Provera or Premarin. Although these two therapies have proven similar in hot flush control,[31] in a factor analysis, Premarin was more strongly associated with negative moods than was Provera.* So how did a natural women's hormone, progesterone, become the poster child for all that is wrong with the aging female body, while the other

---

*Unpublished communication, C. L. Hitchcock, E. Kingwell, W. Mercer, and J. C. Prior, 2008.

hormone—the one known to cause migraines, endometrial hyperplasia, breast cancer, blood clots, stroke, and more—retain its halo? Clearly, neither physiology nor logic had anything to do with it.

HOPE, HABIT, BELIEF, AND EPIDEMIOLOGY

Hope, habit, and staunch belief in the ultimate goodness of estrogen were fused, not only in medical practice, where the belief was reinforced through medical training and drug advertising, but as a social belief and practice. So positive was the ethos with respect to estrogen that from there it was only a short step to deciding it must also prevent disease. After all, because many diseases appear with advancing age, and because menopause occurs around age fifty, then everything from heart disease to osteoporosis could be saddled with the adjective *postmenopausal*: postmenopausal osteoporosis, postmenopausal cardiac disease, and so on. A few voices did urge caution, but, overall, they were ignored or unheard in the cacophony of estrogen support, led by the drug companies and gynecologists (and later also cardiologists) for whom women's midlife equaled estrogen deficiency.

Because what we believe also determines our hypotheses and our field of study, various researchers began testing the idea that women who took estrogen had health advantages over those who did not. Various observational and survey-type trials were undertaken to confirm just how marvelous estrogen was. The most comprehensive of these was the Nurses Health Study, in which a huge cohort of married nurses (more than 120,000) were sent questionnaires biennially checking on their health and on the status of their chronic disease(s) such as coronary artery disease.[32] And lo and behold, as with a number of smaller studies along the same lines, researchers found that women who took estrogen suffered fewer heart attacks and were generally healthier. The researchers did make cursory attempts not to trumpet the estrogen horn too loudly and acknowledge the shortcomings of their research, but their belief in the inherent ability of estrogen to keep women healthy was so powerful that their heart just wasn't in it; the overwhelming tone was ecstatic and positive, with the majority stressing just how "significant" estrogen was as a "public health advance."[33]

There is, of course, an inherent problem in attempting to deduce cause from mere association, which is all that an observational study can observe (so to speak), or in using epidemiological data, which, again, cannot determine causality. Questionnaires are particularly problematic, for not only do people forget, lie, or otherwise dissemble in their self-reporting, there is also what is called the *healthy user bias*, which means that people who tend to join such studies are already prone to taking better care of themselves. They are also people who are literate and have the time to fill out forms, which means they are probably also relatively well-off: all of which correlate with better health. People who readily respond to even a telephone survey tend to be white, married, and younger.[34] Such considerations never stopped anyone from drawing broad conclusions, however. Soon, women were being advised to take hormones to ward off the possibility of *future* ill health. The climate was ripe for this advice, for, as we cover in later chapters, the notion of taking a drug today to ward off the possibility of disease tomorrow had taken off in the 1970s with the conceptualization of disease in terms of so-called risk factors. And for women, menopause had to be the biggest risk factor of all because they were no longer at their peak, fertile years—which, as far as society was concerned, equaled normalcy for a woman.

There is an enormous presumption in all this—telling healthy people they need to take a pill to ward off future illness (or the risk of future illness)—what David Sackett, the physician associated with the term *evidence-based medicine*, has called the "arrogance of preventive medicine": it is not only "aggressively assertive," but "overbearing."[35] But from hormones to drugs to lower cholesterol, prevention became the word of the day. So convinced was everyone of the benefits of hormones that

> by the mid-1990's, the American Heart Association, the American College of Physicians and the American College of Obstetricians and Gynecologists had all concluded that the beneficial effects of H.R.T. were sufficiently well established that it could be recommended to older women as a means of warding off heart disease and osteoporosis.[36]

THE WOMEN'S HEALTH INITIATIVE

Thankfully, a large National Institutes of Health (NIH) clinical study (the WHI) had begun some years before (at a time when the director of the NIH was a woman) of 160,000 women between the ages of fifty and seventy-nine. The WHI would finally determine, through multiple individual studies and two placebo-controlled trials comparing women who took hormones with those who did not, whether hormones were A Good Thing (with the expectation fully being that of course they would be).

Then, in 2002, the other shoe finally dropped. Vindicating the (few) estrogen critics, the trial had to be stopped early: estrogen-progestin hormone "replacement" therapy compared to placebo in a large group of women (16,608 to be exact) turned out not only to *not* be cardioprotective but culminated in net *harm* for the women taking it. "This treatment should not be prescribed for the prevention of cardiovascular disease," the researchers baldly stated.[37] Plus, the hormone therapy caused an unacceptable rise in breast cancer, blood clots, and stroke. Even the incidence of dementia and Alzheimer's disease, which hormones had been supposed to prevent, were higher in women who took hormones. In short, hormone therapy was a disaster.

The news made international headlines with the discomfiting—and unexpected—news that estrogen (with a smidge of progestin) was not the panacea it had been thought to be. Finally, the people screaming at the sidelines, calling for caution, were heard—but alas, not for long. After a brief flurry of negative news about estrogen, the excuses and the justifications began pouring in, in both the lay and the medical press. Surely there had been some mistake. One really should not be hasty; the fault could not have been with estrogen, the good hormone. It was probably the progesterone (well, progestin). Maybe if women took hormones at a younger age, closer to menopause, and for a shorter length of time? The women recruited for the WHI were somewhat older (average age sixty-three and "more than a decade after menopause," according to the North American Menopause Society), so what if hormones were started earlier, perhaps closer to menopause? Then there should be little to worry about.[38] The *timing* was surely the problem. This was, of course, precisely the same rhetoric that had led to the estrogen debacle in the first place, the same misguided logic that had used flawed data from the Nurse's Health Study and other observational studies, ignored any outliers or conflicting evidence, and was used to convince women to take "HRT" in the first place.*

Women were understandably confused in the face of this conflicting advice, as were their primary care doctors, who no longer knew what to suggest. For years, hormones had been the holy grail of prevention: "HRT" was said to reduce cardiac risk by up to 50 percent and estrogen was touted as a preventive for osteoporosis, ovarian, and colon cancer, and was even supposed to push back the onset of dementia. Hormones ostensibly kept women youthful and unwrinkled; their skin supple and their minds sharp. Plus, for those women who had difficult symptoms in what persistently was called the menopausal transition, there was little else to offer in terms of symptom relief. But, as we saw earlier in this chapter, in perimenopause, when estrogen levels are already high, the last thing a woman needs is *more* estrogen. The hormone that is diminished is progesterone. Unfortunately, the pro-estrogen and anti-progesterone biases are so strong that this idea still has not made any inroads—and cognitive dissonance being what it is, probably will not for a long time. (*Cognitive dissonance* is the term used in psychology to describe our inability to believe and engage in contradictory activities, so if we already believe—and have gone on record as

---

*It was probably no accident that a great many of the authors—although not all—had links to the pharmaceutical companies. But even without those drug company connections, the ideological and historical bias in favor of estrogen was and is so powerful that researchers seem incapable of letting go of it.

saying—that hormones are good, then that belief remains stubbornly resistant to new information.)

BACK TO BASICS

In general, the passage of time is not something we notice. Only rarely do we realize that, imperceptibly, the years have gone by—when we run into someone we haven't seen since high school or meet a young person we last remember seeing as an infant. Yet age, becoming older, is universal within living systems; even microbes grow old. For years, it was believed that bacteria, being simpler forms of life, went on forever, but microbiologists have recently found that even organisms that reproduce by dividing into two halves eventually become less efficient at the process. It turns out that even *E. coli* does not enjoy eternal youth. Over time, it, too, loses the ability to make quick, flawless copies of itself, suggesting that aging is a common property of life. This has not prevented us from doing all we can to turn the clock back, spending untold amounts of money on cosmetic surgeries, cosmetics, creams, potions, and other miracle cures promising to keep us young and beautiful. Botox and other substances that can be injected to "iron out" wrinkles are a booming business, and the spike in the numbers of such procedures has meant that fairly rare side effects and adverse consequences are now increasingly common, visible on the Internet and in gossip magazines, should one care to look.

Given our social and cultural disdain for anything other than youth and vigor, there is no question that menopause can be a devastating blow, psychically, socially, and psychologically. What we hear, perhaps subliminally, is that we are getting old—in this culture, not an easy message to accept. We are also told that menopause is a medical liability, leading to disease and dysfunction (or at least the elevated *risk* of disease, whatever that means), and also that our estrogen levels have dropped below some magical, desirable level. So menopause equals "estrogen deficiency." (No doubt this makes some kind of warped sense, given how easy our culture finds it to blame women's reproductive hormones for disease.) These ideas linking the change in reproductive capability with age, and making menopause a point in time, rather than a process, then labeling it an estrogen-deficiency disease, all add up to a powerful rationale for estrogen. But menopause is not a disease, estrogen deficiency or otherwise; it is a natural phase of life for all women. The last thing women need is medicine and adjunct professions insisting they are somehow deficient or diseased in some way simply because time has passed—particularly during perimenopause, when cycles are often still regular and it is the balance of hormones that is off, with high levels of estrogen leading to hot flushes, night sweats, and other symptoms, all of which can be disturbing and even a bit scary.

Moreover, we are so inundated with stories about disease symptoms and risk factors (and so-called health stories) that some women may become genuinely frightened at this time, believing they might have some terrible illness. The night sweats could be leukemia; their sore breasts might be breast cancer; their headaches could mean a brain tumor. They are, after all, only in their forties, too young for menopause. Plus, the sleep disturbance alone creates anxiety, fatigue, and an inability to focus, adding to the potential stress. One woman felt sure she was developing Alzheimer's disease; she could not remember a phone number or the previous line of text she had read two minutes before. Other women become violently emotional, angry, depressed, or just stressed and fragile. For many women, this is also a time of life when children are growing up and they are starting to care for aging parents; as the late Erma Bombeck wryly observed, we have adjusted "the timetable for childbearing so that menopause and teaching a 16-year-old to drive" both fall at the same time.

This is why it is so important that midlife women realize what perimenopause is and how differently it plays out in different women. But as Janine O. Cobb, the founder and editor of a newsletter on menopause, speaking at a presentation to the North American Menopause Society in the early 1990s, pointed out, women rarely receive the information or the support they need:

> What do midlife women expect from their gynecologists? Too much. The average midlife woman believes that her gynecologist is familiar with the whole gamut of complaints associated with natural menopause and that he or she could (if only they would) explain exactly what is going on in that woman's body right now, as well as what she might expect in the future. Since it is impossible to predict the course of a natural menopause, this would call for unusual prescience on the part of her physician. And it is no big secret that the training of gynecologists allots very little time to natural menopause.[39]

Cobb is correct to say that gynecology is the specialty women usually rely on during this time; it is the discipline they connect with what used to be euphemistically called "women's problems." Plus, many women already have an obstetrician-gynecologist, who was there for them when they were pregnant. Gynecologists, however, are trained in surgery, not hormone physiology, and too many of them respond to symptoms with a prescription for "HRT" or a recommendation to have a hysterectomy—since, from the perspective of obstetrics and gynecology, the womb is no longer useful—as ridiculous as that might seem. (We have an alarming tendency to disregard any organ or body part we don't understand too well, from tonsils to the uterus, and a blithe disregard for the damage surgically removing the aforesaid part subsequently might have.)

Although a small proportion of midlife women might end up needing a hysterectomy, that surgery should really be the very final option, the last recourse.

All surgeries create scar tissue, and this is a site often already scarred for other reasons, ranging from a previous appendectomy, to endometriosis, fibroids, Caesarian deliveries, or even surgery for cancer. There are horrifying tales of women with such previous surgeries for whom the resultant scarring from the hysterectomy caused extensive damage, to the point where they could no longer void naturally. Whenever possible, surgery is best avoided.

What women need at midlife is reassurance, support, and good information, none of which they currently receive—and unfortunately, endocrinologists whose specialty is hormones (like one of the authors of this book) are few and far between. The few there are more frequently deal with possibly more high-profile conditions such as diabetes, or the thyroid, not women's hormones. Given that gynecologists (i.e., surgeons) are designated by society as *the* experts in women's health, the result is that too much of what has been called fact around midlife and menopause actually comes from surgical menopause (hysterectomy and/or ovariectomy), not the natural menopause most of us experience. Surgically removing the uterus and ovaries causes an abrupt change in hormone status (not to mention creating a giant shock to the system) and leads to major symptoms. This is not how a gradual, natural menopause happens. Surgically removing any organ, furthermore, is physiologically traumatic and causes enormous physical stress and a surge in stress hormones, not to mention scar tissue, as discussed earlier. Additionally, even though more and more damning data have been found for estrogen, the general tenor of the discussion remains focused on the erroneous assumption that being a woman equals high levels of estrogen. As a result, even today, women are considered hormonally vulnerable; in essence, baby factories in whom interest wanes once they are no longer fertile.

The delicate balance of hormones and their relationship to health—the impact of life stressors and our modern environment on hormone levels, and the natural changes that occur with the passage of time—are neither well understood nor particularly interesting to medical researchers, biologists, or scientists in general. It is far more glamorous to map some bacterial genome—at least that will put you on the cover of a glossy magazine and let you buy a yacht. Yet the solution for those women (approximately 20%, give or take) who experience troubling symptoms during perimenopause is as simple as a small, round capsule containing oral micronized progesterone (bioidentical progesterone) at bedtime, which not only helps with sleep[40] and night sweats, but also can decrease anxiety and promote bone gain[41] and may well reduce the risk of heart disease and breast cancer. Most important, progesterone reduces those disabling and onerous perimenopausal symptoms, as both authors discovered.*

*The authors were astonished and dismayed at their difficulties with perimenopause; both had become used to regular, easy periods.

AN AMBIGUOUS WORLD VERSUS THE CERTAINTIES OF FACT

The pronouncements of medical science have a tendency to be authoritative, authoritarian, and, all too often, dead wrong—particularly when they only too neatly reflect the biases and discriminatory ideas of the culture at large. The workings of the natural world, biology, human physiology, and endocrinology are simply too complex to reduce to a sentence, metaphor, or aphorism, and inevitably, our own worldview leaches into the science we do. How we envision the behavior of a cell or primate or galaxy depends on who we are and how we see the world—and many scientific descriptions have had to be modified over time as their shortcomings became obvious. For instance, as biologist and philosopher of science Evelyn Fox-Keller has pointed out, fifty years ago in vitro fertilization was described in ways that evoked the Sleeping Beauty myth with the "penetration, vanquishing, or awakening of the egg by the sperm."[42] At the time, both image and metaphor matched the available technology and the prevailing sexual wisdom. Today, the metaphor is cast more in the language of equal opportunity, and the egg is no longer considered a purely passive recipient. This does not mean that we still do not regularly hear of the egg "being fertilized" or of sperm having characteristics more appropriate to an Olympic athlete than a miniscule active particle contained in an aqueous solution.

When medical science takes on the metaphorical assurances of socially determined facts to make therapeutic recommendations, however, the consequences can be dire. What we consider "normal" ovarian or cardiac or neuronal function may be a mere statistic, gleaned from studies with a particular slant often peculiar and specific to a certain time and place—but its incorporation into clinical practice has very real consequences.

Too many so-called truths, whether on women and hormones or anything else, are unexamined assumptions. Everybody knows these things because, well, everybody knows them. Numeric reasoning, in particular, has singular cachet—if we can phrase things in terms of numbers, then somehow they must be true.[43] Repetition adds to the credibility of the claims, no matter how unscientific or illogical, and eventually, regardless of the actual data on which they are based, they become accepted, things that are known because they are known. So, if we keep repeating that one in four of us will suffer from osteoporosis or one in nine will have breast cancer, it ends up feeling true, even if it is not. But facts, as the Harvard biologist and feminist writer Ruth Hubbard wrote in *The Politics of Women's Biology* nearly twenty years ago, are contextual.[44] They depend not only on who we are (and where and when), but also on the direction in which we want those facts to take us. It cannot be incidental that the Latin root of the word *fact*, as Hubbard reminds us, is *facere*, meaning "to make and/or make function."

Science has had a great deal to do with the medical and social making of women as biological and social organisms, particularly because human nature has been defined, essentially, by a small enclave of predominantly white men who have had the authority to declare what is normal and what is not, what is dysfunctional and what is right. As Hubbard writes:

> As women, we have been not only scientifically misdefined but mistreated. Gyne-cologists and surgeons remove our female organs with a lack of concern that is in marked contrast to the respect they display for men's private parts. Indeed . . . a sci-entific/medical profession that has tried to exclude women from public life, lest our participation disturb the natural ebb and flow of our hormones, has not been equally hesitant to manipulate those very hormones—all, of course, in order to "help" us conceive or abort, or prevent conception or abortion, or keep from showing signs of advancing age.[45]

Hubbard's position is particularly impressive given that from the 1940s to the late 1960s, she was, in her own words, a "devout" scientist who never questioned how her work as a scientist and researcher fit into the culture, assuming that she was "probing nature" in true scientific fashion. It was only much later, after she and other longtime women scientists classified as research associates were granted tenure (through the activities of feminists at Harvard), that she came to appreciate that science was part of the arsenal used to "maintain differences in wealth and power" between nations and ethnic, racial, economic, and gender groups.

The metaphors and language we use to describe what we study, furthermore, alter what we observe and how we feel. In Japan, for instance, there is no word for *hot flush*, and women in other cultures describe symptoms, such as backache, that Western culture does not associate with hormones.[46] In 1995, George Annas, writing in the prestigious *New England Journal of Medicine*, succinctly described how our metaphors create our attitudes.[47] Annas, a jurist, described how American language, permeated with military and market metaphors, affects our perceptions of medicine. The overriding implication is that ill health is an invader of some kind, hence diseases *attack* the body, and we *fight* cancer with chemotherapy that *destroys* the rogue cells. The newspaper today describes how officials review their *battle plan* in a mumps outbreak. Substitute *terrorist cells* or *enemy*, and the sentences still make sense. In some medical articles, drugs are even referred to as missiles or other types of weapon. Market metaphors have also begun to make inroads; presently, we invoke the health care *industry* (which makes acute care sound like a factory) or managed care, and we refer to the changes in the workings of the medical system in terms more common to the factory floor or business such as *productivity* and *waste*. Even though economists tell us that health care is not a commodity (nobody gives up a Caribbean holiday to check themselves into the hospital for a quadruple bypass unless they feel they absolutely must) and that patients are not consumers, direct-to-consumer ads (illegal everywhere except the United States and New Zealand) imply otherwise. Ideally, what we need, suggests Annas, is an ecological metaphor—a prescient comment in 1995, although to date nobody seems to have taken him up on it.

ACCEPTING AMBIGUITY

When a physicist describes a distant galaxy, an entomologist describes insect behavior, or a biologist describes a cell, the terms, metaphors, and ideas they use to frame their hypotheses come from the language and ideas they already have. Emily Martin, in *The Woman in the Body*, describes ways in which Western medical descriptions of women's bodies are suffused with "metaphors of production"— revealing that she herself had enormous problems once she moved her research from China, where she was an outsider, to the United States, where, as a white, middle-class academic, she felt she belonged.[48] As she studied reproduction and women's health issues, Martin often found herself at a loss when attempting to critique her interviews with American women because so much of what they said seemed like ordinary "common sense" to her. For instance, her understanding of uterine contractions during pregnancy came from medical texts, where they are described as involuntary, so it made perfect sense to her that women described them as "separate and distinct" from themselves. She "anguished" that what she was hearing made good, scientific, factual sense; seemed "obvious." It was only later, as she remembered the "facts" that women in China had told her (certain diseases were "hot" and others, "cold"; other times, the yin and the yang were out of balance), facts that made no sense to her but were absolute truths to the Chinese interviewees, that it all fell into place. She had so internalized the American perspective that to her, *these* were the facts, what she knew and believed. Martin came to recognize her own subconscious biases only with extreme difficulty, often in speaking to women who were unlike her, for example, poor or uneducated.

Very little in life can genuinely be said to be a given. Even that most common of all verbal shortcuts, the binary or oppositional phrase, which we use to describe all manner of things—men/women, estrogen/testosterone, up/down, left/right, north/south—is simply a reflection of the universe that Western thinkers such as Plato and Pascal bequeathed us. If we stop to consider, it is our vantage point that determines our position and therefore how we see the world. Take, for instance, that most basic of geographical directions, north versus south. It seems perfectly normal for us to think of the northern hemisphere as the top of the globe and the southern hemisphere as what is below. But the earth is a sphere, which means it is round—and by definition it cannot have an up or down, or north or south. We are the ones determining those distinctions; we are the ones deciding which way is up, so to speak.

Even medical classification systems, to which we tend to give considerably more weight, are neither unchanging nor obvious. How we define illness and dysfunction, how we categorize disease, has ramifications far beyond the personal. And as this book shows, women's cycles and the time they stop, what we call menopause, rely not only on the simple physical phenomenon of a woman having a monthly period (and then not), but on everything from the environment in which she lives to the cultural and linguistic milieu. In the following chapters, we will continue the topics we touched in this chapter, from the menstrual cycle and perimenopause to the so-called preventive power of hormones in reducing our risk of heart disease, osteoporosis, and so on. As the reader will see, nothing is as simple as it might seem.

2

CIRCADIAN RHYTHMS, MENSTRUAL CYCLES, AND CULTURE

The scientist . . . decides what the research question is, whose answers to it are relevant, the precise form in which the question should be asked and the "correct" interpretation of the responses. No matter whether the person being researched is called a "participant" or a "respondent," they are still a "subject" in this power relationship, with no influence over how the data are collected or interpreted and, in many cases, no knowledge of the outcome of the research. Similarly women's experiences are rarely of interest in their own right but only as a secondary phenomenon. In menstrual cycle research, for example, women's premenstrual experiences are investigated because they are thought to be symptoms of disease or to interfere with work or domestic functions, not because how women feel is of intrinsic interest.

—Anne Walker[1]

What is it about the menstrual cycle that is so fundamental, so essential, to being a woman—so much so that the time when it permanently stops, menopause, has been called pathological and even a "deficiency" disease? Menstruation, after all, is simply a natural, ordinary part of being a woman.

"What's there to discuss?" asks a woman interviewed in British psychologist Anne Walker's comprehensive book, *The Menstrual Cycle*. "It's like fingernails, hair—they grow. It's just a fact of life." And, when you come right down to it, what *is* there to discuss? Or rather, what would there be to discuss if our cultural worldview accepted women's physiology as being as commonplace and as normal as a man's?[2] For if we think about menstruation without all the social, cultural, emotional, and personal overlay with which we inevitably saddle it, menstruation is simply part and parcel of being a woman, an essential part of our biology and who we are.

As girls, we barely know anything about our menstrual cycle and have little sense that at some point it will start; then it does. That first period often does lead to strong feelings—relief that it has started, consternation, joy, fear, and a kind of proud embarrassment—but over the next few years, after the tumult of puberty, both the idea of menstruation and menstruation itself normalize, and we learn how our body's cyclic nature works. As that woman interviewee said, then it is just a fact of life.* After several decades, usually in our forties, menstruation begins to change, becoming less predictable, and eventually, our periods stop. For most adult women, this is neither extraordinary nor anything to write home about, so to speak.

But we do not inhabit a world that appreciates, accommodates, or understands women or women's bodies, whether it is pregnancy and motherhood, or menstruation and menopause; on the contrary, our natural biological rhythms are things we hide, along with our tampons, only speaking of menstruation in hushed voices. "In Western [and many other] cultures, menstruation is a private and usually hidden experience," writes Walker.[3] We use euphemisms to describe our monthly cycle and engage in a "subtle menstrual 'etiquette'" that reflects the overwhelmingly negative attitudes we have internalized on the subject. The medical literature is particularly disagreeable about menstruation, frequently describing it as a "loss" or "failure" of reproduction. Plus, the bulk of medical writing refers to *problems* with menstruation, and few, if any, references are made to the majority of women for whom this is a natural part of who they are, not a burden.

The media further emphasize the need for discretion and secrecy, and the overt discourse on menstruation consists primarily of television and print advertisements touting a particular brand of tampon or pad as the one that will "prevent embarrassing leaks" and allow us to function "normally" (implying that menstruation is somehow abnormal for a competent woman in today's world). As Walker ironically adds,

> Although adverts for menstrual products appear to be breaking this bond of silence surrounding menstruation, they in fact reinforce secrecy and shame by working from an assumed shared knowledge of the anxieties and taboos related to it.† While they seem to promise an active, liberated lifestyle, [they] never mention menstruation itself. They fuel concern that our secret will be found out, emphasising the possibility of "leakage" or bulky towels showing through tight trousers, telling us that we can

---

*Unfortunately, we are increasingly altering our normal cycles, and a regrettable consequence of giving a thirteen-year-old girl the birth control pill for her cramps is that as she matures, she may never really know what her own normal cycle is or what it feels like.

†A recent ad does exhort having a "happy" period, but only in the context of hiding it better.

even wear white shorts.... [These in turn] make us increasingly anxious about menstruation and unable to acknowledge the reality.... With all these wonderful products to help us, what possible excuse could there be for leaking or being incapacitated by menstruation? In other words, shame sells, and will continue to sell whilst the taboo around menstruation persists.[4]

Then there is menopause, when menstruation ends, where the message turns downright nasty, and we are led to believe that this is The End—of womanhood, of youth and vigor, of life as we know it. From here on in it is downhill all the way. Again, if we strip away the emotive imagery and language (inasmuch as we can, since we are all products of this culture and our own biases are notoriously difficult to discern) and simply regard premenopausal menstruation and postmenopausal lack of flow as normal parts of every woman's life—just as we all went through life as children without menstruation—then, to paraphrase H. L. Mencken, it is what it is. What's there to talk about? (Of course, perimenopause *is* a whole other story, but more on that later.)

All life changes with time, whether we are speaking of a man or a woman, a dog or a kangaroo, an insect or an amoeba. With repeated cellular change comes an eventual slowing down, and as our lives continue, our physiology evolves; immune function becomes less reactive (a seven-year-old will heal from a cut or scrape with amazing speed, whereas even for a person of thirty, it will take longer), bones become less dense for both men and women, and, for all of us, hair loses its pigment and skin decreases in thickness and elasticity. The fingers of a seven-year-old will wrinkle in a bath; those of a seventy-year-old will not. Susceptibility to toxic and viral insults changes. Nothing is static. Yet we place so much weight and extraordinary focus on women's *fertility* (which is associated with hormone "strength" and presence), that it appears to be the only sign of female value we recognize. We see this reflected in the powerful emotions the pro-choice movement arouses, and even in adjunct areas such as birth control for women in developing countries. In some ways, this deflection of attention onto the physiological and physical is a stroke of genius, for as long as women, along with everyone else, believe that it is their menstrual cycle that makes them real women, and that menopause is to be dreaded, then the centrality of fertility and hormones to our identity remains the same.

BLOOD, SWEAT, AND TEARS

The menstrual cycle can be likened to an orchestra, one with many instruments all playing different parts of the same score, all taking their tempo and direction from the conductor, in this instance, the brain—or, more specifically, the hypothalamus—from which all the other sections take their cue. Each woman is different, so, in each woman, the volume and combinations of instruments that play simultaneously (the hormones) are different. Nutrition, age, and the emotional and physical health of the woman all have an effect on the character of the music, and thus, although the score may be the same, the music is endlessly varied. During childhood, it is as though that orchestra conductor is satisfied with small pulses of the reproductive hormones, like a quiet humming. But during early puberty, the conductor signals the pituitary (a small nubbin of co-ordinating hormonal tissue that sits just behind and between the eyes) to start increasing the pulses of luteinizing hormone (LH, or progesterone) and follicle-stimulating hormone (FSH, estrogen). These pituitary hormones have the job of awakening the cells of the ovaries, the walnut-sized organs hiding behind the hip-bones containing follicles—hormone-producing cells—which surround an egg. (The term *luteinizing* comes from "making yellowness"—the color of the corpus luteum, or "yellow body," left after release of an egg that early barber surgeons saw under the microscope when they dissected an ovary after ovulation.) Each woman is born with about 1 million of these follicles and their internal eggs, but by puberty, there are only some one hundred thousand left; the rest partially mature and are absorbed back into the body.

At first, these hormonal swings occur only during sleep as they are connected to circadian rhythms, or sleep–wake cycles (those same rhythms that fall out of kilter when we are jetlagged), and for many women, this hormonal connection to sleep becomes sharply obvious during perimenopause, as sleep becomes fitful and disturbed. Once these nocturnal hormonal spikes move to the daytime, however, we really begin the process of pubertal maturation. In the West, this usually happens between the ages of eight and ten. The adrenal glands become more active, and this enhances sweat gland activity and causes more and darker limb hair. As these new nighttime brain hormone surges increase, the ovaries enlarge, the follicles mature and produce more estrogen, and this, in turn, stimulates breast development. Testosterone levels also rise, leading to pubic hair. Meanwhile, the increasing estrogen levels have stimulated the endometrial lining of the uterus, and it thickens and then sheds. This is *menarche*, or a girl's first period.

The first cycles after menarche are often hit or miss, out of sync, as though only some of the instruments in the orchestra play the right notes and the music is occasionally discordant. (Think of it as a slightly atonal high school band.) Those first cycles make sufficient or even high levels of estrogen, but it is as though the conductor is unsure, as if the pituitary hormones are awkward and uncoordinated. It is only after many months, in fact, usually a year, that the orchestra gains the confidence and skill to create an *ovulatory* cycle. From menarche onward, monthly, several of the outermost follicles of one ovary grow and make estrogen; then, one of these gets more pituitary signals and becomes the dominant follicle, growing to some 18 mm in size (about the size of a fingernail). This chosen follicle then gets to play a solo, making all the estrogen for that single cycle as well as releasing its egg and making progesterone and estrogen after ovulation. So each period results from a single follicle with its egg, which, if you come right down to it, is quite extraordinary. Every period is different and involves one follicle, and if ovulatory, one egg.

Before ovulation can happen, however, estrogen has to reach a crescendo, becoming loud and intense and reaching a peak of 220 percent above its low level during flow. This, in turn, signals the brain and pituitary gland to create an LH peak that—to continue the orchestra metaphor—rings out and signals the rupture of the fluid-filled cyst that the dominant follicle has become, thus releasing the egg into the great pelvic unknown. This is ovulation.

Once the egg is released from its bed of estrogen-producing cells, those cells change their color and character, and after ovulation, progesterone is made by the same cells that formerly only made estrogen. Progesterone floods the region, rising clear and loud over the rest of the orchestra and reaching a peak that increases to more than fourteen hundred times higher than during the menstrual period itself. While the egg is being enveloped by the fingerlike projections of the fallopian tube and progressing toward the uterus, progesterone is creating orchestra-wide change. Its essential task, and the one for which it is known (and the role for which it may even be valued), is to create a moist, mature, and nurturing endometrium (uterine lining) so that, should the egg, on its travels, meet up with a sperm, the fertilized egg can find a home and make a baby.* Progesterone also changes that formerly slippery cervical mucus† making a sperm freeway into a dry, sticky route through which sperm cannot travel. In the breasts, high progesterone stops the estrogen-stimulated growth of breast cells and makes the cells more mature and ready to make milk,[5] as well as stimulating new bone formation.[6] In the arteries, progesterone modulates blood flow throughout the body.[7] So it may well be progesterone alone, or perhaps estrogen and progesterone together—but certainly not estrogen alone, as most believe—that keeps blood vessels healthy and responsive and makes the heart resilient and strong.

OVULATION: EXTRAORDINARY, UNIQUE—AND MISUNDERSTOOD

The menstrual cycle is a unique glandular secretion. Generally, it is the permanent cells of the entire gland that are engaged in making hormones—for instance,

---

*Other progesterone-related changes are a 0.2 degree Celsius increase in the whole body's core temperature, a minuscule rise in breathing rate (although not enough for the woman to notice), and a desire to eat more to keep weight stable (which is fundamental to all organisms) because even that slight increase in temperature uses up energy (about three hundred more calories a day).

†The cervical glands, under the influence of high levels of estrogen, secrete a mucus that is clear, like egg white and has a characteristic fern-like pattern when dried under a slide and viewed through a microscope. This estrogenized mucus creates an ideal passage for sperm to get from the vagina to the uterus.

all thyroid cells or all pancreatic islet beta cells join to make, respectively, thyroxine or insulin. Each follicle in the ovary, however, has the potential to create a menstrual cycle, and all the high hormone levels during each cycle emanate from the specific cells surrounding a single egg.

Such exquisite differentiation is simply extraordinary, although perhaps what is truly amazing is that any of us manages to have regular, ovulatory menstrual cycles at all. Nevertheless, if a woman is emotionally distraught (if, for instance, her child dies or she is forced to flee her home because of war), if she is starving and undernourished, if her physical body is exhausted (if she is an anxious, overtrained teenage track-and-field champion), or if she is seriously ill, then the stress response and the hormones it engenders will suppress pituitary LH and FSH. The preservation of the organism takes priority over the menstrual cycle and reproduction. This makes perfect physiologic sense: better to conserve energy and survive without menstruating, and live to menstruate and ovulate another day, than use up what energy there is in maintaining a normal cycle and compromising continued life. Lesser stressors may inhibit ovulation (called an anovulatory cycle) but not the menstrual cycle. This means that there is sufficient estrogen to thicken the endometrium and allow it to shed, but no release of an egg and no progesterone (or release of an egg with too short a duration of progesterone to support pregnancy). Strangely, the cycle length may be, and often is, perfectly normal, and a woman may not have a clue that her body is reacting so profoundly to stress; her cycles are regular, but what is lacking are ovulation and progesterone. Alternatively, the anovulatory cycle may be too short or too long. But in the long term, normal ovulatory cycles are important for good health, and when we focus exclusively on flow (as too often gynecology does), we lose sight of this.

With more minor stressors (family conflicts, problems at work), or with adaptation to stress, the cycle does take place and ovulation does occur, but the time between the release of the egg and the menstrual flow is shorter than it ideally should be. So although the cycle length may be normal and estrogen levels fine, progesterone is only secreted for a few days causing too much estrogen for the amount of progesterone and depriving the woman of the benefits of optimal hormone balance. This short luteal phase cycle is ovulatory and has some progesterone, but is not long enough to allow the endometrium to support a fertilized egg. A combination of stressors (such as a partnership breakdown or abruptly beginning to train for a marathon) in a woman in her early twenties, or even one stressor (being jilted in first love as a teenager), may plunge the entire orchestra into near silence, with only the nighttime LH and FSH peaks taking place, resembling puberty before menarche. The cycle regresses to an earlier era.

The two main hormones that the ovary produces, and the complicated brain, pituitary, and life-balance assessment (of stress, of nutrition, of everything) that makes up each and every ovulatory menstrual cycle, have been consistently misunderstood and badly described. Perhaps it is because endocrinology is hard, and women's hormones contain an extra layer of complexity. For example, to gynecologists, *anovulation* simply means irregular or absent menstrual cycles,[8] rather than what we just described: a cycle of normal or abnormal length but without an egg being released or sufficient levels of progesterone being produced. This erroneous notion—that we require ovulation and progesterone to trigger menstrual flow (so if your periods are regular then everything is fine)—is one that dates back to the early 1900s when it was believed that it was the unfertilized egg that brought down the menstrual flow. Again, this description fits social, not physiologic parameters.

MISLEADING DIAGRAMS

Furthermore, estrogen levels (which are, without question, obvious and important), have long been overemphasized, to the detriment of the second hormone, progesterone. The normal estrogen increase (of two hundred plus times above the baseline during menstruation) that occurs at midcycle is generally clearly defined and reasonably well understood, but the second important player in this cyclic dance, progesterone, is not, even though, during the second half of a normal cycle, progesterone levels increase to fourteen hundred times higher than their menstrual baseline. This makes estrogen's 220 percent increase look miniscule—but somehow this enormous difference, this vast discrepancy between the maximum amounts of progesterone compared with estrogen that are secreted during each menstrual cycle, remains unacknowledged and virtually ignored.

More insidiously, the graph that is commonly used to pictorially describe the menstrual cycle to sixth-grade students or medical students (as well as in the medical or health literature) shows the two hormones rising, at their appropriately different times, to levels that look nearly identical making this graph essentially false, if not fraudulent. Either way, it is just plain wrong.

Yet nobody—not statisticians, medical editors, doctors—appears to have noticed. Medical textbooks all perpetuate the error, with this so-called standard description of hormone levels during the menstrual cycle appearing over and over as well as in self-help books, on the Internet, and elsewhere. Figure 2.1 shows the diagram as it is ordinarily shown and taught. Figure 2.2 shows estrogen and progesterone both drawn as percentage change from their low baseline levels during menstrual flow. In fact, progesterone levels end up so much higher that, were estrogen and progesterone drawn to the same scale in the standard textbook graph, the estrogen molehill would sit as it does in the figure, while the progesterone mountain would fly as high as the floor above our heads in whatever room we are in. Because it would be difficult to draw such a graph accurately, the two hormones are expressed in different units, breaking the cardinal rule of statistical communication; namely, that all items being compared must be expressed in the same units.

Figure 2.1

This line drawing is the typical representation of the estradiol (estrogen, solid line) and progesterone (dashed line) changes across a normal menstrual cycle. Note that there are no units listed and that estradiol peak appears to be higher than the progesterone peak. This figure was redrawn by J. C. Prior from a diagram shown at http://embryology.med.unsw.edu.au/wwwhuman/MCycle/SmLSec.htm.

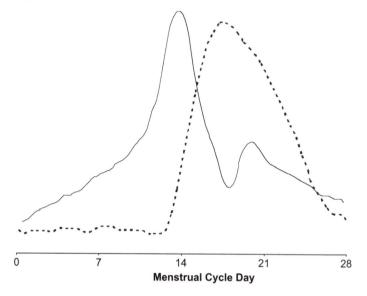

Menstrual Cycle Day

Figure 2.2

This line drawing of the menstrual cycle hormones across one normal cycle shows the percentage changes of estradiol (estrogen, solid line) from the low baseline during flow and the percentage changes of progesterone (dashed line) from the low baseline during the whole first half of the menstrual cycle. This figure was redrawn by J. C. Prior from data in Nielsen, H. K., *Journal of Clinical Endocrinology and Metabolism 70*, 1431–7 (1990).

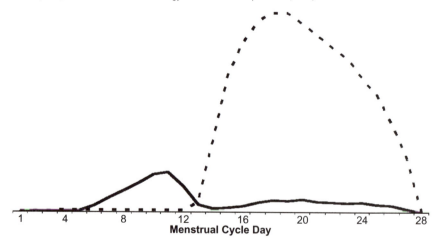

Menstrual Cycle Day

To better understand the errors in drawing estrogen and progesterone during the menstrual cycle, consider the following example: if we were to ask you to compare two people's weights, but were to give you one of those weights in kilograms and the other in pounds, what do you think would happen? A kilogram is roughly two pounds, so if we asked you who is heavier, the person who weighs 132 or the one who weighs 60, naturally, you would pick the former. But both people would be exactly the same weight, since 60 kilograms is exactly 132 pounds. This is what has happened with the two primary menstrual hormones. Estrogen is expressed in picograms (pg, or picomols) and progesterone in nanograms (ng, or nanomols). (Any unit that is *nano* is one thousand times bigger than one that is *pico*.) This may explain, in part at least, why our medicine and our culture are so eager to emphasize estrogen and to ignore progesterone: fundamental ignorance of their true balance within the ovulatory menstrual cycle.

PERFECT B-CUP BREASTS

In every young woman's life, before and following menarche, comes breast development: the transformation of our breasts from flat, unisex models into larger mounds during those years around our first period. Most women remember some angst about their breasts in sixth or seventh grade: wondering if they would ever grow, or if they were growing too fast or were too lopsided or were just not right. We also may remember our first bra, with either embarrassment or pride, our first intimation that we were moving into the transition our mothers would sometimes call "becoming a woman."

Breast development initially involves only estrogen because, as we pointed out earlier, the brain–pituitary–ovary system takes a while to learn to make ovulation and settle into healthy ovulatory cycles that generate an ideal balance of both estrogen and progesterone. In fact, at menarche, the Tanner scale, the scoring system used to evaluate pubertal breast and pubic hair development, commonly gives young women's breasts a score of three (out of a possible five).

Developed by two male pediatricians in the late 1950s and early 1960s, the Tanner scale is an archetypal example of medical science as it has pertained to women's health: simultaneously amazing, systematic, and vaguely vile. Every three months, the British physicians Marshall and Tanner photographed 192 naked foundling girls from a British orphanage—something that would never get past an ethics committee today (at least, we hope it wouldn't). To look at photographs of these skinny kids in successive stages of maturity today is to cringe with embarrassment, yet also to marvel at the detail and complexity of breast maturation.[9] These photos record a diverse set of changes that advance in a reasonably orderly (yet not consistently symmetrical) fashion, as maturation alters the size of the mound of breast tissue itself, the areolae (the darker, bull's-eye circle in the middle of each breast), and the nipple.

What the two pediatricians did not know (having no expertise in hormones), and the majority of physicians also remain unaware of, is that although estrogen is involved in the size and voluptuousness of breasts, by itself, it cannot create "grown-up" or Tanner stage five breasts. It takes more than estrogen to make the areolae and nipple mature beyond the infantile size of boys and babies. It takes progesterone for that final stage of development of the areola and, more important, to create the milk ducts beneath—which, of course, is their raison d'être. By comparison, in a teenaged boy or adult man, the areolae are the size of a quarter, but a fully developed adult woman (scoring five out of five on the Tanner scale) would have areolae at least the size of a silver dollar. One of the authors (J.C.P.) first realized this in a rather unusual way, years ago, at a clinic that treated (male to female) transsexuals. Typically, when these patients first came for evaluation, these biological men (who felt like women) were all taking high doses of estrogen. This made their breasts grow into sexy B or C cups, yet, incongruously, their areolae and nipples stayed tiny and male. Adding progesterone to their estrogen therapy allowed their breasts to mature into fully grown-up female models.[10] So clearly, as in other aspects of physiology, it takes both estrogen and progesterone, working in tandem, for normal development.

Is this terribly important? Well yes, it is, at least when it comes to the breasts' ability to produce milk: clear evidence of the importance of progesterone within the entire spectrum of female development.* It may also be important in decreasing the risk for breast cancer, as we discuss later.

ESTROGEN AND THE PARADIGM OF HEALTHY FERTILITY

Since the 1920s, "the assumption that sex hormones were the agents of masculinity and femininity functioned as a paradigm," writes University of Amsterdam sociologist and feminist professor Nelly Oudshoorn, and what had formerly been scattered bits of research zeroed in on this single subject.[11] Gynecologists, she adds, particularly, "fell under the spell of the glands because of their therapeutic promises," for they quickly perceived the benefit it would provide for them in maintaining medical control over the "complex of disorders in their female patients"—disorders that they connected to the ovaries, to hormones, and to the menstrual cycle.

By 1929, within three years of the chemical isolation of estrogen, a book had already been published called *The Female Sex Hormone*.[12] Thus, estrogen became *the* female hormone, testosterone the quintessentially male one, whereas progesterone really did not figure in the discussion at all. Yet anatomists had

---

*If you have not been on the birth control pill (and thus exposed to progestin), look in the mirror and see what size your areolae are.

known for centuries that there were two female hormones, both made by the ovary—one, the hormone of the follicle (estrogen), was followed by a second made by the corpus luteum after the release of the egg (progesterone). Although it was 1934 before progesterone was isolated and chemically purified, by 1929, the actions of the "corpus luteum hormone" (progesterone) had been well described using bioassays and yet even early on these data were ignored.

Pharmaceutical companies were quick to jump on board with this new female hormone. Even at the turn of the twentieth century, as Oudshoorn points out, "the advertising pages of medical journals were full of recommendations" for doctors to prescribe the new ovarian and testicular preparations the drug companies had quickly begun producing.[13] The practice was so profitable that it never ceased—at least in terms of women, who were, and continue to be, told—from the first night sweat or hint of menstrual irregularity—to take estrogen to restore health. Men were never quite as good a market. Even today, although some older men are prescribed androgens/testosterone to treat sexual dysfunction or decreased libido, and some athletes of both sexes do take androgenic steroids to increase musculature and performance, the primary target for hormones remains the female half of the population. Hormones and the menstrual cycle, furthermore, not only have been superb for drug company sales but, given their iconic status in fertility, a cause all men could support. And because menstruation is the only visible sign of a woman's fertility, the only external or observable indication that she could bear a child, it remains pivotal and inexorably connected to womanhood.

Even today, when hormone levels can (more or less) be measured—although not as reliably or accurately as most people believe—and scanning techniques have made the ovaries, fallopian tubes, uterus, bones, and so on more visible,[14] when we are (somewhat) more savvy as to the anatomic and physiologic nature of women's sexual and reproductive selves—again, nowhere to the extent that our popular culture implies—the menstrual cycle and estrogen retain their iconic status. They are perceived as being central to, and the cause, of fertility, while the symphony of changes that must be appropriately coordinated to produce an ovulatory menstrual cycle are virtually ignored. Witness the inordinate focus we have maintained on the birth control pill for contraception rather than the practical and proven barrier and vaginal spermicide methods that are equally effective and also prevent sexually transmitted diseases. Instead, over the last fifty years, it has been considered important to somehow improve on women's own hormonal cycles, while also controlling their fertility. Today, 86 percent of North American women have used the Pill for a minimum of three months and for an average of six years.[15] In fact, the oral contraceptive is so much a part of our culture that the U.S. Food and Drug Administration (FDA) and Canada's Health Protection Branch have both maintained that the standard contraceptive schedule (twenty-one days on with seven days off) constitutes a perfectly adequate control group for research on extended contraceptive schedules that stretch from three to twelve months.*

In addition to preventing pregnancy, hormones are prescribed to streamline, change, or otherwise alter the course and nature of women's menstrual cycles, used to treat heavy periods and premenstrual syndrome (PMS)—what is called premenstrual tension, or PMT, outside North America—as well as "fix" whatever time frame has been deemed as infertility. (Given the enormous physiologic variability that exists between people, and the many factors involved in reproduction, who is to say what time period is the appropriate one in which to become pregnant?) Under the guise of good therapeutic practice, medicine—notably gynecology—has taken on itself the role of guardian of such measures, and with immeasurable insouciance, given the dearth of data and the lack of logic behind many such practices, convinced women to take powerful drugs or go under the knife. Women, in essence, have become guinea pigs for untested therapies and skewed theories not based on any hard science, but primarily used to confirm prejudicial sociocultural concepts that equate fertility with being a woman. Neither the long-term impact of such interventions nor their consequences have seemed to unduly concern either medical researchers or gynecologists—or the majority of women for that matter, although this last is more understandable. When everyone and everything around you stresses the authority and importance of medical science and its trustworthiness, not to mention the centrality of hormones (especially estrogen) to health, it is difficult to argue.

On closer examination, however, it is clear that a culture that continues to refer to menstruation as the "curse" is simply not neutral on the subject.

MENSTRUAL BASICS

In its most basic definition, menstruation is characterized by what we think of as blood and its temporal—and cyclic—elements, which are obvious from the descriptive terms we use. For example, many people in the English-speaking world use the word *period* or, in England, the *monthlies*, whereas in French, it is *les regles*, and in German, *das Regule*. In fact, the word *menses* comes from Latin and means "month." In Gaelic, the words for menstruation and calendar are the same. But as clear as this may seem to individual women who understand their own rhythms, creating definite borders for the menstrual cycle is more complicated. There is, again, enormous variability between individual women and between

---

*This statement is based on several negative reviews J.C.P. and colleagues received on a still-unpublished critical review of the data on hormonal contraceptive schedules with durations longer than the standard twenty-one days on high-dose estrogen and progestin, and on the fact that the FDA and the Canadian Health Protection Branch have not required placebo-controlled trials.

groups of women. One of the most detailed studies of normal menstruation was commissioned by the World Health Organization (WHO) in the late 1970s and included 5,322 women from ten countries. Approximately fifty women in each country kept a daily diary. There was variation in flow within countries, ranging from one to three days (in Egypt, Mexico, and India) to six or more (in England), with the norm being four to five days. Some women reported heavy flow at the start, which then tapered off; others reported light bleeding at the start, followed by two or three days of heavy flow, which then tapered off. Most women said their flow was moderate. In a more recent attempt to describe flow,[16] primarily motivated by a standard against which to compare bleeding while taking the Pill, data were collected from more than one thousand American women university students who took part in a study that began in the 1930s.[17] Women recorded the start and end of flow of every cycle for many years, sometimes from menarche to menopause, with the upshot being that the original WHO standards should be modified—and that flow lasting over one week is too long.*

Another question arises with respect to menstrual cycle length (not to mention who gets to make that decision and determine what is normal).† Everyone knows that a so-called normal cycle is four weeks long (the classical twenty-eight days), or so we are told, with ovulation occurring on day fourteen. This mythical cycle length (much like the norm of the 70-kg man used as the template in pharmacotherapy) may be a reasonable statistical average, but who can say what cycle is too long or too short in a particular person? Over the last century, this question has been repeatedly asked and answered; in the 1970s, a gynecologist decided, based on a few observational studies, that a menstrual cycle could be anywhere from twenty-one to thirty-five days (which was very neat arithmetic: precisely three to five weeks).[18] Anything shorter would be *polymenorrhea*, which means periods that are too frequent (as in *polygamy*, which means too many spouses) and anything longer would be *oligomenorrhea*, which refers to too few periods. However, the sample used to determine this so-called normal cycle was not random and only included white women.

A subsequent random population-based sample of more than 3,500 women of various ages from a single Danish county (also largely, although not exclusively, white) that looked at menstrual cycle lengths found that normal waxed and waned and depended on the woman.‡ Throughout a single year, approximately one-fifth of the women surveyed had a cycle of less than three weeks, whereas one-third had a cycle that went on for as long as five weeks. The Danish researchers found that the woman's age made a difference: between ages fifteen and nineteen, cycles

---

*See Notes.

†Defined by the start of one period up until the day before the next flow.

‡Postal questionnaires were sent out to women; some 78 percent chose to answer. Most of these women were asked during the eighth grade to keep a one-year record, and many continued to keep this record. This was therefore more accurate than if the women had relied on memory alone.

tended to be twenty-three to thirty-five days, but by age forty to forty-four, these had decreased to twenty-three to thirty days.[19] In other words, our individual cycles get shorter as we get older—which makes sense because most women are approaching perimenopause, the transition into menopause, by their forties. So as in most things, there are differences, not only between women, but also within a single woman across her life cycle.

REGULATING MENSTRUATION PHARMACOLOGICALLY

Oral contraceptives are said to decrease cramps, improve menstrual flow, prevent ovarian cancer, and of course, make it possible for a woman to have sex at any time. They have also become the new way to get rid of the "curse" outright, by taking the Pill every day. Full-page advertisements in women's magazines show models in white trousers, ecstatic at the thought. Unfortunately, this therapy of "cycle stopping," or menstrual suppression, will indeed stop a regular, *predictable* flow, but what the advertisements and promotional material omit to mention is that this regimen translates into just as many days of bleeding, except that the flow is unexpected and comes without warning.[20] So much for trying to fool Mother Nature.

In contrast to the subtext of the white-clad nymphs whirling about in delight in the current advertisements, what this actually turns out to be is a boon for the manufacturers of panty liners (which one can be persuaded to wear every single day). In fact, Proctor and Gamble, makers of sanitary products, now co-market Seasonale (the every-three-month Pill) in Canada. Moreover, the dubious benefit of stopping periods altogether comes at a high physiologic price: higher total estrogen exposure, which could potentially lead to blood clots and the other catastrophic consequences of high estrogen load, with absolutely no long-term evidence that this will not cause bone loss.[21] This is assuming that we will not find out, down the road, about other benefits a normal, ovulatory cycle could have and what other conditions it might potentially prevent, ranging from breast cancer to osteoporosis. Additionally, this menstrual suppression could also lead to a delayed return of fertility.[22] Of course this, in turn, would be excellent for fertility clinics and expensive in vitro fertilization (IVF) therapies. Additionally, such pharmacological manipulation of menstruation and obliteration of the five- to seven-day break from high hormones that both the normal cycle and the twenty-one-days-on-seven-days-off Pill provide could cause potentially harmful changes in breast tissue (which in turn might become cancerous). For younger women, these Pills also could cause significant disruptions in their fragile adolescent reproductive and hormonal development.[23]

In short, menstrual suppression is a disaster waiting to happen.

PMS: THE *DSM* VERSION

Given the continuous cyclic nature of menstruation throughout most of an adult woman's life, one might think that the menstrual cycle would have lent itself to thoughtful analysis and study throughout the years, and as Walker suggests, any most conceivable emotional or physical states relating to menstruation would have been investigated, or at least reported on—but this has not even remotely been the case.[24] Only a very narrow range of experiences, notably negative ones, have attracted attention—in other words, PMS or PMT. This focus has remained perennial, even though for most women, their menstrual cycle is not problematic: fewer than 1 percent of randomly sampled Canadian women from a medium-sized city reported being disturbed by negative premenstrual experiences in a well-designed study that minimized cultural expectation.[25]

In other words, when we are not primed to expect pain or discomfort, or handed a questionnaire that insists on it, we tend not to focus that much on negative premenstrual problems—perhaps the majority of us even forget we have them. In a way, this emphasis on all that is painful and uncomfortable about menstruation is analogous to the research on abuse: although the vast majority of children who are abused do not grow up to be abusers themselves, the research has exclusively focused on that minority (by some estimates, fewer than 20 percent) who do grow up to be monsters. Perhaps this speaks to our society's penchant for focusing on the negative and our ghoulish preference for reading bad news. Similarly, it is those women who have indicated they do suffer from their period on whom researchers, both behavioral and medical, have focused. As far back as the 1930s, R. Franks, the author of the 1929 book *The Female Sex Hormone*, who coined the term *premenstrual syndrome,* advocated ovarian irradiation for PMS,[26] a process that even he should have realized increased the risk of ovarian cancer or caused a pathologically early menopause.

Mood and emotional state have been of particular interest since ancient times, when, it is thought, menstruation inspired dread (again, insofar as we can know what anybody centuries ago believed) because it involves blood. It was even more mysterious given that it was the only natural instance in which blood occurred without injury. Given that the phases of the moon are often linked to the timing of menstruation, the connection also was often made with madness. Yet both these interpretations, as recent feminist slants on older anthropological literature have suggested, are more a reflection of current social norms than what early beliefs actually were, given that one could just as easily translate primitive or early ideologies on menstruation in a positive way—as being life enhancing and a blessing, a sign of health. Of course, our modern medical literature and lexicon do not tend to stress blessings or focus overmuch on anything positive. In fact, the current *Diagnostic and Statistical Manual of Mental Disorders, Fourth Edition*, or *DSM-IV,* used throughout much of the Western world and beyond to categorize the degrees and permutations of psychiatric disorders (which presupposes that we actually understand what *normal* means), categorizes PMS as "Premenstrual Dysphoric Disorder," with symptoms ranging from "markedly depressed mood, marked anxiety" and "marked affective lability" (emotional instability) to "decreased interest in activities."[27] What activities, the *DSM-IV* does not specify. Neither does it explain who decides at what point a woman's emotions may be considered "labile" or by whose standards. Given that, what would constitute a perfectly normal display of emotion in a Francophone culture, such as in Quebec, or a Hispanic one, such as in Mexico or Spain, would probably seem like crazy excess in a more restrained social climate, such as in New England or Great Britain, it is obvious from the first sentence that the category is steeped in sociocultural norms. The influence of society is very real when we see, from a controlled study in Mexico, how quickly women without the cultural concept of premenstrual symptoms learn to describe themselves as having troubling premenstrual symptoms—it only takes a single short videotape.[28] Focusing on somatic problems is incredibly easy once these issues have been pointed out.*

Nevertheless, women themselves have been influential in declaring PMS a real and occasionally distressing phenomenon. (Of course, this also might be the only sanctioned time women are able to express anger and say what they mean.) It does, nevertheless, appear that during this time in one's cycle, for reasons that are unclear, a woman's ability to absorb stress and conflict is somewhat eroded; a woman tends to be more sensitive at this time to stressors that she might shrug off at others. Once defined as a medical problem, however, the field is then thrown wide open for pharmaceutical solutions, although there is evidence that those women who are troubled by premenstrual experiences (such as feeling bloated, having a runaway appetite, sore breasts, or feeling irritable and frustrated) can be helped by charting their menstrual cycle experiences,† discussions with a sympathetic nurse,[29] increasing exercise,[30] or taking vitamin B_6.[31]

Official medical sanction and an acceptance of PMS as a genuine problem has nonetheless been considered valuable in legitimizing the problems some women do experience. There is little question that in a world like ours, where it is difficult to concede that anything exists unless there is a category or a name for it, a medical diagnosis will reduce the stress of having to prove that one is experiencing problems.[32] The issue then becomes what type of diagnostic categorization and corresponding therapeutic treatment is deemed appropriate. As Walker writes,

---

*Try it some time. Focus on your elbow, and think about how it feels when you push on it a certain way. It will start to hurt.

†The daily Menstrual Cycle Diary, a self-help instrument that includes positives such as "feeling of self-worth, energy, interest in sex" as well as physiological experiences like sore breasts, fluid retention, and headaches, is available for free on the CeMCOR Web site http://www.cemcor.ubc.ca/files/uploads/Menstrual_Cycle_Diary.pdf.

It means that women may receive a medical or psychiatric diagnosis and be exposed to a wide variety of treatments, ranging from vitamin supplements to hysterectomy and ovariectomy. For some, this is a positive step—acknowledging at least that women's distress is important and offering treatment. For others, the risk of medicalisation and psychologisation of women's experiences outweighs any benefit.[33]

And from many of these labels or solutions, there is no going back.

WOMEN'S ATTITUDES

Little wonder then that women have such contradictory and often negative feelings about their menstrual cycle. We rarely, if ever, hear anything positive, and the bulk of social references made to our cycle consist of being told we need to keep this monthly event under wraps.

The first empirical study of attitudes toward menstruation was reported in 1959. Two hundred students from two women's colleges were asked to complete an open-ended questionnaire. Unfortunately, the authors did not record the frequency of the responses or "consider their factor structure," which set the tone (and methodological sloppiness) that continues to permeate the field.[34] At least this once—versus the majority of the time—the study authors who were examining women's attitudes toward menstruation did not generate the statements themselves and then ask women to indicate whether or not they agreed, but allowed participants to generate their own statements. Eventually, one such study evolved into the Menstrual Attitudes Questionnaire, in the late 1970s. Conceptualized on a single positive/negative dimension (we really do love our binary classification systems), what emerged was that women's attitudes were considerably more complex than the researchers had anticipated and were more multidimensional than researchers had believed they would be. The majority of women (77%) expressed positive attitudes and agreed with statements such as "menstruation provides a way for me to keep in touch with my body" and "menstruation is a reoccurring affirmation of womanhood."[35]

Women slightly older than those at university, who are the standard test subjects in most psychology research, in particular, were more prone to reporting that their experiences with their cycles were predominantly positive. Walker posits that this may be in part because the early years after menarche, one's first period, are often tumultuous—much like the perimenopausal years—and the younger women were still experiencing some menstrual difficulties when they were asked about their attitudes. Interestingly, attitudes toward menstruation were not affected by religious beliefs, and few differences were found between groups of practicing Orthodox Jewish, Protestant, or Roman Catholic women. This suggests that women are stronger-minded than researchers give them credit for, particularly because the Jewish faith considers a woman unclean when she is having her period, and at the end, she is required to immerse her body in a stream or a special bath called the *Mikweh* (at least, according to Leviticus in the Old Testament, a passage to which Orthodox Jews continue to refer).

THE LEGITIMIZING ROLE OF SCIENCE

It is not surprising that as women, we have, by and large, believed what medicine and science have told us, given their position and authority within our collective Western imagination. Overall, we have exquisite faith in scientific knowledge, believing it to be vast and painstakingly discovered, brick by brick, bit by bit, by dedicated men (and women, although that is a phrase that is usually an afterthought, if it is mentioned at all) who labored to discover the "truths" of nature. After all, it is thanks to science that we currently enjoy so many marvelous advances in the health sciences, agriculture (like genetic engineering), and so on; it is science, and the technologies to which it has led, that allows us to enjoy such novel experiences as walking down the street talking to someone on the other side of the planet with a tiny, handheld device or seeing pictures sent back by a spaceship from Mars. Science and technology have brought us stealth bombers, video games, and the Internet.* Science, moreover, is purportedly objective (as we are repeatedly told, usually by scientists themselves), so what science relays is above petty human concerns. So, by definition, science cannot be sullied by such unseemly issues as prejudice or sexism.

Nonsense, retorts professor and geneticist Richard Lewontin, "Science is a social institution."[36] In a series of radio lectures later written up as a book, *Biology as Ideology*, Lewontin points out that like the state, the family, sport, and every other activity in which human beings engage, science is part and parcel of the world, integrated into our beliefs and values. And women, women's health, and women's cycles (and hormones) not only have been the subject of biased thinking, but are, in and of themselves, proof of it. Science and scientific beliefs matter, he adds, not only because science affects our lives on a daily basis, by manipulating the external, material world through various techniques and inventions (such as the research and development that led to that mobile telephone device), but because of its *potential*. This means that science allows us to imagine what is possible and likely, affecting how we think, our templates, about the world and the future. When geneticists or biologists refer to having discovered or "mapped" the human genome or some incredible new type of radio wave that may someday

---

*The Internet actually relies on a large network of cables running for hundreds of miles beneath the oceans, where it was submerged over fifty years ago; many of the so-called scientific advances we enjoy are actually the result of hard work and the painstaking building of infrastructure.

lead to new and improved therapies (or medicines or time travel), they not only create the illusion of magical new technologies that will transform our lives, but also provide us with a means of visualizing the possibilities these technologies might create.

When that vision is one of biological destiny, such as the one the DNA hypothesis involves, it predisposes us into believing that innate, inborn biological, factors outside our control—like our genes or our hormones—matter more than our social environment or culture or nationality or neighborhood (or ourselves), thus changing our perspective of the world. It is this function of science, says Lewontin, that is the more insidious: science explains our world to us, and, in doing so, creates the metaphors and mental shortcuts we use to describe and explain how the world works:

> It is not at all clear that a correct understanding of how the world works is basic to a successful manipulation of the world. But explanations of how the world really works serve another purpose, one in which there has been a remarkable success, irrespective of the practical truth of scientific claims. The purpose is that of *legitimation*.[37]

Science provides social legitimacy, in other words, a kind of official sanction for the worldview it espouses. For example, if science says that three-fourths of women are disabled in the week before their periods, then it must be true. If science says that our genes contain the blueprint for what we will become and what diseases we will get, then who will argue? Our mental picture of human development, therefore, resembles that of an actual blueprint: one of those purplish drawings that most of us have seen but few of us understand, the plan for what ends up being built, showing where the walls and staircases are and how many rooms the structure will hold. (Of course, even an architectural blueprint is rarely an exact abstract replica of what ends up being built, but that is another story.) As this idea of genes-as-blueprint takes hold, those voices that urge caution in taking that blueprint analogy too far, or point out that such a metaphor for human development is reductionist and simplistic, are simply not heard. Meanwhile, television and newspapers and magazine covers trumpet the extraordinary achievements of these researchers mapping the human genome, further firing up our cultural imagination toward this ostensibly "correct" scientific view of human beings. So we begin to believe that biology is destiny.

With time, the pendulum inevitably does swing, and today, nearly a decade since the Human Genome Project, with none—zero—of those early promises of extraordinary new gene therapies and drugs having come to fruition, we are beginning to hear alternate views expressed more openly. But, for most people, it is too late: the die is cast and this idea, this vision, has been set in stone—who we become was determined long ago by the structure of our genes.

Hormones, by definition biological, are then subsumed into this picture, and even the lopsided view of female hormones and the overemphasis on estrogen simply become part and parcel of this worldview—and we believe that our fate is indeed determined by our hormones, or estrogen, or our menstrual cycle, or its cessation, menopause. The problem is that such beliefs have consequences. Whether it is a disease or the sky at night, in creating these ideas we also narrow the range of possible solutions—whether it is the impact of fossil fuels on climate or how hormones work within our body or even what factors might lead to heart disease. After all, it is one thing to say that women (or Blacks or Asians, or Martians, for that matter) are not cut out for the competitive business of law or medicine or what-have-you; it is quite another to say that *science* has found this to be true. In fact, just about any nonsense can be spouted as long as it is prefaced by the phrase "science has shown." Nevertheless, the grand, universalistic assumptions and conclusions that science makes—whether it is the gene containing the blueprint to life or women's innate physiology being the reason they are the "weaker" sex—inevitably create the impression that what is being framed is a fundamental, biological truth. And nobody wants to argue with that.

DIFFERENT BUT NOT EQUAL

We do not need science to demonstrate that men and women have obvious anatomic and physiologic differences—small children playing doctor can figure that out. What matters is whether these differences are significant with respect to our ability to learn or do math or anything else that is valued in our world. In the context of this book, what is at issue is whether the medical definition and description of menstruation or menopause are the right ones, the only ones we need consider. Simply being different vis-à-vis reproductive roles is not particularly useful information in terms of cognitive or intellectual abilities, behaviorally or otherwise. All mammalian reproduction is similar to that of humans and requires a similar confluence of male and female—even though the mammals themselves do not necessarily fall into two neat categories but are ranged along a continuum, given that one's sex is not determined by one factor but many: genital, reproductive, hormonal, and psychological. In any event, from chimps to Chihuahuas, it is impossible to determine the sex of an animal one observes wandering about in its natural habitat. (If you hear a small dog barking by a park bench, it is impossible to tell, just by looking at it, whether it is male or female, regardless of what the ridiculous pseudo-science that calls itself sociobiology professes.)

When it comes to people, however, all bets are off. From the moment a baby is born and it is announced that it's a girl or a boy, the gender stereotyping begins, from pink and blue diapers to the types of toys toddlers are steered toward. Knowledge of who we are, "our femaleness or our maleness, of who we are to be, and knowledge of others' expectations of us" is reflected back to us from the moment we are born, as neurophysiologist Ruth Bleier writes in *Science and Gender*. Then, having persistently focused on the differences, society and science further classify and codify them, extending them into the social, economic, political, and even domestic spheres, where they are used as proof for the hierarchies we see all around.[38]

When a young woman is labeled as "premenstrual" if she is angry, when an older woman is dismissed as "hormonal" if she is a feminist, when even women believe that hormones are a fundamental determinant of who they are, then their options and choices are automatically narrowed, their opportunities reduced. In a hierarchical culture where, even today, only one class of person—the white male— truly seems to have lasting and genuine value, this further handicaps women's capacity for growth, change, and creativity. And because women, by definition, have been classified biologically through their ability to bear children, it remains a circular argument: what is a woman? A woman is a human being who is able to be a mother. And it is because woman's nature has been defined biologically "to *be* a mother and wife that the rest of the social construct of woman 'naturally' follows: nurturing, passive, dependent, weak, intuitive, non-intellectual" and whatever else happens to make sense for the time.[39]

Science, which evolved within this binary, hierarchic belief system, therefore, has taken on a distinctly masculine tone and developed a pervasive male bias in which women's biology, from their hormones to their menstrual cycle, became proof of women's inability to function equally: women were too fragile, too easily governed by their hormones, too prone to cyclic influences that made them unable to work or study, and in terms of medicine, this has had devastating consequences—weirdly, because these restrictions did not apply to lower socioeconomic classes, in other words, to women who had to work for a living.

As the biologist Ruth Hubbard points out in *The Politics of Women's Biology*, it was middle-class women, the wives and mothers and sisters of the scientists and researchers coming up with the theories, who were the focus of the women-are-the-weaker-sex perspective:

> The ideology of women's nature that is invoked . . . posits that a woman's capacity to become pregnant leaves her always physically disabled in comparison with men. The scientific underpinnings for these ideas were produced in the nineteenth century by the white, university-educated, mainly upper-class men who make up the bulk of the new professions of obstetrics and gynecology, biology, psychology, sociology, and anthropology. These professionals (perhaps unconsciously) realized that they might lose the kinds of personal attention they were accustomed to getting from their mothers, wives, and sisters if women of their own class gained access to the professions. They therefore used theories about women's innate frailty to disqualify girls and women . . . who might compete with them for education and professional status. But they did not invoke women's weakness to protest the long hours poor

women worked in the homes and factories belonging to members of their own class nor to protest the labor black slave women were forced to do.[40]

Women's brains, according to these experts on women's health, were smaller and their "ovaries and uteruses required much energy and rest in order to function" properly. It was, moreover, simply a fact that girls could not pursue higher education once they began menstruating—in fact, without enormous care, women's ovaries would simply shrivel up and die, and so (for sure) the human race would die out. In true contrarian fashion, these men also stated that poor women had far too many children, which was proof positive that they were not genteel enough to be real women. Whatever contradictions such statements held did not seem to bother anyone; these were, after all, the Voices of Authority: respected experts on the subject, men of science.

Today, safely ensconced in the advanced twenty-first century, much as we would like to think things have fundamentally changed, in too many ways they have not. Professional, well-off women flock to gynecologists during perimenopause and are given hysterectomies, whereas poor women, whether in the West or in the developing world, have no access to basic health care or the time to worry about their menstrual cycle. They put up with the flooding and anemia of perimenopause, or PMS, which make it more difficult for them to work at jobs they need to make ends meet. Meanwhile, all women are unwitting guinea pigs for whatever theories of female endocrinology happen to be fashionable at the time.[41] From the birth control they are assured is "safe" and "tested" to the drugs they are given while pregnant, which experts assure them could not possibly harm the developing fetus, women and children worldwide suffer disproportionately as a result of this medical nonchalance. Note that the new birth control pill for continuous use was approved last year without any evidence of its long-term safety with respect to bones, blood clots, or even fertility.[42]

Meanwhile, HIV-AIDS continues to be passed on to women via promiscuous men who refuse to wear condoms, and vaccines are federally mandated and tested out on young girls years before the long-term effects are known. Of course, men, too, are subject to medical theories and given untested drugs (particularly in the developing world, which is often a convenient dumping ground for drugs banned in the West), but the history of meddling in women's health began long before there were any genuine drugs that actually *did* anything for anybody. Gynecology has been a specialty since before the germ theory of disease. Since their isolation and chemical characterization, sex hormones were primarily targeted to women. The surgical removal of women's ovaries and uteruses, furthermore, was performed even hundreds of years ago, although this surgery did not become routine until the late nineteenth century.

The first time a woman's ovaries were successfully removed was in 1809, writes medical historian Jaclyn Duffin in *History of Medicine: A Scandalously Short*

Introduction. In that year, Kentucky doctor Ephraim McDowell operated on a woman with severe abdominal swelling and pain, removing a cancerous "ten-kilogram ovary." He did not use an anesthetic (because it did not exist at the time). Not only did the woman survive, but she outlived him by many years. McDowell repeated the procedure a few more times, later using alcohol and laudanum (a preparation containing opium) for pain relief. His success was probably due to his preoccupation with cleanliness and his concern for the well-being of his patients, even though he later admitted he really had not expected his patients to live. Some seventy or so years later, however, removing the ovaries had become "an antidote for many female ailments, including psychiatric disorders." Gynecologists then, as now, insisted they were acting in their patients' best interests and "called upon their colleagues to sympathize with the tyranny of female biology."

For uterine problems, hysterectomies and amputation of the cervix were rarely attempted prior to 1900, and then only through the vagina. However, in 1878, a German physician introduced the abdominal approach (for malignancy), and it soon became a common feature of gynecological practice. Duffin adds,

> By 1900 the Austrian Ernst Wertheim had treated uterine cancer with radical extirpation combined with oophorectomy and node dissection. The operation, [once] dubbed "utterly unjustifiable," soon became a standard treatment for cervical cancer, fibroid tumors, and prolapse; however these conditions were also used as a pretext for surgical birth control.[43]

METAPHORS OF PRODUCTION

In the early history of the West, the Greeks did not believe that men's and women's sex organs differed much—women merely had on the inside what men had on the outside. But from the seventeenth century and the Industrial Revolution onward, everything from the Western ideals of economic production and efficiency to concepts on the workings of physiology became blended with the factory floor, and women's bodies and their capacity to give birth took on the metaphor of industrial production. As anthropologist Emily Martin writes in her cultural analysis of reproduction, *The Woman in the Body*, "this mechanical metaphor" moved from the hospital, where the womb and uterus were spoken of as though they consisted of a "pump" that pushed the fetus out, to the term *labor*, which implies an equivalence with the burgeoning idea of factory production that was gaining currency at the time. The development of actual mechanical tools in obstetrics, such as forceps, further emphasized this metaphor, even as male physicians gradually took over from female midwives. As Martin writes, "The woman's body is [therefore] the machine and the doctor is the mechanic or technician who 'fixes' it."[44] By the same token, this metaphor of factory production became so prevalent that it dominates the way we describe most physiologic functions, from the cellular level on up, right from the start of life, as the chromosomal head that is DNA gives its subordinate RNA instructions on what to do within the cell (the metaphor being that of a corporation or plant), whereupon things happen—much as the workers on the plant floor comply with the orders they are given.[45] Within this belief system is the tacit understanding that hierarchical systems are part and parcel of the natural order of things, from a microscopic level upward. There are those who rule and those who are ruled, those who govern and those are governed—this is natural law, and we merely abide by it. The question then becomes, how do we know?

More to the point, how *can* we know?

These are not questions with which medical science concerns itself, especially since modern medical practice has managed to incorporate the majority of prejudicial gender assumptions and did so right from the start. Perhaps unsurprisingly, given that the template for normal remains fixed at that of a forty-year-old, 70-kg white man for everything from blood pressure to ideal percentage of body fat, women's physiology easily and blatantly falls into the realm of the pathological because it deviates from the (male) norm. Culture and language happily picked up the concept without skipping a beat. Hence, men are strong, equal to the task nature has meant them for: power and status come naturally to them because they are meant to be at the top. Women, meanwhile, are victims of their biology, hormonally and reproductively challenged, and over their lifetimes, even the one hormone, estrogen, that appears to provide them with a certain ability to get on, diminishes with time. Testosterone rules. The occasional woman may be allowed into the corridors of power or into the army, the odd female may buck expectation and become prime minister or CEO or a university professor, but these are not natural female roles. Reinforced in subtle and covert ways, this message is so fundamental that it has become invisible. In short, men are men, women are women, and anyone who rocks that boat will get eaten by sharks or right-wing commentators.

MENSTRUATION AS A FAILED PRODUCTION

Menstrual flow is the most visible sign that women are not men's equals. Medicine, therefore, keeping to the metaphor of factory production obligingly provided in earlier centuries (why give up a good metaphor when it is so useful?), is able to declare menstruation to be the archetypal instance of failed production. For what is menstruation but proof that a fetus has not been implanted? And, as written in a medical text that Emily Martin cites, "when fertilization fails to occur, the endometrium is shed, and a new cycle starts. That is why it used to be taught that 'menstruation is the uterus crying for lack of a baby'" (p. 45). (When one has stopped spluttering at the sheer effrontery of this, one also could note how a word like *fails* stresses the metaphor of production.) The effect of being told that menopause is a kind of "failure of the authority structure in the body," as Martin points out, cannot help but have negative connotations because not only do we value humming factories churning out cars and chocolate bars, and so on, but we are all only too painfully aware of the economic and personal fallout of failed production: plants shut down and boarded over leave disused and rusting machines and an unemployed, often unemployable, workforce.

This metaphor of failure may not mean the same thing today as it did 150 years ago, but the psychological impact remains perennial. Lest anyone think that these metaphors are out of date, consider a recent text (2001) on endocrinology that describes the complex interactions preceding menstruation by explaining that "in the absence of pregnancy, the corpus luteum *regresses* [italics added]" and "a *degenerative* [italics added] phase follows" that results in menstruation.[46] Why the corpus luteum could not merely alter its course or rid itself of unwanted secretions is not clear. By the same token, that same modern text insists that the "sole function of the uterus is to accommodate and support a fetus," rather than to create hormones (like prolactin and prostaglandins), the functions of which we have no real clue about, or carefully expand to accommodate the placenta, amniotic fluid, and fetus, plus be ready for the hard work of expelling a baby at birth. The idea that a woman could be somehow cleaned out by a hysterectomy and that the uterus is useless are precisely the kinds of thinking that make hysterectomies such a commonplace event, in North America especially.[47]

This language and the blinkered assumptions it makes have resulted in an entire phase of a woman's life, the years leading up to the end of menstruation, being ignored, misrepresented, and disregarded. Worse, perimenopause and its symptoms have been conflated with menopause—by ordinary women and official and medical statements—with such blithe certainty that women for whom this phase is a difficult one, like the authors, both of whom experienced near-disabling perimenopausal problems, frequently believe what they are experiencing will continue for the rest of their natural lives.[48] After all, if this is menopause, where else is there to go from here?

In the next chapter, we describe and explain perimenopause in detail. The reader will be able to judge for herself whether she is experiencing this transition, bearing in mind that the majority of women have no problems at all. Nevertheless, perimenopause is excruciatingly confusing because often we are told (and feel) that we are far too young for menopause, and yet we *know* that something is changing. But the menstrual cycle, like most things physiological, is neither static nor unchanging, and nothing goes from simply being there to not, especially not for such a complex sequence of events as the ovulatory menstrual cycle.

3

PERIMENOPAUSE: THE FORGOTTEN TRANSITION

For the last 10 years, we have known that estrogen levels are higher and less predictable in perimenopause. . . . I feel a profound sense of personal outrage that "experts" can deny the existence of perimenopause or portray it as dropping estrogen levels when estrogen is really high and unpredictable. For me, perimenopause was an extremely difficult time, made worse because I was experiencing the opposite of what I had expected. I experienced more than 12 years of sore, swollen and nodular breasts. The premenstrual fluid and mood symptoms I had learned to control with increased exercise when I was premenopausal no longer relented no matter how far I ran or walked. And I dreamed I was pregnant! Both my rational and my unconscious mind knew I was experiencing high estrogen levels. However, the medical literature at the time asserted the opposite. Therefore, I was jubilant when I first saw the data from an excellent population-based study showing higher-than-premenopausal-normal estrogen levels in perimenopause. . . . My excitement at seeing scientific validation of my high estrogen perimenopausal experiences, however, was dashed when I read the conclusion for that paper [which was that estrogen levels were decreased].

—Jerilynn C. Prior[1]

At the turn of the twentieth century, Freud and his contemporaries believed that adulthood was a peaceful time; that once childhood and adolescence had passed, it was smooth sailing all the way. But by the 1970s, this perspective had changed. Such enormous social, political, cultural, and economic changes had taken place over the course of the previous sixty-five years that adulthood no longer seemed quite so simple, at least for people in the affluent West. Life had become more complicated and, by extension, so had midlife. In many ways this notion harkened back several centuries; the fourteenth-century Italian poet Dante, for instance, had described his own experiences with middle age in *The Inferno* as "wild, rugged" and "harsh."[2] Dante (who died at the ripe old age of fifty-six) was describing himself, during an era when women did not figure highly, but for many women today, Dante's description could well describe their midlife years and the stage that has euphemistically been called the *menopausal transition*.

Given that the official definition of menopause is simply one's last period, defined retrospectively as a year without flow, the word *menopause* makes no sense here; the proper term is *perimenopause*. Yet not only was this more precise term not even a blip on the medical, social, or even linguistic radar, the word *perimenopause* did not actually exist until the 1990s, even though for many women this is a time fraught with disruptive and tumultuous physical symptoms and onerous, often cyclic, problems with mood, sleep, concentration, relationships—and life.

WHAT IS PERIMENOPAUSE?

Perimenopause is the transition between the normal, adult menstrual years (premenopause) and menopause, the time when menstruation stops. It can be a chaotic and confusing time, with bodily changes and symptoms that range from the relatively benign, albeit disturbing (weird dreams, itching of the vulva, frequent urination, weight gain), to distressing (breathlessness, vertigo, migraines, thinning hair) and outright terrifying (mysterious bruising, panic attacks, memory lapses, chest pain and palpitations).[3] As Sylvia,* a level-headed medical editor, describes,

> I well remember my own struggles with perimenopause. Like you, I had never had even a touch of PMS [premenstrual syndrome], and the only hint I ever had that a period might be approaching was a tiny tenderness in my breasts. But my perimenopause was horrendous—my breasts felt like bruised cantaloupes two weeks out of the month, to the point that I crossed my arms under them when I walked down the hall; I woke up drenched several times during the night, virtually every night, and often couldn't sleep at all after 4:00 A.M.; I had hot flushes at the most embarrassing moments; and, perhaps worst of all, I started having migrainous auras without the headaches: blind spots, speech disturbances, and peripheral light flashes. My family physician kept testing me for TIAs [transient ischemic attacks, often the precursors of a stroke], but it was simply migrainous auras. (I had had migraines in my teens and outgrown them in my late twenties—apparently hormonally linked. My mother had them from puberty until menopause and then had nearly thirty years migraine-free.) And oh, was I a bitch. My husband had just endured my nicotine

---

*All names have been changed.

withdrawal for six months, and my irritability had just begun to wane, when my estrogen levels started to roller-coaster. I'm amazed he didn't leave right then and there. You'll laugh to hear the comment made to me by a friend, a newspaper editor who had borne five children: "You really didn't expect Mother Nature to let you off scot-free, did you?"*

Thankfully, it appears that only some 15 to 20 percent of women experience symptoms of this magnitude; for the majority of women, perimenopause is only mildly disruptive if at all.

As social psychologists Bernice Neugarten and Ruth Kraines wrote in an influential, often quoted article in 1965, where they detailed painstaking research into "menopausal" (i.e., perimenopausal) symptoms, most women report that this period in their lives does not create any "major discontinuity." Even though they are "cognizant of the underlying biologic changes," they fully expect to have a "relative degree of control" over any symptoms they might have. In contrast to pubescent girls (between ages thirteen and eighteen), in whom Neugarten and Kraines found a similar pattern of hormonal instability and change, women in their forties had enough "experience and maturity" to cope with whatever complications they experienced.[4] This parallel between perimenopause and puberty that the psychologists noted was remarkable not only for its time, but in its perspicacity— not to mention the accurate hormonal observations the authors gleaned from the interviews. There are indeed endocrinological similarities between these two stages in a woman's life; similarities that the medical and gynecological community, completely caught up in its "estrogen deficiency" paradigm, has largely ignored. But as Neugarten and Kraines noticed, both these stages, puberty and perimenopause, are often characterized by a "heightened sensitivity to and an increased frequency of reported symptoms" that bear a striking resemblance to those of *high* estrogen levels. What puberty and perimenopause have in common hormonally is higher estrogen levels and lower progesterone production.[5]

Unfortunately, perimenopause has remained the orphan child of the menstrual years. Physiologically and semantically ambiguous, it is the transition that time and everyone else forgot. Everyone, that is except those women for whom this transitional phase is problematic—and, speaking from experience, we can say that they are not likely to forget.

Perimenopause can be a lonely and confusing time, not least because even although a woman may *feel* something is changing and *knows* that there has been a physical shift somewhere, neither she nor her physician have the language, the metaphors, to describe what is going on; neither do they have the endocrinological framework to comprehend the hormonal nuances of the transition. The perimenopausal woman is fully aware that this is not menopause: for one thing,

---

*This is a personal communication.

her periods are still regular, but there are perceptible differences. Like Sylvia, she may find that for the first time in her life, she is developing premenstrual symptoms (or, if she always had PMS, it is getting worse). She is waking up at night feeling strange, panicked, often desperately hot. Her pillow feels like a stove, emanating heat. She has to urinate more frequently, especially at night, waking up again and again. Many women find the changes minor, barely noticeable, but for others, the symptoms are debilitating and mystifyingly hard to pin down. Perhaps she feels queasy, or itchy. During the day, she feels uncomfortable, fat, old, dull. She may have trouble concentrating in a way she never has before, as though there is a thin film between her and the world. And none of it makes sense. So she asks her doctor, for whom these mysterious symptoms are just as perplexing.

A common complaint of perimenopausal women is that their physicians do not listen, or if they do, they dismiss their concerns by saying, "You're too young to be menopausal." The problem is that most doctors simply have no template for this complex pattern of symptoms and no idea how to fit them into a coherent picture or differential diagnosis. When a physician hears that menstrual flow is heavy but regular, that breasts are sore and PMS has worsened—at the same time as the woman is complaining of hot flushes and vaginal dryness—it simply does not compute. It doesn't match what they were taught in medical school or fit the descriptions in journals or textbooks because they are a mixture that medicine ordinarily associates with *high* estrogen (heavy flow,[6] tender breasts, and PMS[7]) but also include the hot flushes and vaginal dryness commonly ascribed to menopause and *low* estrogen. And not having been taught about perimenopause, the doctor will conclude that the woman is either dramatizing—or has to decide which hormonal extreme to diagnose and treat.

There is no simple fit for perimenopause. As Jerome Groopman, the Harvard hematologist and author, writes in *How Doctors Think:* "Clinical algorithms . . . quickly fall apart when a doctor needs to think outside their boxes, when symptoms are vague or multiple and confusing, or when test results are inexact."[8] Unfortunately for both patient and doctor, vague, multiple, confusing symptoms are the hallmark of perimenopause—and are part of the reason high estrogen is not suspected. Additionally, gynecology (the de facto specialty on women's health) has authoritatively told family doctors that those pesky hot flushes are the cornerstone of *menopause* and are due to estrogen deficiency. So the majority of the time, the doctor will decide that this forty-something woman is going through "premature ovarian failure" (early menopause), that she is estrogen "deficient" and will reach for the prescription pad to recommend "HRT."

Of course there could be other reasons for these symptoms, and some doctors will indeed investigate, as Sylvia's doctor did, but were physicians versed in the signs of perimenopause and its higher-than-normal estrogen levels, other telltale symptoms would soon become obvious: shorter cycles with heavier flow and increased PMS, night sweats and nausea, perhaps migraines. The easiest, least interventionist solution would be a clinical course of progesterone at bedtime.* This is called a *therapeutic trial*, and many experienced clinicians will choose this course; if the drug works, then they know their suspicion was correct. It is an easier, cheaper, and often less invasive means of confirming a diagnosis than costly (and often inconclusive) investigations and tests, plus it is easily reversible if it is not effective—you stop the drug. Particularly if the treatment is simple and has no major side effects, it is a pragmatic and sensible solution. Unfortunately, most doctors do not know enough about perimenopause, or progesterone, to give this option a try.

Even though medical education ostensibly teaches trainees the basics about women's reproductive changes as they age, most doctors neither know how to identify perimenopause nor how to manage it because what they were taught implied a clear-cut, definite break between the two recognized stages of a woman's reproductive cycle—as though women magically switch from fertile to post-menopausal overnight, which makes no sense physiologically. Nothing works like that, not even a simple viral illness. No biological phenomenon takes a quantum leap from zero to one without some intervening indication(s). There's a reason lab results and blood tests are presented along a continuum, with normal being somewhere between the two numbers of a reference range. There is no such thing as a "normal" that applies to every person. "The menopausal process is not a discrete event," write social scientists Naughton, Jones, and Shumaker in their analysis of stakeholder differences in the hormone debate, "but rather a gradual process that occurs over a period of years as hormone levels involved in ovulatory cycles fluctuate."[9] All of us intuitively know that about physiology: even with a cold, one person may be miserably snuffling, whereas another, whose immune system differs in its response, may have a mild sore throat or perhaps imperceptible symptoms, even with the same virus making the office rounds.

Hormones and their regulatory functions in the body, furthermore, are devilishly complicated and not particularly well understood; the subtle interplay of different hormones is involved in all our systems and physiologic processes, from how much energy we have and how well we sleep to our weight and height, ability to conceive, and so on. A woman's menstrual cycle, as we saw in the previous chapter, is a subtle dance between the brain (hypothalamus), pituitary gland, ovaries, follicles, and more. So although it may be more expedient for medicine not to get too caught up in perimenopause and to resort to reductionist thinking, to consider fertility and its cessation as having finite borders is not an option for the women in question.

---

*Prometrium (bioidentical oral micronized progesterone), 300 mg, at bedtime from day fourteen to twenty-seven of the cycle (see Appendix A for details).

SYSTEMIC PROBLEMS

Part of the problem in terms of medicine's lack of recognition of perimenopause has to do with the giant tentacles that we call the health care industry. Ironically, the more advanced we have become technologically, pharmacologically, epidemiologically, surgically, and otherwise, it seems that in our collective minds the mechanics of health and health care have overwhelmed physiology and its complexities. Perhaps because we can do more than we could fifty years ago, medical thinking does not concern itself with the underlying processes involved, but tends to be more focused on best administering of clinical guidelines or working from decision trees or algorithms derived from statistics and randomized clinical trials—the gold standard of medicine.[10] This tends to result in static, step-by-step diagnostic measures and linear reasoning (more on this later), with few physicians genuinely interested in or capable of lateral or creative clinical analysis. This, along with their medical training, has instilled in the majority of doctors a tendency to reduce the (often) muddled narratives and vague descriptions the person/patient brings to the visit into a series of yes/no boxes.[11]

Cardiac disease, for instance, is no longer thought of as a poorly understood chronic disease, as it once was—a condition specific to the person (who would be advised in general terms to reduce their stress, change their diet, modify their lifestyle)—but has become a technical checklist of numbers (blood pressure, cholesterol, glucose levels, etc.), which, once past a specific, often arbitrary point, puts the person "at risk" and in line for treatment, usually with drugs and sometimes surgery. The identification, prevention, or "cure" of disease takes precedence over the care of the patient, which has fundamentally altered the clinician's role.[12] Today, statistical and numeric reasoning reigns supreme.[13] The "proliferation of these boilerplate schemes," as Groopman politely phrases it, often causes doctors to ignore the individual, whereas the overreliance on evidence and algorithms risks turning them into "well-programmed computers" working within what Groopman calls a "strict binary framework."[14] And perimenopause, the diagnosis of which requires attention to detail and an ability to think outside those preprinted boxes (and which has few, if any, consistent or ostensibly objective findings), would be a challenge to even the most thoughtful or creative of physicians. Disentangling the hodgepodge of aches and pains, vague mood and sleep changes, and cyclic disturbances requires finesse and at least a rudimentary understanding of endocrinology and the hormonal mechanisms involved.

Diagnosing perimenopause means understanding that estrogen levels are high and erratic, often dropping from the stratospheric to normal. It is this abrupt change that causes the body to generate that sudden heat we call a hot flash or flush. The hypothalamus in the brain, having been exposed to higher estrogen levels, reacts when there is any decrease at all. Such swings are common during the hormonal chaos of perimenopause.[15] Stress also increases hot flushes and, in addition, there are the intricate endocrine interactions to consider: higher estrogen levels amplify the levels of stress hormones[16] (similar to puberty, as Neugarten and Kraines realized just by talking to girls and women), notably the all-encompassing adrenocorticotropic hormone (ACTH) that leads to higher cortisol levels, and the flight-fight response (noradrenaline/adrenaline) we so often hear about.[17] The result is a "heightened sensitivity to and an increased frequency"[18] of reported symptoms such as headaches, fatigue, irritability, and vertigo. This was demonstrated physiologically when researchers assessed the effect estrogen had on a standardized experimental stress test in young *men,* randomized to placebo or an estrogen patch. What they found was that estrogen-treated men had higher levels of stress hormones (ACTH, cortisol, and noradrenaline) when doing math in front of a heckling audience than those treated with placebo.[19]

There is also the *balance* of hormones to consider and what happens when progesterone levels dip too low to be able to offset the tissue effects of the high estrogen levels, with synergistic results that affect other parts of the body and other hormones (or their reuptake)—in short, entire bodily systems. Comparisons between women have shown that premenstrual symptoms (though poorly understood) are worse when estrogen levels are higher and progesterone, lower.[20] Although in earlier years, PMS could be kept at bay by exercise, during perimenopause, this no longer holds true.[21] Further complicating the picture, and proving what perimenopausal women know only too well—given that weight loss becomes next to impossible during this time—is that the delicate balancing act of body metabolism goes off kilter as the combination of stress hormones, higher estrogen, and poor sleep often further results in insulin resistance (a term recently popularized in connection to weight loss and diets to explain why some people have such trouble losing weight). This leads to a commensurate rise in appetite and weight.

Take Marie,* a thirty-nine-year-old physiotherapist with three young children, who is waking up several times a night to urinate and who is struggling with various mysterious symptoms, including an inability to focus:

> It was my day off and I was at home with my two youngest, trying to do our taxes, but I just couldn't concentrate. Without realizing how it happened, I went through a bag of corn chips and a box of cookies—and felt bloated and totally disgusted at myself. My clothes are all getting tight and two of my work skirts don't button up anymore. There's diabetes in my family, but I'm really good with diet usually and exercise (I typically walk the forty minutes to work) and my blood sugar is normal. Plus I'm starting to get these horrible headaches. I've been back and forth to my family doctor, trying to find out what's wrong, but everything seemed fine. I went in because I was scared: I was walking home one evening—really fast because I was running late—when I suddenly felt weak and just drenched in perspiration.

---

*"Marie" is a composite of several women.

I thought I might be hypoglycemic because I drank a whole carton of chocolate milk before I felt better. This time my blood pressure was a bit high, so my doctor referred me to an internal medicine specialist.

The internist checked Marie's blood pressure (she had to wear an automated blood pressure monitor for a week), hemoglobin A1C (an amazing test that measures average blood sugars over the previous three months), fasting cholesterol, lipids, and waist circumference. Marie's blood pressure was a bit high (146/94), as were her lipids, but fasting blood sugar was normal, and the internist told Marie that she had "metabolic syndrome," that she was at risk for heart disease, stroke, and diabetes, and gave her prescriptions for a statin (a drug that lowers cholesterol), an expensive blood pressure medication, and a diabetic weight loss diet to follow. Marie took the pills, but the blood pressure medication made her cough day and night (a common side effect of ACE inhibitors), and she still felt hungry all the time:

> I still couldn't lose weight even though I cut out sugar; in fact, I gained weight. I was achy and tired all the time. We tried some different blood pressure medications (each more expensive than the next) 'til we found one that worked—except my feet would swell by the end of the day. We do more tests and my blood pressure is higher than it was (151/97) and my good cholesterol is down and all the other lipids are up. My family doctor finally decides to send me to an endocrinologist, except this one is only interested in diabetes and we're back on the merry-go-round. This one changes the cholesterol medication, sends me to the Diabetes Education Program (that he assures me will help me lose weight), and gives me a drug that helps with insulin resistance and blood sugar (rosiglitazone). It doesn't, and my feet swell more. Finally, something good happens—one of my work colleagues says she went through something similar when she was in perimenopause and tells me about this other endocrinologist she's seeing, one who understands women's hormones.

Marie finally saw an endocrinologist who understands that the high estrogen levels of perimenopause (and the corresponding lack of progesterone) make weight loss, for all practical purposes, impossible, and, in Marie's case, were also causing her insulin resistance, hunger, and weight gain:

> It was such a relief to talk to someone who understood what I was going through. Dr. Prior told me not to try to lose weight for the time being, just to increase my protein intake, exercise a bit more, eat more fruits and vegetables instead of chips and things—and eat a bigger breakfast to get me going. (Maybe my kids will do the same if they see me doing it.) She stopped the rosiglitazone because it was causing my lower legs to swell up and gave me metformin instead; that's an old, safe drug that helps my body use insulin more effectively. I started gradually, with half a 500 mg pill at lunch and dinner and working up to a whole tablet. We also agreed that I would stop the expensive blood pressure medication and take an old diuretic (spironolactone) that is used to lower blood pressure (and costs pennies a day), 100

mg at night. I also stopped the statin (that other endocrinologist had already found I had elevated muscle enzymes, and that could lead to a dangerous side effect of cholesterol-lowering drugs); Dr. Prior told me that there's really no good evidence that total high cholesterol or LDL cholesterol caused heart attacks in women. And my triglycerides came down as my insulin resistance improved.

In fact, lowering cholesterol levels does not seem to lower heart attack risk in anyone who has not already had a heart attack. Although there is some evidence that as secondary prevention (to prevent a second heart attack), particularly in those people who have had a heart attack at a young age, cholesterol-lowering drugs, such as the statins, could reduce the risk of another heart attack.[22] When it comes to preventing that first heart attack, the data are underwhelming. For instance, 10,000 asymptomatic individuals would need to take pravastatin (a cholesterol-lowering drug) to prevent some 245 cardiac events in the future (and 9,755 people would see no benefit at all).[23] For women, there is even less evidence that lowering cholesterol is beneficial in the long term.[24]

Marie's story illustrates the extent to which perimenopause is misunderstood and misdiagnosed, particularly when the picture is blurred by something like a family history of diabetes. But at present, not only is this knowledge not in the usual (or even outstanding) doctor's repertoire, it is not something most doctors *could* know. Perimenopause is not covered in continuing medical education luncheons or at conferences; the gynecologist doing the Family Practice grand rounds (lecture) typically does not mention it, and neither do the journals the doctor reads. In fact, when the journal *American Family Physician* did run a comprehensive article on night sweats, perimenopause was not mentioned at all. Doctors were merely advised to evaluate for "ovarian failure" by checking for elevated levels of follicle-stimulating hormone (FSH).[25] Yet, according to a comprehensive clinical review of perimenopause (one of the few times the term *perimenopause* actually figured in a prominent journal) in the *Journal of the American Medical Association* (*JAMA*), FSH levels can go up *or* down during perimenopause, depending on when during the cycle the test is done, with this "hormonal variability" creating major clinical "difficulties" and making this lab test of dubious value, as the *JAMA* review authors obliquely suggest.[26] In fact, more often than not, during perimenopause, tests like FSH turn out to be normal, particularly when the clinical picture is confusing (as it often is).

As valiant an attempt as the *JAMA* article is in describing what is known of perimenopause, and in spite of the authors' painstaking analysis of more than twelve hundred articles, even this ostensibly comprehensive review makes it next to impossible for clinicians to answer the authors' title question, "Is This Woman Perimenopausal?" In fact, trying to pinpoint how the diagnosis might be made using this review is enough to make one vertiginous, so circuitous are the attempts to arrive at an absolute description of perimenopause—not least because of

Figure 3.1

This diagram depicts various aspects of women's midlife as the menopausal transition, menopause, final menstrual period (FMP), postmenopause, and perimenopause. Note that postmenopause and perimenopause overlap. Redrawn by J. C. Prior from research on menopause in the 1990s. A report of the WHO Scientific Group, *866*, 1–107 (1996). World Health Organization: Geneva, Switzerland.

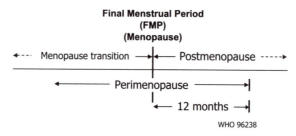

WHO 96238

the semantic and diagnostic confusion inherent in trying to synthesize information from studies that seem to use the terms *perimenopause* and *menopause* interchangeably. Of course comparability in medicine is no simple matter, whether the topic is cancer, congestive heart failure, or perimenopause. Researchers define their own preset limits, and these often differ from study to study and researcher to researcher, as does terminology.

SQUARE PEGS INTO ROUND HOLES

The World Health Organization (WHO) has defined natural (versus surgical) menopause as the "permanent cessation of menstruation, determined retrospectively after 12 continuous months of amenorrhea (no periods) without any other pathological or physiological cause"[27] (see Figure 3.1). Menopause, then, is literally that last period. But the question then becomes, how does one know that this *is* the last menstrual period? Particularly because the only way we can know is to wait a year and then look backward. For many of us, that last flow is not easy to pinpoint—just as we think "that's it" and start to relax, eight months later we get another period and have to start all over again.* According to the WHO, once this retrospective point in time has been determined, then anything after that is defined as *postmenopause*, a term so vague and redundant as to be completely useless clinically, diagnostically, sociologically, or personally. How can we be *post* something that is already a year past? In this book, therefore, we use a more straightforward definition, more in keeping with women's own perceptions

---

*For women who take progesterone, menopause is considered to start two years after their last period because progesterone makes flow less likely by thinning the endometrium.

and hormone changes: menopause is simply the normal phase of a woman's life that begins after one year has passed since her final menstrual flow; menopause continues for the rest of her life.* There is no point in attempting to create precise classification systems and names for life phases that are not only different for every woman, but that have no clear borders to begin with.

This attachment to and insistence on finite classifications (defining borders between perimenopause and menopause, e.g., or what precisely constitutes the "correct" blood pressure or glucose level) as well as the various guidelines and policies currently in vogue medically not only powerfully affect the way(s) we frame whatever diagnostic issues there are, but are instrumental in creating a sense of what fits diagnostically and therapeutically. The implication, simplistic as it might be, is that at its root, medicine is quantifiable and manageable. As physician Robert Arnowitz writes in *Making Sense of Illness*,

> Proponents of... [such classification systems] assume that variation in medical practice generally reflects poor quality care, as is generally held to be true *in industrial production* [italics added]. The success and practicality of such guidelines, typically formulated as an algorithmic approach to patients with a specific problem, ultimately depends on the degree to which clinical reality can be adequately understood as a set of uniform and predictable encounters between patients suffering specific ailments and physicians who apply specific diagnostic and therapeutic technology and practices.[28]

Yet people are not units of production, and it is impossible to separate the disease or symptom complex from the person having them. Individuals vary physiologically, socially, culturally, and in countless other ways; what is normal for one person can be completely wrong for another, whether it is their waking time or menstrual cycle. Although it is true that we can statistically describe what the average is, there is no way that a numeric average provides any meaningful information about any individual. Perimenopause, which is variable, confusing, and chaotic, is therefore nearly impossible to understand within these types of rigid parameters.

For the rare woman, menopause can occur as early as age forty; in others, menopause can occur at fifty-nine or sixty. The statistically computed average age for menopause in the West is around fifty-one, which simply means that in general, somewhere around age fifty, most women will graduate from the storm of perimenopause into the calm of menopause. Some women will find that the upheaval continues for a few more years, because bodies don't know how to tell time and rarely adhere to the schedules we set, no matter how august the panel members of the consensus conference determining those preset boundaries. Furthermore, in trying to create specific definitions for menopause, perimenopause, premenopause, and whatever else a woman might experience, we straitjacket

---

*We use the definition that J.C.P. and her colleagues use at the Centre for Menstrual Cycle and Ovulation Research (see http://www.cemcor.ubc.ca/).

ourselves. We know that perimenopause is indeed a transitional phase between premenopause and menopause, but when it actually begins, at what point it stops, and how long it takes are all vague and ephemeral and as different as the women experiencing it.

Attempting to codify and create strict criteria only creates the kind of confusion that is present in the *JAMA* review, in which perimenopause is either the year before the final flow (which means that one can only identify this two years later, since nobody knows when the final flow was until a year after that) or the time preceding menopause during which a woman has had skipped or irregular periods within the previous three to eleven months.[29] Then again, other studies suggest that perhaps perimenopause is when a woman has had changes in menstrual regularity during the previous twelve months.[30] (Note the awkward past tense constructs of these last sentences.) Apparently, all of these, according to the different researchers the *JAMA* authors cite, are the signs "most predictive of menopause within the following 3 years."[31] (Whew.) Average age for perimenopause is 45.5 years, with a mean duration of six years and three months.[32] Or mean age could also be 47.5 years, with perimenopause lasting closer to four (3.8) years.[33] So, to summarize, perimenopause precedes menopause by a year, or three years, or maybe four; it can last just under four years or over six years; it is a time of menstrual irregularity—whatever that means—and skipped periods. Or not. Doctors should check FSH levels, but really, those are not particularly useful, as clinicians have long known and many researchers do concede. Women can have hot flushes, but those also happen during menopause, so it is difficult to know which is which without a detailed history and a thorough analysis of what the symptoms might suggest, none of which medicine is currently all that good at. Is it any wonder doctors are confused and have no idea what to tell their patients or that women have no clue as to what might be going on?

UNDERSTANDING AMBIGUITY

Problems with diagnosing perimenopause highlight the current weakness of modern medicine, particularly as it has evolved in North America: spurious accuracy and rigid classification systems warp the doctor-patient relationship and juxtapose the gaze of both physician and patient away from the patient and her life circumstances and onto rigid categorizations (as previously decided) and/or the diagnosis, even if it bears no relationship to what may actually be taking place. In addition, medicine is increasingly driven by economic models that rely on strict categorizations of disease—for instance, for a physician to be paid in the United States, the HMO must have a diagnosis, a category, in which the patient can be slotted—further reducing the doctor's options.

Perimenopause, which will not fit into the menopause category unless several of the woman's complaints are ignored or glossed over, therefore becomes a figment of the woman's imagination, instead of a genuine transition stage with which some women need help to cope. Already suffering from high levels of estrogen, she is commonly given even more estrogen, which then leads to a thickening of the endometrial lining (hyperplasia), for which she is then told she must have a dilation and curettage (D&C) or a hysterectomy. Various epidemiological studies have shown that early perimenopausal women between the ages of forty-two and forty-six are the most likely to have hysterectomies, with "disorders of menstruations" making up the bulk.[34] When British clinical epidemiologist Angela Coulter and her colleagues examined the increasing number of hysterectomies in parts of the United Kingdom (which has always had lower rates of all surgeries, including hysterectomies, than the United States), the characteristic abnormal uterine bleeding of perimenopause was cited as the primary presenting symptom. Yet

> fibroids, endometriosis and other conditions for which hysterectomy is done can produce disruptions in bleeding patterns. However, fibroids are known to be very common and can be asymptomatic, so a post-operative diagnosis of fibroids may not be an adequate explanation for the perceived increase in blood loss. In common with the findings from other [American and Scottish] studies, only around 10% of these operations . . . were carried out in response to diagnosed malignancies.[35]

In other words, although a hysterectomy may be necessary for a minority of women, far too many perimenopausal women end up with an unnecessary surgery, for reasons that may have more to do with expedience or cognitive shortcuts than good medical care.*

Take, for instance, a frequently cited problem associated with perimenopause such as missed or skipped menstrual periods, which in and of themselves are neither particularly enlightening diagnostically nor indicative of anything when considered outside the history. There are several potential explanations for a skipped period, depending on the age, health, and circumstances of the woman. Gaining or losing weight can lead to a skipped period, as can pregnancy or perimenopause. But if it is the latter, then it is important to see if other, characteristic symptoms of perimenopause are also present such as heavier flow, PMS, and cyclic night sweats. Skipped periods may also be a result of stress, and for women of perimenopausal age, it is not unusual for there to be simultaneous and major life stressors present. In our forties, often, our parents are getting older and more frail; some of us will be dealing with the loss of a parent. Our children are also older by now, and some of them are leaving (or returning) home. Economic and

---

*The CeMCOR Web site, in the health care providers' practitioners section, includes an article titled "Managing Menorrhagia (heavy menstrual flow) Without Surgery" http://www.cemcor.ubc.ca/help_yourself/articles/managing_menorrhagia.

housing downturns affect us all, and it is never easy keeping on top of everything when one is feeling suboptimal, as can happen during perimenopause.

Those women who experience an early menopause (before forty) often will also have had multiple, confusing perimenopausal symptoms for at least ten years by the time their periods start to skip. In the real world, versus that of the medical journal or textbook, the chance that a younger perimenopausal woman will have a further menstrual flow after several skipped periods is more than 20 percent.[36] But none of these women's other symptoms will have been associated with perimenopause because they were considered too young. Perimenopause, the inception of which is similarly difficult to pinpoint, also creates confusion, as was the case with Brenda:

> Brenda, a thirty-six-year-old librarian with severe monthly night sweats, wakes up several times a night totally soaked. The next day, she's groggy and "not like myself." Her periods are regular, about thirty days apart, and not too heavy. Her doctor refers Brenda to specialists, who test for gastric reflux, lymphoma, and sleep apnea. She has X-rays, abdominal ultrasounds, a gastroscopy, and waits six months for the "privilege of trying to sleep wired up like an astronaut" at a sleep clinic. She even has a bone marrow biopsy (to test for leukemia). Her FSH is normal and nobody suspects perimenopause because her periods are regular. She is treated with H_2 blockers (to prevent stomach acid), sleeping pills, and antidepressants, which she says make her "feel weird and wired," but still the night sweats continue. Thankfully, Brenda is referred to an endocrinologist (J.C.P.), who recognizes that she is in early perimenopause. A thorough history reveals that Brenda's night sweats are happening just before and during menstruation and that Brenda has been having worse PMS over the last year. Brenda is understandably relieved that she has nothing seriously wrong and begins taking micronized progesterone (300 mg) at bedtime on days sixteen to thirty or up until her flow has started. Brenda's PMS and night sweats improve, and she is sleeping better.

Brenda was lucky; many women who go into perimenopause relatively early also carry the baggage of multiple medical and psychiatric diagnoses such as fibromyalgia, spastic colon, depression, irritable bowel, chronic insomnia, and premenstrual dysphoric disorder.[37] Almost none of them will trust that a physician, any physician, can make sense of what is happening or be able to help, and many of them will feel demoralized and depressed because they believe that their symptoms will go on forever. After all, if this is "menopause," then this is it, for the rest of your life. Additionally, current medical practice, with its overt focus on surrogate end points and biomarkers (measurable signs such as blood pressure or cholesterol levels) that are easily tested and then compared to some predetermined "ideal" level, cloud the issue even further. When a perimenopausal woman (like Marie, with a family history of diabetes) arrives at a specialist's office, she is already primed for diabetes and its attendant risks. Unfortunately, what this too often translates into is poor *individual* care, whether you are a woman or a man. The idea that insulin resistance, weight gain, and irrational food binges are caused by the (temporary) hormonal fluctuations of perimenopause is simply not acknowledged.

THE VAGUE SYMPTOMS OF PERIMENOPAUSE

The reality is that whatever *JAMA* and various and sundry panels may agree on, perimenopause is as unique as the woman experiencing it. (Certainly for the authors, both of whom had perimenopausal symptoms for well over a decade, those glib estimates of perimenopause expressed in months, rather than years, seem absurd.) In any event, that final retrospectively defined menstrual flow (a magical point where things are supposed to shift from one state to the next, quickly and cleanly) is rarely as easy to identify as the WHO and other sources make out. Those of us (S.B. being a case in point) who forget to jot it down and rely on our faulty memories, simply forget and have to estimate the time that has passed, and even those women who are meticulous in recording their periods (such as J.C.P.) will often find that the transition into menopause is fluid and dynamic, a moving point in space and not a fixed period on a graph. Often, just as one breathes easy that menopause is around the corner, another period shows up and throws off the calculation—and this starts the twelve-month clock ticking again. And simply hitting that magical final-period mark does not guarantee the end of migraines and hot flushes, although by this point, breast tenderness and bloating are abating.[38]

Hot flushes in particular are hard to pinpoint, being symptomatic of both perimenopause and menopause, and not that simple to differentiate during the transitional phase. Perhaps it would make more sense to consider perimenopause in its true etymological sense, where *peri* refers to what is "around" something. For instance, the *pericardium* is the sac around the heart and a *periscope* can enhance one's view up and around our direct field of vision—so it makes sense to think of perimenopause as simply the time around, encircling, the final menstrual flow, which is what older gynecologists refer to as the day of menopause. (Of course, one could also go with the other dictionary definition of *peri* as an evil spirit or fairy in Persian mythology.) In any event, biology and physiology do not deal in precise, finite points (of time or anything else)—ever—and variability between individuals goes well beyond the visible, such as body shape, to internal mechanisms, such as susceptibility to illness. We are not the result of our genes, or environment, or diet, or past, or culture, or nationality, or career, or personality, but of *all* those things together in differing degrees.

For that minority of women whose symptoms are disruptive and difficult, the invisibility of perimenopause as a term or concept becomes part of the problem. Women like Sylvia, who suddenly find themselves beset by insomnia, panic attacks, migraines, and other debilitating symptoms, have no clue what is going on, and doctors are often of little help, throwing out diagnoses like stroke (and scaring her to death). Even a physician and expert on women's health, like one of the authors of this book (J.C.P.), can find perimenopause a shock to the system:

> When I was forty-four, I believed that the changes of midlife would be gradual, with estrogen levels drifting downward, a few skipped periods and then, suddenly, I would ask myself, when was my last period? Lo and behold, it would have been over a year and I would be menopausal. I was so bold as to say in *Is It Hot in Here?* (a Canadian National Film Board video) that I was looking forward to menopause! A few years later, and for ten long, miserable years, I desperately longed for menopause. Why? Because there was nothing gentle, gradual, or likeable about my transition to menopause! When I made that brash, looking-forward-to-menopause statement, although I had been a physician for twenty years and was a recognized expert in women's menstrual cycles, I didn't yet know about perimenopause—the cruel irony of the so-called dropping and deficient estrogen story. Perimenopause is the forgotten phase of women's midlife and is important because it is long, it is misunderstood, it is mistreated, and it makes 10 to 20 percent of us, Susan Baxter and myself being two examples of those unlucky few, bloody miserable.

Perimenopausal symptoms run the gamut, from those we associate with menopause to those we think of as more premenstrual. The checklist includes those golden oldies always cited: vasomotor symptoms (medical shorthand for hot flashes/flushes and night sweats and all their attendant discomforts), vaginal dryness (always mentioned, yet, according to the *JAMA* review, only about one-fifth of women experience this), "variable" sexual interest (shorthand for less interest, although the majority of women studied indicated that perimenopause had no effect on their interest in sex—and for many women, any disinterest in sex is often more related to sociocultural and psychological factors connected to fears of aging than biology), urinary incontinence (which *JAMA*, despite subsequent evidence from randomized controlled WHI trials to the contrary,* attributes to low estrogen levels), depressed mood, nervous tension, and irritability. These last, highly ambiguous terms are always included on menopause checklists but have never been defined—the *JAMA* authors admit that "the relevance" of these symptoms are not clear but are probably the result of lack of sleep.[39]

Less frequently listed, but common, as an address over ten years ago to the North American Menopause Society[40] pointed out, are migraines and headaches; insomnia (both trouble falling asleep and waking up too soon); electric shock–type

---

*The Women's Health Initiative randomized controlled hormone therapy trials asked women about incontinence before they began therapy and then again at one year. The results showed that estrogen and estrogen/progestin *cause* incontinence or make it worse in those who initially experienced it. S. L. Hendrix, B. B. Cochrane, I. E. Nygaard, V. L. Handa, V. M. Barnabei, C. Iglesia. Effects of estrogen with and without progestin on urinary incontinence. *Journal of the American Medical Association*; **293**(8):935–48 (2005).

sensations in the head; lower back pain; itching of the vulva; bloating, indigestion, and gas; thinning scalp and rogue chin whiskers; aching knees, ankles, wrists, or shoulders; bruising; a sudden inability to breathe ("air hunger"); dizzy spells and vertigo; panic attacks; and a general, heightened sensitivity—to other people, to sensory stimuli, to perceived slights, and anything else that hits one the wrong way. Tempers and patience can be short.

In spite of the epidemiological stress on irregular cycles, for most women, perimenopause often begins surreptitiously, with regular cycles, without fanfare or anything particularly obvious or measurable.[41] In fact, given that there are virtually no truly objective signs or lab tests that can conclusively prove that a woman is perimenopausal throughout this stage (although longitudinal studies, such as the one described at the start of this chapter, do note higher estrogen levels), the best the average women can hope for is to ask herself if anything has changed. When she is sure it has, and the changes fit with higher estrogen and lower progesterone, she is in perimenopause.

IRREGULARLY REGULAR

Usually, perimenopause begins in women whose periods are still regular but who find that they are experiencing either increased PMS or are having PMS for the first time in their lives—which commonly means that their breasts feel sore, tender, and enlarged. Or they may experience mood swings, retain fluid, and feel hungry all the time. Women prone to migraines find they are having them with increasing intensity and more frequently (one of the authors, S.B., had a migraine virtually every day for several years), and others will find that they are suddenly developing them, often with classic symptoms, including altered vision and an insane sensitivity to smell and sound. Cycles tend to grow shorter than normal, but they can also intermittently be longer, and often, the flow is heavier. Commonly, cramps will return and be similar to what they were in the teens (or before the first baby). There are cyclic flow-related night sweats, often accompanied by sudden waking in the middle of the night. Women may find themselves inexplicably gaining weight and cannot lose the weight even if they diet and exercise. And every single one of these symptoms, when parsed in terms of the hormonal storm happening, as well as clinically, leads us straight to often dramatically higher and sometimes fluctuating levels of estrogen—and a concurrent decrease in progesterone.

It is not entirely clear why, but the normal complex interplay of brain, pituitary, and ovary is showing signs of wear as a woman moves into perimenopause. During a normal cycle throughout most of her adult life, the estrogen peak leading up to ovulation always made that surge of luteinizing hormone (LH)—but now that doesn't always seem to happen. Conversely, a woman can have perfectly fine estrogen and LH peaks, but release no egg. Even if normal ovulation does occur, the corpus luteum (the yellow substance in the ovary that makes progesterone) seems fatigued and not able to crank out enough progesterone, long enough to balance out the estrogen. Just when it is most needed, progesterone is not around. (Ovulation can and does occur in perimenopausal women, and there are surprise pregnancies for women in their forties. Not unexpectedly, perimenopausal women with nausea, sore and swollen breasts, weight gain, and bloating who are not expecting a regular flow anyway may not have a clue a baby is on the way.) When estrogen levels are high and progesterone lacking, the uterine lining thickens and causes heavy flow, for which women often are prescribed birth control pills. Although this eventually does seem to improve flow, it does not appreciably improve hot flushes or enhance how women feel or their quality of life[42]:

> Freya, a sturdy woman of forty-four, is the executive director for the local Red Cross. Since her mid-thirties, her periods have been regular. Over the past months, she has been experiencing heavy flow and clots with increasing cramps. Freya, who had her first period at eleven, always suffered from unwanted facial hair (which she removed with laser treatment). Her physician suggested Freya take a so-called low-dose birth control pill (low dose only by comparison with the 1960s; even 20–30 μg of ethinyl estradiol is some four times the body's normal). The Pill made Freya nauseous and bloated, and her periods became painful, irregular, and more frequent: two periods a month, rather than one. Already stressed, one day at work, she developed chest pain and breathlessness. Rushed to the emergency room, she was told her heart enzymes and electrocardiogram were fine—perhaps she had been hyperventilating. She was also told she was anemic. She was referred to a gynecologist, who said the heavy bleeding was due to fibroids since a low FSH test "proved she wasn't in menopause." He added that an I.U.D. (intrauterine device) might help, but she would eventually need a hysterectomy. Freya, a strong woman not accustomed to taking orders, said she didn't want a hysterectomy. She canceled the appointment the gynecologist had made for an endometrial biopsy. She did agree to take an iron tablet three times a day, as her family doctor suggested, but when a repeat blood test showed her iron levels to be normal, she stopped. Her doctor asked her to keep taking one iron tablet a day; taking iron quickly made her blood count normal, but it took time (and low-dose iron) for bone marrow reserve iron stores to normalize. Her doctor also suggested taking ibuprofen every four hours on the days she had heavy flow; this would decrease flow somewhat. Her doctor, somewhat reluctantly, also prescribed 100 mg of Prometrium for ten days per cycle.* Freya told her doctor to write whatever dosage she felt comfortable with; she (Freya) was convinced she was in perimenopause and needed a higher dose: 300 mg of Prometrium (a bioidentical progesterone) at bedtime, from day six of her cycle to day twenty-five (day one being the first day of her period). Freya's next flow was normal (starting on time the day after she stopped the progesterone), and her cramps went away.

---

*See "Managing Menorrhagia without Surgery" at http://www.cemcor.ubc.ca/help_yourself/articles/managing_menorrhagia.

The accepted medical wisdom, derived from a consensus conference in 2001, to which one of the authors (J.C.P.) was invited,[43] is that the menopausal transition begins with cycles that vary in length by plus or minus seven days plus a high FSH level. But these so-called high FSH levels have not been defined, and even if they were, are simply not a reliable predictor of symptoms of perimenopause.[44] Most researchers reluctantly concede that although measuring FSH levels might come in handy, most researchers and clinicians doubt that they are of any value "as FSH levels fluctuate considerably" each month.[45] In the end, and as the authors of the *JAMA* review (to give them credit) do suggest, the doctor's ultimate task is simple: *listen* to the woman. Her self-assessment will be based on "awareness of the subtle changes taking place" in her body, which she knows better than anybody else, and this, they flatly write, is a far better clinical indicator of perimenopause than FSH or anything else. This dovetails with research in other areas of medicine—notably chronic illness, where the patient's self-knowledge is often highly sophisticated—and it has been found that patients' self-assessments and subjective feelings about the progression of their own disorder or disease, be it diabetes or asthma or anything else, are often a far better indicator (and predictor) of their health status than so-called objective laboratory tests or scans.[46]

Regardless of what the scant literature on this transition, with its overfocus on declining estrogen, insists, women alert to or aware of what high estrogen feels like know that low estrogen is not the problem. For instance, often women will dream they are pregnant (a time when estrogen is high). Hot flushes, which during menopause are due to lower estrogen levels, are extrapolated to perimenopause but in and of themselves are not particularly indicative of anything other than a sudden drop in estrogen levels and of the complex interaction between brain, pituitary, and ovary. Perimenopause is characterized by high endogenous estrogen; menopause is a time when the ovaries gradually stop producing estrogen. This may be exacerbated by body fat, which also may add to endogenous estrogen, and diet (hormone-fed cows, for instance). Logically then, perimenopausal symptoms are related to higher, swinging estrogen levels and the lack of balance between estrogen and progesterone, providing too-low progesterone levels.[47]

Progesterone, as we saw in the previous chapter, is essential to the normal, cyclic hormone balance and is normally present after ovulation in levels far higher than those reached by estrogen at its peak. Yet progesterone, for inexplicable reasons, simply does not resonate or even register with researchers and others experts on women's reproduction. Even feminist thinkers who decry the medicalization of menopause and espouse woman-centered care at all stages of life equate perimenopause primarily with the psychosocial effects that midlife has on women who feel that their value and status are disappearing along with their youth. They doubt hormone levels, whether estrogen or progesterone, have anything to do with it.

This is not to say that these psychosocial effects do not matter; they matter in all physical symptoms. Furthermore, how one interprets one's symptoms certainly plays a part in their severity and intensity. All pain, all physical symptoms, are affected by the value afforded them—it has long been known, for instance, that soldiers wounded on the battlefield report less pain from similar injuries than civilians, possibly because, for the soldier, this is his or her ticket home. But the hormones generated by the stress of the battlefield also play a part in pain awareness, and this interaction between the person, his or her circumstances, as well as physiology is also important to consider and include in the differential. There would be no psychosocial overlay without a symptom to attach it to. Although appropriately mistrustful of doctors and scientists who construe menopause as a deficiency disease, women's collectives and feminist groups have often been slow to question the dropping estrogen orthodoxy and have not pushed for holistic answers that deal with the entire woman along with her biologic, sociocultural, psychogenic, and other factors.

THE TROUBLE WITH AMBIGUOUS SYMPTOMS

It is important to remember, however, that simply because women have reported having these sensations and symptoms does not mean (1) that all women will have them or (2) that they will always be related to perimenopause. There are, at any given time, "a large pool of bodily symptoms available" that can be attributed to a host of factors from normal fatigue or stress to medication side effects or illness. And to what one attributes these symptoms makes a large difference not only to the severity with which they are perceived but also to the distress they cause.[48] There is, in addition, considerable tension between the complex narrative that the person—the patient—brings and how this is interpreted by the clinician. In addition to diagnostic criteria, medicine today is also driven by a model that no longer places any appreciable value on the person and who she is (work, family, stresses, etc.), but rather, on what she is, so when a woman in her forties arrives at a doctor's office complaining of vague pains and ill-defined symptoms, what the doctor sees is a woman nearing that famous "menopausal transition" (with its attendant lack of estrogen that was so drummed into him or her at medical school), and reacts accordingly.[49] For many women, it will indeed be perimenopause, but for some, it might not be—or there could be more than one process involved. Simply because one is going through perimenopause does not automatically exclude everything else:

> Emma, a vibrant, healthy woman in her seventies, recalls only too well her symptoms before she hit menopause at fifty-three. She wasn't having hot flushes, but she found that she was blushing easily, just as she had when she was a teenager. (There's that

puberty-perimenopause connection again.) All she knows is that she just didn't feel right. It was a nebulous thing, but she felt robbed of her self-confidence and sense of well-being. She was given "HRT" (Premarin and progestin, to the best of her recollection), which did seem to help for a time, but she bled on and off through the month, which she hated, and once she was told she needed a D&C, she decided to stop. She was tired of having periods. But she had other upheavals in her life—like teenagers—and kept having vague symptoms. Eventually, she was diagnosed with gallstones and had surgery, after which her symptoms resolved.

It is therefore important that women, particularly those for whom perimenopause is long and difficult, ensure that nothing else is concurrently evolving—or that they are not dismissed as merely menopausal or overdramatic. Groopman relates a similar story about a woman called Ellen who was having "menopausal" symptoms but also insisted that she felt like "bombs" were going off in her body, making her hot and her skin crawl. Five doctors dismissed her symptoms as menopause, but she persisted. She finally found a thorough, caring physician who did not think she was crazy (even though she was, by her own admission, a bit "kooky"). A urine test with sky-high levels of catecholamine (chemicals similar to the hormone adrenaline) alerted the physician to a tumor in her left adrenal gland, above her kidney. Once removed, Ellen's symptoms returned to normal (for a perimenopausal woman). Such diagnoses are nevertheless rare, so women with vague symptoms who believe they are perimenopausal need to exercise caution and not rush headlong into unnecessary surgeries or procedures that may have long-term consequences. In the earlier case of Emma, those hormones she took might also have exacerbated her gallbladder, as "HRT" was later found to do.[50]

A possible solution for those women who, like the authors of this book, have overwhelming difficulties (although they are still menstruating) during this time might be to try a course of cyclic progesterone at bedtime and see whether this clears up their symptoms—before doing anything too drastic.

Everything in medicine has consequences: every drug has side effects, every surgery, potentially disastrous consequences. The only truly safe surgery is the one they do on someone else, as doctors used to say. Even procedures ostensibly intended for diagnostic purposes should be closely questioned: CT scans, depending on the machine, can subject a person to up to four times as much radiation as an X-ray; as for magnetic resonance imaging, any machine that can make your watch fly about the room willy-nilly is bound to have *some* physiologic impact. Simply because a test is high-tech and modern and cool does not mean it is a good idea or that there might not be long-term consequences. It is therefore important for women to use their common sense. In the search for answers, it is easy to fall victim to inaccurate diagnoses, surgeries, or other potentially harmful interventions they do not need.

Perimenopause does end, but by not clarifying that this is a stage in and of itself, separate and distinct from menopause—worse, by calling this stage "menopause" or "being menopausal" and insisting that low or deficient estrogen is the problem—gynecologists and others depress and terrify women who are led to believe that these demoralizing symptoms will go on for the rest of their lives, symptoms that often are, in turn, exacerbated by the ostensible solution, which is to add more estrogen to already high levels. Too many women at midlife do not know that perimenopause does end and that the next phase is the kinder, gentler menopause (the real one), where hormones do settle and, just as when one was a girl, are no longer an issue. Instead, women at midlife seeking help are unhelpfully and inaccurately told that they are going through "menopause" and are prescribed estrogen alone if they have had a hysterectomy and estrogen with a smidgeon of a synthetic form of progesterone, progestin, if they have not. This strong hint that the *balance* of hormones matters is not that difficult to figure out; when estrogen levels rise during the time preceding ovulation during the normal menstrual cycle, the endometrium (uterine lining) becomes thick and proliferative. At that point, progesterone increases, creating an endometrium that is full of glands to prepare the uterus for a potential pregnancy. Then, when that is not forthcoming, the dropping of the high levels of progesterone remove that lining. Without progesterone, however, that estrogen-related thickening carries a high risk for becoming pathological. Hence, were one to consider the biology, the endocrinology, of a woman who is still having her period, as women during perimenopause usually are, then it makes sense that not adding some form of progesterone will lead to an excess of endometrial tissue and a risk for endometrial cancer.[51] Indeed, the lives of perimenopausal women, and everyone else, would be much improved if, as a society, we practiced mindful medicine.

COPING WITH COMPLEXITY

Despite the general acceptance of (and lip service paid to) the complexity of physiology and medical treatment, our corresponding sociocultural and medical template for illness or onerous symptoms and their treatment is simple, even simplistic: normal, healthy functioning goes awry for some reason, whereupon medical advice is sought. Through a series of investigations, scans, blood tests, and the like, experts zero in on the problem, diagnose what is at fault, and devise a treatment plan. Once engaged, the process fulfills its promise, life returns to normal, and homeostasis is restored. Unfortunately, this parable, like most, bears little relation to reality and is as inaccurate as other parables we hold dear, from fairy tales to television commercials (ask anyone who's lost a wallet in a foreign country about the truth of the Parable of the Lost Traveler's Checks). What it reflects is the social narrative we have constructed around medicine and health care and—as the many sufferers of chronic illness can attest—is less about the reality of medicine than our faith in progress, technology, and science; our trust in the power of expertise; and our belief in those snippets of medical news that assure us daily that advances in biology, genetics, pharmaceutical science, and informatics are expanding our knowledge by leaps and bounds. Particularly in North America, where our media tend to focus on personalities and celebrities, sensationalist and dramatic events, and in terms of health and medicine, "magical," quick-fix solutions, we tend to forget just what an intricate and complex blend each person is of individual physiology and psychology within a broader social and cultural milieu—not to mention all the historical, economic, social, and *human* reasons medicine has evolved as it has.

During the early part of the twentieth century, what medicine had to offer was sparse. But World War II, the rise of technology, and the economic power of the United States at that time blended with many other realities (the formation of the FDA, the rise of drug companies and sophisticated marketing strategies, etc.) to create the medicine we know today. In later chapters, we discuss some of these patterns and influences on the so-called objective practice of medicine; for now, it is important to remember that symptoms do not occur in a vacuum: how we think, feel, eat, and otherwise exist in the world has an effect on everything from our health to our hormones. Personal factors ranging from our sleep, nutrition, exercise, and so on to our socioeconomic status; how we function within our social milieu; and whether we are happy at our work, in our family lives, and in ourselves (what the French call feeling well in one's own skin) matter. Furthermore, as living organisms, just like fish or polar bears, our ability to thrive depends not only on our own individual characteristics, but on our physical environment, which, in turn, exists within a much larger sphere and includes the quality of the air we breathe, what is in the water we drink, and whatever remnants of pesticides or minerals or what have you that have leeched into our fruits and vegetables and the meat we eat. Not all of these may be harmful, but they will have an impact. Add to this picture the synthetics, plastics, and various additives (some of which mimic our own hormones[52] and whose long-term effects we simply do not know) we ingest and breathe and touch, and the result is a giant feedback loop in which health and well-being tie in with all facets of our lives. So complicated is this whole process that it is impossible to tease out precisely what might tilt one person over into having symptoms or feeling unwell and not another—or to know exactly what factors might be involved in one woman's experience of menstruation or perimenopause versus another's.

Sadly, not recognizing perimenopause as a stage preceding menopause has the unfortunate effect of further clouding the picture, and those women with the most onerous symptoms—particularly those with migraines or who are at risk for blood clots or heart disease, all contraindicated for estrogen—then end up vainly searching for answers to their physical problems. Women who are already stressed and anxious from not sleeping, who are worried that they are unable to focus or concentrate (the lack of sleep naturally has a lot to do with that), and who experience aches and pains feel certain there is something wrong, but medical science offers little but templates, tests, scans, and labels, which often have little to do with the individual and confuse more than they enlighten. Is it any wonder so many women find themselves seeking out medical advice or end up having unnecessary tests and surgeries? Women at midlife are also the demographic most likely to seek help from alternative practitioners—not surprising when traditional allopathic medicine ignores their concerns. Other women will end up finding legitimation for their distress in labels such as fibromyalgia or chronic fatigue syndrome, accompanied by medications that may or may not help, may be harmful, and could well have unpleasant side effects. Medical labels, furthermore, once applied, are nearly impossible to shake off and follow the person like the sword of Damocles.

Hormones have been used to define the core essence of women's physiology and health for more than one hundred years—to our detriment. In the next chapters, we examine the myriad factors that have gone into making up those myths modern medicine too often takes for granted and examine the adjunct reasons women have been told "HRT" is A Good Thing. Hormones, notably estrogen, have been associated with youth and vigor, cardiac health, and strong bones; they have been recommended as a preventive against cancer, dementia, Alzheimer's disease, and a host of other ailments women fear—yet nothing could be further from the truth. As Germaine Greer writes in her angry denunciation of estrogen supplementation at midlife in *The Whole Woman*, "Sex steroids [hormones] can hardly be expected to be neutral. . . . The more expert the endocrinologist, the more respect s/he has for the synergistic interactions of body chemicals; unfortunately most health practitioners have only an elementary understanding of endocrinology and are far too ready to believe in quick-fix remedies for perceived malfunction."[53] It behooves women to be far more cautious in their acceptance of these so-called hormonal panaceas. In the next chapters, we examine how societal norms, commercial interests, our cultural attachment to technological and scientific cures, and a compendium of other complicating factors have built on the belief that women *are* their hormones to convince an entire sector of the population that they need to take hormones to feel well and remain healthy.

Part 2

HORMONES AND HEALTH

Once upon a time, women took estrogen only to relieve the hot flashes, sweating, vaginal dryness and the other discomforting symptoms of menopause. In the late 1960's, thanks in part to the efforts of Robert Wilson, a Brooklyn gynecologist, in his 1966 best seller, "Feminine Forever," this began to change, and estrogen therapy evolved into a long-term remedy for the chronic ills of aging.... By the mid-1990's, the American Heart Association, the American College of Physicians and the American College of Obstetricians and Gynecologists had all concluded that the beneficial effects of H.R.T. were sufficiently well established that it could be recommended to older women as a means of warding off heart disease and osteoporosis. By 2001, 15 million women were filling H.R.T. prescriptions annually; perhaps 5 million were older women taking the drug solely with the expectation that it would allow them to lead a longer and healthier life. A year later, the tide would turn. In the summer of 2002, estrogen therapy was exposed as a hazard to health rather than a benefit, and its story became what Jerry Avorn, a Harvard epidemiologist, has called the "estrogen debacle" and a "case study waiting to be written" on the elusive search for truth.

—*Gary Taubes*, The New York Times[1]

4

THE MEDICALIZATION OF MENOPAUSE

The use of exogenous estrogens, and more recently, progestins, for women in their peri- and postmenopausal years has gone through a series of transformations over the past 100 years. The history of these drugs serves as an excellent example of how different constituencies with competing objectives often collide and produce health practices and policies with questionable benefits and potential harm. Interestingly, in this complex historical drama, the "patients," women in their fifties and beyond, emerge as both willing participants and unwilling victims of the unintended consequences of these drugs.
—Michelle Naughton et al.[1]

Nothing occurs in a vacuum—even the Greeks recognized that. If Athena sprang, fully formed (and fully armed, apparently), from the forehead of Zeus, then it had to be the work of the gods. The medicalization of menopause similarly did not spring up, fully formed, in the twentieth century, but had roots going back several centuries. Although the term *medicalization* (meaning "to make medical") was only coined in 1972 by the American sociologist Irving Zola, medicalization as a concept had begun to evolve during the seventeenth and eighteenth centuries, alongside science and engineering, as the natural world increasingly became the subject of inquiry and manipulation. The human body, and therefore health, also became something to control and improve. By the nineteenth century, as medical discourse became increasingly allied with the observational techniques of the burgeoning sciences, the body, as Foucault later remarked, had fundamentally changed; conceptually, it had become "part of nature and thus part of the project to identify and classify the workings of nature."[2]

Previously, the body had been considered holistically, in its entirety: the model for illness or dysfunction was that of a body out of balance with nature. The role of the physician or healer, therefore, was one that restored equilibrium. As the physical sciences changed, however, so did medicine—and physicians began to concern themselves not only with individual pathology and sickness, but also with life-cycle events such as birth and menopause. As anthropologist Margaret Lock writes,

> Birth had been entirely the provenance of women, but from the early eighteenth century, in both Europe and North America, male midwives trained and worked at the lying-in hospitals located in major urban centers to deliver the babies of well-off women. These *accoucheurs* later consolidated themselves as the profession of obstetrics. By the mid-nineteenth century, other life cycle transitions, including adolescence, menopause, aging, and death had been medicalized, followed by infancy in the first years of the twentieth century. In practice however, large segments of the population remained unaffected by these changes until the mid-twentieth century.[3]

One could argue, of course, that it makes a certain amount of sense, when those life transitions, such as birth or death, of which Lock speaks are difficult or painful that they might come under medical jurisdiction, for instance, a breach birth. After all, if childbirth can kill you, then perhaps it makes sense to have expert medical help standing by, at least under some circumstances. But have we gone too far? As sociologists Simon Williams and Michael Calnan write:

> Essentially . . . medicalization refers to the ways in which medical jurisdiction has expanded in recent years and now encompasses many problems which hitherto were not defined as medical. . . . A broad range of behaviours from homosexuality to alcoholism have been subsumed under the medical rubric and the current obsession with locating the genetic precursors of illness, diseases, disabilities and behaviours, means that the knowledge base of scientific medicine has encroached still further into defining the limits of "normality" and the proper functioning, deportment and control of the human body.[4]

Women, in particular, as feminist writers have stressed, are particularly subject to medicalization, sometimes coerced into accepting obstetric and gynecological techniques ranging from fetal monitoring to induction and forceps—or hysterectomies in perimenopause or hormones at menopause—without necessarily being told, or fully understanding, the reasons why.[5]

AT RISK FOR DISEASE

For centuries, medicine has been the art (and to some extent, the science) of healing, along with the practice of bringing comfort and succor to the sick. Health and illness were obvious, subjective states: your grandmother *knew* when she was ill or needed to go to the hospital. Today, the medical repertoire has expanded and definitions of pathology have broadened to include (at least in the West) a vast array of asymptomatic diagnoses that are invisible and imperceptible to the individual in question. For instance, today, we use drugs and therapies not only when we feel unwell, but because we are "at risk" of disease—our blood pressure is high or our glucose level does not match some previously agreed standard or benchmark. The numbers themselves do not correspond with disease, but are biomarkers: statistically derived measures that are considered predictive with regard to one condition or another such as diabetes or coronary artery disease.

Today, as modern medicine attempts to predict and prevent illness, increasing numbers of us are said to suffer from such invisible and asymptomatic conditions—what critics have called *numbers-created* diseases.[6] There are even such bizarre constructs as being told one is "pre" diabetic when glucose levels are looming too close to some magical cutoff point.* So ubiquitous has this at-risk discourse become that few people realize that until the 1960s this peculiar construct, in which we focus on measuring individual factors believed to contribute to disease, did not exist.[7] This piecemeal, reductionist approach—in which focus has shifted onto biomarkers (surrogate end points) such as lipid levels versus the person as a whole—has therefore completely altered the face of medicine, medical research, and education. Not only has individual care been affected, but by the late 1980s, as the late Yale physician Alvan Feinstein warned, such efforts had converged on a taxonomy of medicine that divided health and health care into what were considered to be its component parts: structure, process, and outcome.[8] In other words, the focus of medicine completely moved *away* from the person and toward pathology and disease.

MENOPAUSE AS RISK FACTOR

The medicalization of menopause fell into this general category, with the promotion of hormones as prevention encouraging "both doctors and women to view their current health status in terms of their risk of future ill health."[9] Such concerns were (and are) exacerbated by playing on women's fears of aging and our general societal preoccupation with how to stave off the diseases of old age. *Guidelines, critical pathways,* and *disease management* have become medical bywords over the past few decades, even as medical care has been transformed into an increasingly impersonal discipline. Today, in some ways, it no longer

---

*Although it makes a certain amount of sense to think of a condition (such as adult-onset diabetes, high blood pressure, or hyperlipidemia) along a continuum, it is currently not presented in those terms, but rather as an either-or proposition. There is also a vaguely threatening, disheartening element to this discourse, which continually places us at the brink of some disaster or disease.

matters *who* you are, but *what*; in other words, nobody cares that you might be a stressed, struggling single mother of two teenagers whose place of work is downsizing and who is frantically trying to hold everything together, or that you are going through perimenopause. What matters is that you are a woman nearing menopause who is overweight and has high blood pressure—which requires treatment of one kind or another. Aside from the obvious and questionable problems with this pithy, modern (some would add peculiarly American) model, defining the so-called norm (against which pathology can be determined), it is not only completely arbitrary much of the time, but is all too often based on statistical, epidemiological, and other types of information that have excluded women altogether. Add into this noxious mix the infatuation with estrogen that has characterized the discussion on women's health and hormones, and the stage is set for potentially disastrous results. Take Barb, a fifty-three-year-old retired teacher:

> Barb has a strong family history of heart disease: her father, a heavy smoker, binge drinker, and alcoholic, had a fatal heart attack at age fifty-one, and her mother, who is in her early seventies (a diabetic and a smoker), has had angina since her fifties. Barb herself has no real risk factors. She plays squash twice a week, walks every day to her volunteer job or to the store, and has a normal body weight. Her doctor checks her blood pressure and tells her it is 128/82, which is terrific. Her cholesterol and other lipids are fine.
>
> Barb's last period was at age fifty, and she was started on "HRT" shortly after, on the advice of a cardiologist. She doesn't like being on estrogen, particularly given the generally negative tone of the studies, but she's afraid of having a heart attack if she stops. The cardiologist also put her on a statin (drugs that lower cholesterol) that had to be changed several times because of side effects, based on some "worrisome changes" on an ECG (electrocardiogram). Then she changed the hormone regimen she was taking from Premarin/Provera to a bioidentical estrogen plus a compounded progesterone cream (at Barb's insistence), 20 mg a day. The cardiologist also suggested that ramipril (a blood pressure medication) would make her blood pressure even lower.
>
> Barb searched the Internet and found that according to the Framingham 10-year Heart Disease Score, her actual risk of heart disease was 1 percent over ten years. She also checked the Centre for Menstrual Cycle and Ovulation Research Web site and read up on heart health. She stopped the statin and didn't fill the ramipril prescription.

The cardiologist, Barb quickly realized, had not been paying attention to *who* she was, but had seen her as a cardboard cutout—a morass of risk factors. Her father's heart attack was related to his weight, smoking, and alcoholism, while her mother's angina was exacerbated by her poorly treated diabetes and smoking. Plus, Barb had been good with exercise all her life.

Barb asked her family physician for full-dose oral micronized progesterone (Prometrium 300 mg at bedtime) to help wean her off the estrogen.* She kept up her exercise, continued her healthy diet with little or no animal fats, and maintained her normal weight.[10]

The cardiologist's advice to Barb demonstrated a fixation with risk factors (as well as a lack of understanding of what they might actually mean), which is fairly typical of current medicine, which is completely preoccupied with the risk factors for heart disease, to which we divert massive amounts of funding, attention, and promotional activity (not to mention drugs). Plus, we are repeatedly told that we must control our five famous risks: blood pressure, cholesterol, diabetes, obesity, and smoking (physical activity occasionally makes it onto more recent lists, but it tends not to garner much attention).

What we tend to forget, however, is that some risks matter more than others (e.g., in women, activity levels[11] and diabetes[12]) and that we are all individuals, not a mishmash of numbers that make up our parts like some complicated machine. Furthermore, our penchant for aggressive treatment requires balancing out with its potential to do harm.[13] Yet our sociocultural fascination with technology, numbers, guidelines, statistics, and other quantitative forms of reasoning (firmly nudged along by pharmaceutical companies eager to sell their drugs) has become so monomaniacal that we rarely even question their veracity. There is increasing evidence, for instance, that lowering cholesterol in individuals who have not had a heart attack (primary prevention) is useless, and even for those who have had that heart attack (secondary prevention), it might not be particularly lifesaving—neither in women nor in men.[14] But it is easier to measure lipids and write a prescription than it is to attempt to understand or explain physiology or come to grips with a person's life situation.

As perimenopause and menopause became part of the risk factor approach, women at midlife found themselves no longer in a *state of nature*, but in a *state of disease*, terms exacerbated by labels like "estrogen deficiency" and "ovarian failure."[15] Even that majority of women for whom the perimenopausal transition and menopause involved few or no symptoms found themselves being labeled "at risk"—an alarming phrase suggesting the need for immediate medical attention. So hormones, even if unnecessary for symptom reduction (since more than 75% of women do not have problems at midlife), needed to be taken to ward off future disease, or at least the *risk* of future disease—a bizarre concept at best. "In women, estrogen and the lack of it are linked to many disorders of aging," insisted a 2001 *JAMA* editorial in an issue in which several articles made the case for estrogen improving cognition as women aged, and even reducing the risk of dementia.[16] (A claim resoundedly disproved by the Women's Health Initiative a few years later.) "What's the matter with

*See "Stopping Estrogen Therapy" on the CeMCOR Web site; http/www.cemcor.ubc.ca.

cardiologists?" scolded an epidemiologist in the *Canadian Medical Association Journal* in 1999. Apparently, contrary to the guidelines (i.e., the truth according to the people writing the guidelines), only a scant 21 percent of women attending a Toronto cardiology clinic were "documented users of HRT."[17] Yet even though it has turned out that hormones' ability to ward off disease in healthy women is a myth,[18] this estrogen-is-good belief is so fundamental that it simply seems to refuse to die, at least in the medical and media imagination.[19]

Ironically, the healthier we have generally become as a society (indicated by what few objective measures there are, such as infant mortality and life expectancy), the lower our general satisfaction with our health and the more concerned we are with risk and preventing future illness. Americans, like Canadians and Britons, report "more frequent and longer-lasting episodes of serious, acute illness now than they did 60 years ago,"[20] and scores on health self-assessment measures hover around the 50 percent mark, hardly a ringing endorsement. Predictably, younger people have higher estimates of their own general health, but as we reach our forties, our perceptions of our physical functioning and well-being decline.[21]

THE SOCIAL CONNECTION

Perceptions of ourselves, in terms of health or anything else, are, of course, contextual and multidimensional, and our notions of what constitutes health emanate from within a horizon of possibilities that changes according to what we believe is possible. As the Nobel Prize–winning economist Amartya Sen described, how we assess our state of health is often the result of what we know, what we hear, and what we think *ought* to be. Sen found, for instance, that in the poorest state in India (Bihar), where medical services and general health are "woeful," people considered themselves to be generally well. Yet in India's richest state (Kerala), with health measures running in the opposite direction, people were dissatisfied and reported their health to be poor, leading Sen to conclude that feeling healthy somehow depends on not knowing what can go wrong—and in comparison to those around us within our community.[22]

Perhaps it is not surprising, then, that in a culture so celebrity- and entertainment-driven as ours—in which the ideal is some hypothetical and terrifically dressed, athletic, exciting, and, above all, youthful person (if she is a woman, always in stiletto heels and a pencil skirt)—the overall belief is that one could always be doing *better*. After all, most of us neither look nor feel anything like those vibrant people in the ads or on TV who get up at six in the morning to run in the park, play tennis or golf, work a full day (at exciting offices with cool technology), and then go out to a restaurant or club (and seem to sleep, on average, three hours a night). Furthermore, as epidemiologist Nortin Hadler writes in

The Last Well Person: How to Stay Well Despite the Health-Care System, our culture predisposes us to frame challenges to everyday coping in medical terms, especially when we feel overwhelmed. (So it is not only medicine medicalizing life, but *us* as well.) For one thing, it is not really socially acceptable to feel exhausted or to hate our job; instead, everything around us, from advertisements and television shows to magazine articles, encourages us to transform our stress or fatigue into "idioms of physical distress."[23] Perhaps we need supplements or vitamins, or antidepressants, or something to help us sleep. Or perhaps the problem is repetitive strain injury—or perhaps we need some arcane nutrient to give us energy.

Then again, it might be our hormones.

Western medicine, notably American medicine—the most advanced in the world, as we are fond of saying—encompasses such extraordinary technologies and presents us with such a continuous barrage of complicated terminologies that we tend to forget just how rudimentary our understanding of physiology and pathology (not to mention human ecology) is. What little we know of the immune or endocrine systems is piecemeal, fragmented, and reductionist,[24] and we know next to nothing about what keeps the whole person healthy—no matter how much we try to manipulate the parts (and imply that the sum of the parts really does add up). We have no idea why one person gets ill and another does not, and we can barely figure out how joints work, never mind more complex systems such as the hypothalamic-pituitary-ovarian axis for women's hormones, particularly if we throw in psychosocial stress.[25] We also blithely forget that the metaphors we use to describe physiology are exactly that: analogies, shortcuts, and heuristics that are expedient, convenient, and not necessarily accurate. Plus, metaphors change with the times (when the telephone was the latest thing, the brain was described as a switchboard; now we prefer to think of it as a computer) and have no real bearing on the workings of the physiologic process involved.

Cardiac function today, for instance, is currently neatly depicted (often in colorful graphics that further reinforce the point) much as our kitchen sink might be: the heart is a pump and the arteries and blood vessels are the pipes, with their plumbing becoming impeded in much the same way. The gunk (plaque) builds up in the arteries, preventing blood flow, and the cardiac surgeon, like the plumber, cleans them out or replaces them. Quick, easy, neat—except that this is so far from the truth as to be laughable. This so-called mechanical pump is self-regulating, affected by everything from how we think to our mother's diet when we were in the womb—with delicate connections, so intricate, to the lungs, kidneys, hormones, emotions, nutrition, and more that at present we could not fathom it if we tried (which we rarely do). Witness the spectacular failure of every artificial heart we have ever tried to build.

Additionally, as anyone who has experienced firsthand some of these "miraculous" treatments, cures, or surgical interventions knows only too well, the reality of medicine is nothing like *House* or those neat bullet points we see on the Internet or in magazines. In that world, as on TV, high-tech drugs (like antivirals and chemotherapies) work beautifully, complicated surgeries happen without a hitch, and recovery moves briskly along, just as the textbooks describe. Nobody gets chronic pain or depressed afterward, and everything goes according to plan. The reality, however, is that even a bad flu can leave us tired, spent, pale, and feeling like death for months, even years. Even the simplest of surgeries under general anesthetic (such as knee cartilage "cleaning") result in scarring and fibrosis, long-term pain, and a long, painful recovery. Many people never recover completely, and those of us who listen to patients probably hear one phrase more than any other: "If only I'd known then what I know now." The harms and long-term side effects of many interventions and drugs are rarely mentioned, and few people appreciate the risks of medicine,[26] even as iatrogenesis (illness *caused* by medical intervention) is on the rise.[27] It behooves us, therefore, to approach any major intervention with caution and approach medical news with skepticism, given that the majority of medical news is disease-oriented.[28]

Conspicuously absent in the discussion on health—or staying free of disease, if you prefer—is any mention of the importance of socioeconomic status (SES) factors: psychosocial issues such as how close we are to loved ones and economics, in other words, how much money we have, and how happy we are in our work, all of which correlate with health more accurately than hormones ever have. Instead of focusing on the ergonomics of our work station (and seeing a physician for our repetitive strain injury), perhaps it would be better to pay closer attention to some basic social and economic factors (such as unemployment insurance, social security, etc.) because these have been shown to have a far larger impact on health than any drug ever could. In fact, even our much-vaunted health and longevity, compared to earlier generations, is far more easily attributed to improvements in hygiene and sanitation, such as clean water and sewage, than anything else.

"What is it about a compromised socioeconomic state . . . that is so malevolent?" asks Hadler.[29] There are multiple factors, of course, not the least of which is the huge physiological and psychological toll that a lower SES takes, including worrying about how to pay the bills or losing your job or your home. Lower SES often implies that one lives in areas without parks for children or good schools (McDonald's fosters a lifelong love of its hamburgers by being the only playground available in many depressed areas), not to mention polluted air or contaminated water and high-priced, suboptimal food. The CEO of the corporation would not allow the plant runoff or the pollutants—whether in the United States or India—to be dumped where he lives; it is the lowly worker whose home abuts such potential toxic sites. Yet the template for health inevitably zeroes in on the person, not on social, economic, or cultural factors.

HORMONES, HISTORY, AND MEDICALIZATION

For women at midlife, this cultural paradigm creates a double-edged sword. Not only have all aspects of our lives become subject to what Foucault called the medical gaze, but over the last fifty years, the medicalization of life in general (and women's experiences in particular) has increased, being highly compatible with what sociologist Susan Bell calls the "values and organizational structure of American society."[30] Different facets of life specific to women, such as childbirth, birth control, menstruation, weight, and mental health, have all become domains for medical input (although why weight, mental health, and birth control should be considered solely women's domain remains a mystery). Women's reproductive health and hormones have therefore lent themselves particularly well to medicalization.

Nevertheless, before the discovery of estrogen and its imagined therapeutic uses, women's midlife voices were at least occasionally heard. A British physician by the name of E. J. Tilt, writing about five hundred French women in 1871, for instance, described the transition to menopause in functional terms, merely saying that it was "clear that the change of life is a time of turbulent activity for the reproductive organs." Without resorting inordinately to judgmental comments, Tilt merely described his clinical findings and commented that women during this phase of their lives appeared to be more prone to "congestion, hemorrhage, mucous flows and neuralgic afflictions."[31] During Tilt's time, physicians viewed menopause as a "physiological crisis" that could lead to "tranquility or disease," as Bell writes,[32] depending on the individual.

This changed with the discovery of hormones. As early as 1896, two Viennese gynecologists (Emil Knauer and Josef Halban) were describing secretions by the ovaries,[33] which they suspected might have therapeutic promise, and by the early twentieth century, in tandem with the pharmaceutical companies,* medical focus had shifted toward defining menopause (and any other problem that could conceivably be linked to reproductive hormones) as a disease. Hormones were powerful substances and, at a time when medicine did not have much to offer, offered enormous potential—for *something*. As the University of Amsterdam's Nelly Oudshoorn wryly notes, right from the start, sex hormones were drugs in search of a disease.†

From the very inception of endocrinology, however, research interest and scientific attention focused on a simplistic idea: too much or too little hormone.

---

*Although midwives and other practitioners prepared pills and powders from dried (presumably animal) ovaries and testes and used these for a variety of disorders.

†Nelly Oudshoorn, "On the Making of Sex Hormones: Research Materials and the Production of Knowledge," *Social Studies of Science* 20(1), 5–33 (1990).

As endocrinologist Jean Wilson described in her plenary address to the Twelfth International Congress of Endocrinology in 2004,

> Two endeavours had dominated endocrinology from the beginning. One concerned the state of hormone deficiency or absence, and the other focused on the effects of hormone excess. Little attention was addressed to the mechanisms by which hormones exert their effects within target tissues.[34]

Although this did prove useful with certain kinds of disorders, such as diabetes (at least the type 1 variety), this mechanistic metaphor generally translated into medical and clinical reductionism, because the majority of physiological mechanisms are considerably more complex. With autoimmune disorders, or even adult-onset diabetes (where it is not the lack of insulin that appears to be the problem, but rather, its effectiveness), moreover, the model loses all utility and metaphoric value— and where it goes spectacularly wrong is in insisting that this simple top-up model applies to all glands, for all people, at all times, particularly because it is not based on the physiology of how the endocrine mechanisms might work, but is based on what we *believe*, usually overt social prejudices and absurd classification systems that devalue certain types of people (e.g., women or people of color) and arbitrarily decide what they may or may not be capable of. Just as important, this too much/too little dichotomy makes a mockery of the importance of balance and interconnectedness, which is central to endocrinology.

As discussed in a previous chapter, in women, the sex hormones are not the result of the *entire* gland's activities (the glands in question being the two ovaries), but result from the follicles that surround each individual egg *within* the ovary. Furthermore, not only is estrogen, the hormone associated with the follicles and leading up to ovulation, not the only female sex hormone, but it is progesterone, the luteal or postovulatory hormone, that is essential to the smooth functioning of the cycle. It is the subtle balance of these two hormones that creates a healthy ovulatory cycle, which—in ways we continue not to understand with any real clarity— plays a role in optimal health (e.g., with respect to bones, the vascular system, and cancer). Like the "feminine forever" myth effectively advertised by Robert Wilson, such ideas of women were based on estrogen being the magical youth-producing hormone. At the same time, as shown in Figure 4.1, his rendering of the natural hormones of the menstrual cycle depicts estrogen as vastly more plentiful than progesterone, although the opposite, as we saw in Figure 2.2, is accurate.

Unfortunately, the medicalization of menopause rested on a theory of etiology (cause) that was, first and foremost, mired in murky sociocultural ideas of hierarchy and women's subordinate roles within that hierarchy. Women's value was irrevocably connected to their biology (fecundity) and was grounded in those peculiarly Western values relating to deficiency and excess (as opposed to the

Figure 4.1
This rather quaint diagram of menstrual cycle estrogen and progesterone levels is reproduced directly from *Feminine Forever* by Robert A. Wilson, M. Evans and Co., New York, NY, 1966.

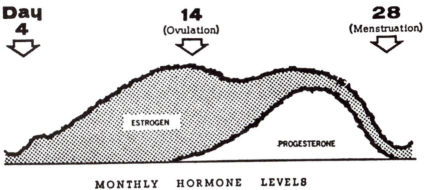

Eastern Tao or First Nations' ideas of balance), as well as political, economic, and commercial interests.

THE GODDESS OF FORTUNE

The discovery of hormones in the late 1800s created high commercial and medical expectations, and Ernst Laqueur, a leading researcher in the 1920s and 1930s and one of the three founders of the Dutch pharmaceutical firm Organon (a company formed in 1923 to make and distribute pancreatic hormone, or insulin, and conduct research on sex hormones) saw female hormones as a golden opportunity to pursue the "goddess of fortune." And by liaising with a slaughterhouse to buy organic remains, the venture quickly evolved into the research and production of estrogen, of which the company remained the major commercial producer worldwide until World War II briefly put a stop to it. (Organon is still in existence, incidentally.) As Oudshoorn describes,

> Laqueur conceptualized sex hormones as sexually specific in origin and function, and he directed female sex hormone therapy strictly toward women. The expectation of manufacturing a medicine for the treatment of all "women's diseases" indicated a very *promising market*, [italics added] because this therapy could be extended to all women.[35]

Although Organon was initially the largest drug company connected to the discovery, research, and manufacture of estrogen, it was by no means the only one. In fact, hormone development worked hand in glove with multiple pharmaceutical companies right from the beginning.

It was the support of the (American) company Parke-Davis that had allowed Takamine and Aldrich's laboratory to purify epinephrine (adrenaline) in 1901 and determine its structure.[36] Later, Parke-Davis was also allied with the work of one of the most famous names in endocrinology, Edward Doisy, the American biochemist whose assay (with Edgar Allen) became the formula in hormone development and who isolated the prevalent menopausal form of estrogen, originally called theelin, later estrone, one of the three estrogen subtypes, for which he won the Nobel Prize in 1943. Simultaneously, in Germany, biochemist Adolf Butenandt also isolated estrone with the support of German pharmaceutical giant Schering, which later developed the synthetic estrogen (ethinyl estradiol) subsequently used in virtually all birth control pills post–World War II.

Closely allied to the laboratory scientists and pharmaceutical firms were the gynecologists, who not only had a wide pool of women patients to draw on, but who also were already comfortable with the idea that women's biology should to be manipulated. Since the 1870s, surgical removal of the ovaries had become fairly common to treat what were ambiguously termed *women's problems*, which were not only related to menstruation but also included "nervous disorders" and "psychoneuroses." Hence there were always, as Oudshoorn explains, three different "groups of actors [who] were interested and actively involved in research into the sex glands: the gynecologists, the pharmaceutical industry and the laboratory scientists."[37]

Estrogen soon demonstrated enormous promise and profit potential. The "disease" had already been identified as *ovarian insufficiency*, as a 1941 Schering booklet on estrogen phrased it (or *estrogen deficiency*, as it later came to be called). Symptoms of this insufficiency were diverse, ranging from menstrual irregularities of one sort or another and menopause to morning sickness and even migraine.[38] (Estrogen actually *causes* both morning sickness and migraine.) The only major drawback was figuring out a nonhuman way to synthesize estrogen. As an article in the *American Journal of Obstetrics and Gynecology* lamented in 1932, estrone could be so useful as a "treatment" for menopausal women, but supplies were simply inadequate.[39]

Neither Organon nor Schering nor anybody else could figure out a reliable source for estrogen. The urine of pregnant women contained estrogen, but there was simply not enough of it available, even with the help of gynecologists. Some scientists nevertheless did manage to become creative at finding solutions to this estrogen supply problem; for instance, a British physiologist wrote that, thanks to the help of the British Museum, he was able to obtain ovaries "in bulk" from a "southern blue whale," which, weighing nearly seventy tons, had correspondingly large ovaries.[40] But because blue whales do not normally swim into laboratories, this was not really a long-term solution. The problem was eventually solved in 1938, across the Atlantic, when two American chemists, Russell Marker and

Thomas Oakwood, figured out how to develop a synthetic chemical that would act like estrogen, known as diethylstilbestrol (DES). Bell writes,

> Until DES was synthesized, estrogen therapy was extremely expensive, since the natural estrogens were difficult to extract, purify and stabilize and most potent when injected. DES was easy to produce and to purify and it was effective orally, so it was cheap to prescribe. If the initial laboratory findings were corroborated, clinical research would no longer be limited to a few financially advantaged patients.[41]

This "cheap and potent hormone substance" could readily be made "available to a large number of women"—and comprised the first wave of the medicalization of menopause.[42]

THE DES DEBACLE

It took some time—and lobbying—before DES was approved for medical use. Many of the physicians of the time, much like today, were ambivalent about this new "science" of medicine, in part because they were not really sure what it implied for the doctor-patient relationship (or whether it undermined their authority as physicians). Most physicians, writes Bell, were of the opinion that ideally, medicine was a blend of clinical judgment and science, and DES, having been concocted in the laboratory, was not, for many doctors, in the best interests of the patient (no matter how much they might have liked a drug with which to treat menstrual and menopausal problems). Given that the prevailing biological model defined menopause as a deficiency in ovarian estrogen production, however, it stood to reason that replacing that lost endogenous estrogen would do the trick, at least in treating vasomotor symptoms like hot flushes and night sweats. "Apart from these two signs, the myriad signs and symptoms associated with menopause presented a confusing and variable puzzle that even the new objective tests could not solve," writes Bell.[43] (The new objective tests consisted of the assays Doisy and Allen had developed to evaluate ovarian preparations; these could assess the estrogen effect from counting the three types of epithelial cells in a vaginal smear. Unfortunately, without appropriately characterizing the normal vaginal smear, what these early physicians considered normal actually was an extremely high level of estrogen.*) These same poorly standardized vaginal smear tests, incidentally, were later used by Robert Wilson (of *Feminine Forever* fame) in the 1960s to justify giving estrogen even to women who were premenopausal, still menstruating, and still having normal estrogen levels.

After World War II, the U.S. government had begun to increase its funding, and organization, of medical research, and in 1938, the same year as DES was

---

*Conjugated equine estrogen at 2.5 to 5.0 mg, compared with the 0.45 or 0.625 mg that are considered appropriate today.

synthesized, the federal Food, Drug, and Cosmetic Act was passed, thus leading to the creation of the FDA.* Companies were now required to submit evidence that their products were safe (when used as directed), although there was no requirement that any particular disease or condition be connected with the product. The FDA approved DES after the concerted efforts of a small group (forty-seven) of "elite" physicians (with the support, naturally, of the pharmaceutical companies), making it the first known, widely used estrogen "replacement" therapy.[†]

The FDA at this point was still in its infancy. The primary impetus behind its formation had been the thalidomide disaster of the 1930s. Thalidomide, a drug used to prevent nausea in pregnancy, had led to gruesome birth defects in Europe and made a heroine of Frances Kelsey, the FDA official who had kept thalidomide out of the U.S. market. Drug approval was a loose and fairly casual process; the randomized clinical trial, or RCT, often considered the gold standard of evidence today, did not exist (more on this later), and the FDA criteria for drug acceptance was essentially based on expert testimony from individuals, usually doctors, who could provide what was called *substantial evidence* of a drug's efficacy. This evidence, as medical historian Marcia Meldrum points out, was in fact a contradiction in terms and consisted of a circular argument, namely, that the substantial evidence, which consisted of "adequate and well-controlled investigations," was provided by "experts qualified by scientific training and experience to *evaluate* the effectiveness of the drug involved."[44] In other words, the evidence was whatever the experts said it was. And experts were the people qualified to assess the evidence. Round and round we go.

In the case of DES, thirty of the forty-seven physicians involved were requested to "complete questionnaires giving clinical evidence of the safety of DES." This information, however tenuous, formed the basis for the 1941 FDA approval of DES for menopausal symptoms, vaginal infections (this was dropped when penicillin appeared on the scene), and lactation suppression—but it took little time for off-label uses to appear. Drug company advertisements showing cute babies promoted DES as a way to prevent miscarriage, avert the possibility of a spontaneous abortion, and reduce the chance of going into premature labor, in particular as a result of maternal (gestational) diabetes, a major problem for some pregnant women. Soon DES was being widely prescribed all over the United States. (Although DES was desultorily used in the United Kingdom and continental Europe, doctors in other Western countries stopped prescribing DES

---

*Although the American Medical Association in 1905 had established a Council on Pharmacy and Chemistry, and Congress had passed the Biologics Control Act in 1902, there was no formal requirement prior to the FDA.

[†]This tactic of using elite physicians (also called *opinion leaders*, or physicians to whom other clinicians would listen) is a common pharmaceutical company strategy. It is still in use today.

by the mid-1940s.[45]) Oddly, no patent was ever taken out on DES, and reportedly, several hundred pharmaceutical companies manufactured (and advertised) it.

Gynecologists extolled the virtues of DES and millions of pregnant women routinely took DES, even though within a very short time, anecdotes and case histories accumulated on harms. A large, randomized, placebo-controlled trial in the 1950s showed that DES was in fact totally useless in preventing miscarriage—in fact, women were *more* likely to abort when taking the synthetic estrogen—yet in spite of this, as late as 1971, a gynecology textbook recommended prescribing DES to pregnant women.[46]

Ominous rumblings also began to rise about the fetal and maternal risks of DES, ranging from birth defects to cancer—and today, we know that not only were the women who took DES more at risk for breast cancer, but their daughters later suffered from clear-cell adenocarcinoma of the vagina (whose growth was exacerbated by puberty). There was even some suggestion that their sons might be more prone to infertility and possibly testicular cancer. Class-action suits were launched, and there are still people around who continue to suffer the consequences of this early estrogen boondoggle because their mothers were prescribed the drug forty years ago.[47]

In terms of follow-up, those women who took DES around menopause got lost in the shuffle; their stories never made it into the headlines or the data. This makes a kind of warped sense; why worry about older women when there are adorable infants and young mothers involved? But without a doubt there were a fair number of older women who did die prematurely of breast, endometrial, or other cancers because of DES. Word finally did trickle out about the harm DES could cause, and by the late 1990s, the only approved use for DES was for prostate cancer in men. In 1997, the last manufacturer of DES, Eli Lilly, stopped making the drug. Bizarrely, given the high toll that DES had and the clear indication that overdosing on estrogen was a *really* bad idea, the whole DES episode sank into oblivion. Barring those families (and their lawyers) who had a direct interest, the DES debacle did not give anyone pause, not even a scant twenty years later, as the second wave of enthusiasm for estrogen hit the United States.

MEDICALIZATION: THE SECOND WAVE

Part of the reason DES did not make as much of an impact in Europe as it did in the United States may have been that since 1930, Organon, the Dutch pharmaceutical company specializing in hormones, had been making estrogen using the urine of pregnant mares. Naturally, America knew nothing about this, what with World War II and all; plus, medical research rarely, if ever, crosses national boundaries (even today, very few researchers or doctors actually read or know about clinical practice in any other country).[48] So in 1943, an American,

James Goodall, was able to have his own epiphany about the urine of pregnant mares in making a pill that would be a marvelous, cheap, readily available estrogen. Plus, this estrogen had the advantage of being *natural* (well, for a horse at least), not a nasty synthetic hormone like DES, which had not worked out so well. The pharmaceutical company Ayerst (now Wyeth) quickly moved to produce and market this estrogen and called it Premarin: an estrogen about half as potent as DES that could be touted as being safe and with fewer side effects.

By 1945, Premarin was big news—and *the* estrogen therapy women were told they needed to keep them well during their menopausal years and beyond. Estrogen "replacement" therapy, or "ERT," became the word of the day, and usage creep being what it is, within a few years, it was implied (then authoritatively stated) that estrogen was no mere solution for hot flushes, not just some short-term option for those women with difficult symptoms, but an überdrug, a magical substance that could keep women young and "stave off the effects of the aging process"[49]: the Fountain of Youth. (Really, aging was so last century; this was the twentieth century, when America ruled and technology reigned supreme.)

This was the perfect environment for the 1966 book *Feminine Forever*, secretly produced by the maker of Premarin, Ayerst (now Wyeth), and couched in the language of a warmly supportive physician providing kindly medical advice. Robert Wilson, the gynecologist who had written the book, turned this blatant piece of propaganda into one of the most effective marketing ploys ever devised. In no time at all, menopause became cemented in the popular imagination as the deficiency disease that estrogen could cure. And now aging itself had been thrown into the equation. (At one point, Wilson wrote that estrogen should be given from "puberty to grave."[50])

Three years later, another best-selling book, *Everything You Wanted to Know about Sex (but Were Afraid to Ask)*, by Dr. David Reuben, reinforced the estrogen orthodoxy even further—arguing (rather rudely) that without estrogen, a woman was, in essence, a man, with facial hair and a deep, booming voice. Her breasts and genitalia would shrink and she would become obese: "Not really a man but no longer a functional woman."[51] Midlife women had outlived their ovaries, and after that, it was downhill all the way without "ERT." Women's magazines also jumped on the bandwagon (bearing in mind that the vast majority of women's publications then—as now—have male publishers). In 1973, *Harper's Bazaar* gushed that "there doesn't seem to be a sexy thing estrogen can't and won't do to keep you flirtatiously feminine."[52] At a time when middle-class women wore kid gloves and hats, housewives were shown in dresses and pearls in television ads as they pushed the new labor-saving devices like vacuum cleaners; a time when women often had to quit their (pink ghetto) jobs once they were married (whether they wanted to or not), at a time when many women attended university to earn what was semi-ironically referred to as their "M.R.S." degree, this cut right to the heart of women's real and subliminal fears. As authors like Updike and Roth (and current shows like *Mad Men*) have shown, men were not necessarily thrilled with the way things were but, unsurprisingly, had no real desire to give up their power and status. Women, on the other hand, were afraid that if they gave up what they had (as the burgeoning women's movement was suggesting), they could end up with nothing at all. Ironically, women's fears were not ill founded; twenty years later, when various laws and statutes were changed so that women and men were considered equal in marriage, no-fault divorce settlements "raised men's standard of living 42% while lowering that of women and children 73%."[53]

Wilson's book was a masterpiece of medicalization. As sociologist Frances McCrea writes,

> From Wilson's own words it is obvious that the disease label [he uses] is not neutral. This label, like any disease label, decreases the status and autonomy of the patient.... By individualizing the problems of menopause... attention [is turned away] from any social structural interpretation of women's conditions. The locus of the solution then becomes the doctor-patient interaction in which the physician is active, instrumental, and authoritative while the patient is passive and dependent.... Such imperialism is independent of the particular motivation of the physician.[54]

Medicine became entrenched as part of the social order.

Wilson subtly played into the upheaval of the times (assassinations, riots, civil rights) even as power remained fixed in the same, conservative hands as before. (Wilson himself was born in the late nineteenth century so would have lived through two world wars and many of those changes.) Women already understood that it was only their fertility, and domestic utility, that gave them what little power they had—and here, in the midst of all this social change, came this doctor telling them it was all about estrogen. They were not losing touch and losing their way; it was just a *disease*. Wilson's true genius, however, lay in his genuine-sounding appreciation for women (at least the ones in his own milieu: white, middle-class women—ladies who lunched) and their fears: "In our civilization, a woman's romantic expectations during her younger years are seldom fully satisfied by the actualities of her life," he sympathetically wrote. "Often her choice of husband was based on a compromise" due to our "social pressures toward marriage."[55] Then, he adds, she approaches menopause and realizes that this knight in shining armor is just not going to appear. Even today, such passages seem almost moving. (Of course, Wilson then says something thuggish, like women have to take estrogen so their husbands won't have to put up with their nagging, and the moment is lost.)

Gynecologists loved Wilson's book, as did geriatricians, and various prominent physicians spoke out in favor of "ERT." Robert Greenblatt, the former president of the American Geriatrics Society, claimed in the early 1970s that up to "75%

of menopausal women are acutely estrogen deficient."[56] Symptoms were not the
point: deficiency was deficiency.

IN SHORT . . .

Two large waves of medicalization with respect to menopause hit the Western
world (and especially the United States) in the twentieth century. First there was
DES, a synthetic estrogen, handed out like candy until the early 1970s, which
caused breast cancer in the mothers and fatal vaginal cancers in their daughters.
Then came estrogen made from pregnant mares' urine, which was soon linked
to endometrial cancer in women with an intact uterus. But, with that peculiarly
American form of 1950s sexism, much of the criticism was pushed aside and
ignored. Eventually, progestin, a synthetic form of progesterone, was added—
turning "ERT" into "HRT"—for women who had not had a hysterectomy. In
no time at all and without missing a step, medicine then moved toward *all*
the diseases of age as being the result of estrogen deficiency in women of a
certain age.

Guidelines and authoritative recommendations for the "treatment" of asymptomatic women at perimenopause and menopause were issued, not for symptom
relief but as *preventive* therapy for heart disease, osteoporosis, dementia, asthma,
cataracts, incontinence, cancer, and anything else they could think of, all of which
dovetailed nicely with the overwhelming focus of medicine on risk reduction and
risk factors as it had evolved over the 1980s. As Canadian physician Stephen
Genuis incredulously writes:

> When it became fashionable to use HRT containing estrogen and progesterone to
> prevent osteoporosis, heart disease, and cognitive decline in women, I considered
> the putative benefits with a somewhat jaundiced eye. During my residency training
> I had read extensively on the relatively recent diethylstilbestrol (DES) estrogen
> therapy fiasco, the resultant birth abnormalities, the reproductive dysfunction and
> the cancerous sequelae. In an environment of mounting pressure to recommend
> widespread use of long-term HRT as preventive therapy for healthy women, I
> reviewed the available information and research. I was astonished to find that
> within a medical paradigm that emphasizes evidence-based medicine, there was
> a remarkable paucity of scientific evidence for long-term preventive HRT as the
> standard-of-care for postmenopausal women. Moreover, I did not understand how
> HRT had catapulted to become the leading drug sold in America.[57]

Frankly, neither can we.

In the next chapters, we examine cardiovascular disease, osteoporosis, and
breast cancer and their putative connection to hormones. We explain how an
entirely new medical focus developed toward the end of the twentieth century with

respect to risk and disease prevention. Much like the estrogen and menopause-is-a-deficiency-disease argument, this new medical focus was based not on science or anything even remotely resembling critical, objective thought but was the result of the peculiar blend of commercial, economic, social, entertainment, historical, linguistic, and other factors American culture exported to the world, along with cars and soap powder.

5

HEARTS AND MINDS

Over the past half-century, a growing belief among women and their physicians held that "replacing" the estrogen lost at menopause would prevent many of the manifestations of aging, including coronary heart disease (CHD), osteoporotic fractures, and a decline in cognitive and sexual function. This attractive and plausible *[italics added] view led to widespread use of hormone therapy after menopause in the era before randomized trials with disease end points were required for proving the effects of new drugs.*
—*Editorial,* JAMA[1]

Robert Wilson's 1966 tract delineating the estrogen-deficiency paradigm of menopause and perimenopause, *Feminine Forever,* had a stunning impact—one that must have shocked even the marketing executives at Ayerst who had supported it. Never in their wildest dreams could they have imagined that within a few years everyone would have jumped on their bandwagon, from best-selling pop culture books to women's magazines and medical schools. "HRT was foisted on the postmenopausal woman under the widely advertised banner of prolonging youthfulness," writes professor of medicine Nortin Hadler scornfully in *The Last Well Person.* "The medicalization of menopause was a goldmine both for gynecologists and for the pharmaceutical firms that manufacture and market estrogen-containing compounds."[2] No matter that proof was less than sparse and entirely based on vague assumptions and observations (gleaned from data from well-off, middle-class white women) that could not and did not indicate causality; estrogen had become the elixir of youth, the magic bullet, the drug that could give women back their health, vigor, smooth skin, and anything else age might take away.

Unfortunately, within a few years, and despite Wilson's assurances (based on nothing but his own conviction and a highly suspect sample of one hundred women from his own practice), came a "fateful bump on the road," as the *JAMA* editorial cited at the start of this chapter put it. Unopposed estrogen treatment caused the endometrium to thicken and become hyperplasic and precancerous—often resulting in endometrial cancer.[3] This makes perfect sense, for as the alert reader has already realized, it is the bath of *progesterone* occurring after ovulation that transforms the thickened endometrial lining: the rapid overgrowth of cells that high levels of estrogen have caused in the days leading up to ovulation in a natural menstrual cycle. Without that important second hormone, progesterone, whose job it is to stop cell growth and promote cell maturation, the scene is set for a potentially pathological situation. This is neither cutting-edge endocrinology nor all that difficult to understand.

Progesterone, originally called the corpus luteum hormone, had been identified in the sixteenth century, and as early as the 1920s the basics of the menstrual cycle were reasonably well understood, even by the drug companies.* In a three-volume set published by the German pharmaceutical firm Schering in 1941, for instance (one small book for each hormone: estrogen, progesterone, and testosterone), the anonymous author describes progesterone first and foremost as the hormone primarily responsible for a safe pregnancy (so much for the DES-estrogen theory of preventing miscarriage), but also explains that it is the hormone important for "chemical equilibria (balance), uterine motility, control of the menstrual cycle, and various systems and organs." Of course, Schering also had a vested interest in that it had developed a synthetic progesterone product, Pranone, which it was promoting—still, this slight volume neatly describes progesterone's role, mid-cycle, after estrogen has built up the endometrium to "up to ten times its original thickness."[4] But somehow, any appreciation that progesterone might also have a part to play in the balance of hormones did not appear to have made it across the Atlantic (perhaps due to World War II and its aftermath—who knows).

In any event, and Schering notwithstanding, throughout the 1960s and 1970s, especially in the United States, the tune was estrogen, and Wilson's unopposed estrogen anthem was the one blaring, the only one anyone wanted to hear. (Wilson does, briefly, mention progesterone in his book, but only as the pregnancy hormone and as an adjunct therapy to be used for younger women whose "femininity" was underdeveloped, which is probably one of the only reasonable physiologic points he makes.) The belief persisted that it was estrogen that was the real deal, *the* female hormone, the seat of all "feminine attraction and wellbeing,"

---

*This "yellow body" (which is what *corpus luteum* means) was named by an Italian, Malpighi, in 1686, although it had been observed in the ovaries of mammals in 1573.

not to mention the reason women would feel optimistic, joyful, and happy, since, according to Wilson, everyone who was anyone realized that emotional states were the sole and direct result of "our blood chemistry"[5]—estrogen, in other words.

By the early 1980s, however, it had become embarrassingly obvious, at least clinically, that unopposed estrogen was no panacea and was causing an unprecedented rise in the incidence of endometrial hyperplasia and cancer in those women who had not had a hysterectomy. The effect of not adding some form of progesterone to the hormone regimen was clearly negative.[6] The *JAMA* editorial writers (in 2004, cited at the start of this chapter) nevertheless took comfort in knowing that the endometrial cancers that were found in women on estrogen therapy were "uncommon and usually curable."[7] The later PEPI randomized, double-blind, placebo-controlled trial found that 12 percent of women on estrogen alone had atypical endometrial hyperplasia versus none in the estrogen plus progestin or placebo groups.[8] Although easily treatable with hysterectomy, it seems doubtful that the women so afflicted with endometrial cancer—when they had merely listened to medical advice—were quite so sanguine. But the good news was that "antagonizing the estrogen with a progestin" appeared to solve the problem, and as a result, various attempts were made to figure out the optimal (and minimal) dose of progesterone (or its synthetic cousin, progestin), one that "preserved the benefits of estrogen."[9] By the late 1980s, various estrogen-progestin preparations had been introduced,[10] and the standard regimen for "HRT" became a mix of equine estrogen (Premarin) and medroxyprogesterone acetate (MPA, or Provera) in a dose relationship that emphasized estrogen and restricted progestin.* Prescriptions for estrogen, which had begun to level off, picked up again.

IMPROVING QUALITY OF LIFE . . . OR NOT

If hormones were the primary determinant of women's health and vitality, then it stood to reason that replacing them at a time when natural levels decreased would make women feel good. But no matter how hard gynecologists pushed "HRT" as a life enhancer and a pill that would make you feel good and keep you young, *adherence* (an odious term used to describe individuals who do not comply with medical advice) to hormone regimens was low. As we touched on in an earlier chapter, predictably, once women had passed through the storm of perimenopause and into the calm of menopause, if they had no (or mild) hot flushes, they no longer felt they needed to take anything. Women simply did not

---

*The standard dose was often 0.625 mg Premarin and 2.5 mg progestin daily, thus representing an approximate 100 percent relative dose of estrogen and a 25 percent relative dose of progestin compared with the normal menstrual cycle.

like taking estrogen, with or without progestin. No matter how much the socio-cultural and medical landscape—the advertisements, the women's magazines, the books, and the gynecologists—insisted that estrogen and femininity (with that reluctant smidgeon of progestin to prevent endometrial cancer) were inextricably linked; no matter how much Wilson and other gynecologists pushed "ERT" and then "HRT"; no matter how many clever advertisements showed happy older women invigorated by hormones, the vast majority of women simply did not agree. As Hadler dryly writes, "the quality-of-life myth" simply proved to be "un-supportable" and attempts to connect being "menopausal" with reduced quality of life simply did not fly.

When British epidemiologists Gita Mishra and Diana Kuh reviewed prospec-tive data from 1,525 British women who had been surveyed annually since birth (1946)* regarding "quality-of-life domains" ("quallies," as they are sometimes called), they found that it was not hormone levels but stress that most affected midlife women's quality of life. In fact, women's experiences around the so-called menopausal transition, although occasionally complicated, were essentially positive.[11] A more recent British trial similarly found that contrary to the re-searchers' expectations, "HRT" only improved *three* out of the nine components of quality of life they compared to placebo—hardly a ringing endorsement.[12] In fact, evidence showed that women who took hormones had "larger declines in physical function" and were more generally fatigued than women who took the placebo.[13] So much for estrogen making women feel good in the real world.

Postmenopausal hormone therapy rates simply were not living up to their promise, or, at least, the promise drug companies and gynecologists deeply felt they should have. Discontinuation rates of hormone therapy in the first years of use were astronomically high.[14] Once any onerous menopausal (i.e., either peri-menopausal or truly menopausal) symptoms resolved—at least in those women who *had* onerous symptoms, bearing in mind that the majority of women do not—women stopped refilling their prescriptions. It seemed that neither of the estrogen/progestin regimens in vogue at the time, whether continuous or sequen-tial, were all that popular, although women disliked sequential therapy (adding progestin to the Premarin for twelve days a month) more, largely because it caused period-like flow.[15] Taking hormones continuously, however, meant irregular and unpredictable bleeding; plus many women also complained of feeling bloated, irritable, anxious, and nervous. (Those of us who experienced difficulties with perimenopause, a time when estrogen levels are high, relate to this and mar-vel that these women managed to take *any* extra estrogen.) Presumably, time, and the placebo effect being what it is, some women who took hormones did

---

*These were data from the Medical Research Council (MRC) National Survey of Health and Develop-ment, also known as the 1946 British Birth Cohort, a longitudinal study of health in England, Scotland, and Wales.

feel better for a while, albeit usually not for long, and even though the majority of women (then, as now) do not see a doctor at midlife, the discourse on perimenopause and menopause remained firmly fixed within the prevailing medical paradigm.

LIFE IN THE DISEASE LANE

The medical model, which had its roots in the early parts of the twentieth century and remains prevalent today, assumes that any symptoms or illness are secondary to *disease*. Hence, by definition, midlife symptoms of any kind had to be related to that famous estrogen-deficiency disease. As an article in the *British Medical Journal* explains,

> The biomedical model of illness, which has dominated health care for the past century [makes] three assumptions: all illness has a single underlying cause; disease (pathology) is always the single cause; and removal or attenuation of the disease will result in a return to health. The model of illness adopted by society can have important consequences. In the first world war, for example, soldiers complaining of symptoms after experiencing severe stresses were sometimes shot as malingerers, but today they are considered victims and eligible for financial settlements. Social acceptance that a behaviour or reported symptom constitutes an illness bestows privileges on an individual and formal duties on society.[16]

Not to mention that such recognition confers status on and power to the medical profession and profits for the pharmaceutical companies.

The medical model also assumes a causal relationship between symptoms and pathology, which turns the patient into a victim of circumstance and the *passive* recipient of treatment—with the assumption being that that person will, of course, cooperate with treatment. Menopause (and perimenopause, although not yet a word), having been defined as an estrogen-deficiency disease, therefore, simply became another focus for medical management. Women's own experiences, perceptions, and feelings about this life transition were of no real concern: menopause was conceptualized as a medical problem even as the data collected were, as in other diseases, primarily quantitative and expressed numerically, with pain or vasomotor symptoms or anything else being reduced to a series of numbers that could subsequently be crunched (or "tortured," as critics suggest).*

The overwhelming implication was that midlife was somehow related to poor health, however little sense it makes to turn a natural transition that occurs in every woman's life into a kind of pathology or a disease. Research findings, being largely based on women who *were* having problems (probably with *peri*menopause, and

---

*This model further assumes that symptoms are universal, yet culture determines how we phrase, perceive, or otherwise pay attention to our bodies.

not menopause, as it was continuously and erroneously called), and who had actively sought out medical treatment (and often received a hysterectomy), provided further impetus for this "poor health" label. Feminist thinkers and others critiqued this dominant medical construction that defined menopause as a pathology as not only wrong, but one that reproduced representations of women as biologically weak[17] and reinforced the sociocultural emphasis on youth and beauty. But much as genetic descriptions point our attention to determinism and essentially imply that biology is destiny, pushing menopause into the domain of medical science continues to identify hormones as the determinants of women's physiological and psychological wellbeing.[18] The bulk of the research on women at midlife, furthermore, had been gleaned from *surgical* menopause—and the women most likely to demand help from physicians (especially from gynecologists) are women who have had a hysterectomy and thus are doubly likely to be suffering a highly symptomatic perimenopause, versus the majority of women who go through a natural menopause and do not seek medical help.

Focus stayed firmly fixed at the level of the pharmacologic and surgical; hormones (well, estrogen) remained center stage, and, because "women's health issues that did not concern reproduction received little attention and little research funding prior to 1986," as a cardiologist writing in the *Archives of Internal Medicine* admitted, modern medicine continued to regard hormones and fertility as central to women's health.[19]

Nevertheless, for years, epidemiologists and gynecologists kept picking away at the associations between "HRT" and clinical outcomes.[20] Unwilling to concede that "HRT" might only be a reasonable solution for *symptomatic* women at midlife as short-term relief for perimenopausal problems (or the menopause transition, as it was called), gynecologists and marketers turned their attention to the other claims Wilson had made for estrogen twenty years before. Maybe hormones really could prevent the ills of aging and reduce the risk of heart disease, osteoporosis, dementia, and cancer, because women were certainly not flocking to take hormones and did not seem to agree that "HRT" improved quality of life.

Fortuitously, heart disease came to the rescue.

TAKING HORMONES TO THE NEXT LEVEL

"Cardiovascular disease is the leading cause of death in the United States, accounting for approximately one half million deaths in women annually," trumpets cardiologist Lori Mosca in the *Archives of Internal Medicine*.[21] Heart disease is "responsible for a third of all deaths of women worldwide and half of all deaths of women over 50 years of age," adds a review of cardiovascular disease.[22] Heart disease, in other words, is dangerous, a scourge, a huge problem. So, when there was a suggestion that taking estrogen could reduce cardiovascular risk by more than one third, it generated enormous excitement. Finally, a good reason to recommend hormones, whether or not women were experiencing troublesome midlife symptoms. Unfortunately, the proof—as with most of the pro-hormone advice—was less than compelling, totally based on observational studies (where people are asked to report on what they did, versus the researcher following and checking their changes into the future), and strongly contaminated by what is known as the *healthy user* bias.

It has long been known that the people who enter studies or clinical trials, of any kind, are not like the rest of us. They tend to be better educated, younger (the cutoff for entry into clinical trials is usually sixty or sixty-four, at the oldest), healthier (no comorbidities), and smarter (better educated, anyway)—heck, they are probably taller and more attractive as well. Until recently, they were all also men, making it impossible to extrapolate study results to women. Selection bias of one sort or another is unavoidable in any clinical trial. Plus, because we rely on the people who enroll in clinical trials giving their (informed) consent, they are, by definition, a "self-selected sample of those eligible to participate."[23] What we glean from examining their lives, the drugs they take, and so on, therefore, may be, and often is, limited. Unfortunately, that rarely stops anyone from drawing broad conclusions, particularly those that bolster their own pet theories. The external validity of a trial, or its ability to be extrapolated outward to the population at large, is often less than compelling. But for those segments of the medical establishment who were, as Harvard physician Jerome Groopman calls them, "believers" in the essential goodness of hormones, even the hint of proof was all they needed. As for the general populace, as Groopman sadly writes, "Many readers do not go beyond an article's headline or its opening paragraph."[24] So when word on the street was that estrogen, initially, and later hormone therapy, was a boon for women's hearts, cardiologists and gynecologists delightedly took it up clinically. By the mid-1990s, the American Heart Association, the American College of Physicians, and the American College of Obstetricians and Gynecologists were all in agreement: "The beneficial effects of H.R.T. were sufficiently well established that it could be recommended to older women as a means of warding off heart disease and osteoporosis."[25]

This idea of taking something to ward off future disease—being at risk—is a peculiar one, one that "encourages both doctors and women to view their current health status in terms of their risk of future ill health," rather than the here and now.[26] A very Western, perhaps American, future-oriented perspective, it is one that ever-so-nicely blames us for what we are, or do, today for what might happen tomorrow—and is the direct result of a major shift in research and clinical focus that occurred after World War II, when *risk factors* became the fashionable term of the day.

THE MONSTER UNDER THE BED

Today, we are so accustomed to the notion of risk factors (and the idea that we can be at risk of disease without even realizing it) that we forget, or just don't know, how recent this thinking is. We take for granted the notion that prevention works, that "catching" a problem early translates into a better prognosis, that we should pay close attention to such things and be "proactive" in health just as we are in taking care of our cars and houses. Such advice, notably on how to avoid coronary artery disease (CAD), is pervasive, the warnings, absolute and authoritative: check your blood pressure because it is, after all, the "silent" killer (one is tempted to ask what the murder weapon is), cholesterol levels (it is essential to have enough of the good kind, not so much of the bad) and glucose (type 2 diabetes, we are warned, is a looming and a major risk for heart disease). Naturally, our weight and fitness level should also concern us, and smoking. In short, it could well be a full-time job, all this checking and testing and scanning and worrying. But the risk factor slant on health is not up for debate, it is simply the way things are, or so we are told. And if our numbers (blood pressure, lipids) are wrong and do not conform to the ideal? Prophylactic (preventive) measures are in order, probably medication. The underlying message is "be afraid; be very afraid."

No wonder, then, that the term is *at risk* and that sense of dangers lurking is always present, from the vaguely threatening tone in the magazine articles to the glib asides in television shows or on Web pages. Yet, as physician Robert Arnowitz reminds us, "Until the 1960's neither lay nor medical people used the term 'risk factor.'"[27] This "set of unquestioned and often unstated assumptions" shared by policymakers, researchers, clinicians, and practically everybody else about how individual factors contribute to disease is so fundamental that risk factors are easily considered as worthy of study and therapeutic action as heart health itself. In other words, research and attention to risk factors supersede basic research into the heart itself, a perspective that simply did not exist prior to the 1950s. For that matter, neither did cardiology as a medical specialty.[28]

Prior to the late 1950s, most clinicians and researchers believed that CAD was a "chronic, degenerative disease, a particular way of aging that did not lend itself to specific, preventive measures."[29] Perhaps it was the Allied victory over Germany and Japan, but somehow the idea that we cannot alter the course of disease began to seem defeatist: surely disease could be vanquished, just like any other enemy? Those military metaphors of which we are so fond, where we fight germs and declare war on cancer, not only permeate the language but affect how we conceptualize medical intervention: the more aggressively we engage in these preventive measures, the better off we are. So why take drugs when you can have quadruple bypass surgery to prevent future heart attacks—as Bill Clinton and David Letterman did? Cardiovascular disease is the enemy, but we shall overcome.

Even the gene for CAD is under consideration. The subtext is that cardiac disease can be broken down into its component parts, with the whole being a simple, mechanistic sum of the pieces. Unfortunately, as our failure to make inroads in curing autoimmune diseases, cancer, and a host of other complex and disabling diseases demonstrates, this model has not been an unqualified success. On the contrary, there is an extensive history of studies with end points using quite plausible surrogate markers, such as cholesterol, for example, rather than heart attacks, but giving the wrong answer.[30] For instance, agents that suppressed ventricular arrhythmias (a kind of irregular heartbeat that is associated with an increased risk of heart attack) were assumed to prevent adverse cardiac events; yet the very opposite was found: suppressing arrhythmias *increased* mortality, an unexpected finding that probably led to the deaths of tens of thousands.[31]*

Yet as with so much else—such as estrogen being the only female hormone worth bothering about—these ideas are deeply rooted in cultural (and medical) ideology and societal norms. For instance, cross-cultural studies demonstrate that Americans undergo nearly double the number of cardiac surgeries compared to other countries in the West, yet outcomes are no better.[32] Aggressive treatment is the cornerstone of American medicine, from birth—which is more likely to be by Caesarian delivery than anywhere else in the world—to death, and as the late medical writer Lynn Payer explained in her popular and often-quoted book *Medicine and Culture*,

> American doctors want to *do* something. . . . [They] perform more diagnostic tests than doctors in France, West Germany, or England. They often eschew drug treatment in favor of more aggressive surgery, but if they do use drugs they are likely to use higher doses and more aggressive drugs. While official recommendations as to dose are often higher than those given in other countries, even when official recommendations drop many doctors continue to believe that higher doses are better. Surgery, too, besides being performed more often, is likely to be more aggressive when it is performed. This seems to be particularly true where surgery on or near the sex organs is performed. An American woman has two or three times the chance of having a hysterectomy as her counterpart in England, France, or West Germany, and foreign doctors joke about American "birthday hysterectomies" perhaps without realizing how young the birthday is: over 60 percent of hysterectomies in the United States are performed in women under forty-four.[33]

Probably, these are women experiencing a difficult perimenopause, and they just don't know it. The explanation for this attitude may well lie in America's frontier mentality, which, since its inception, has made it a country of extremes, suggests Payer. America is a country where heroic practice is admired, and disease, illness, and symptoms are not to be borne. Benjamin Rush, one of the signatories of the Declaration of Independence, truly believed that American diseases were

---

*For more on surrogate end points being spectacularly wrong, see Notes.

tougher and meaner than those effete pathologies Europeans suffered, just like Americans. Unfortunately, human bodies, wherever they reside, are fragile, and aggressive drugs and surgeries exert a high physical price, particularly as we get older. It is difficult to predict what, if any, impact taking strong drugs or having all those tests and scans today will have on our health tomorrow. It is therefore important to remember that this risk factor perspective is simply a hypothesis, an idea, with respect to the etiology (cause) of cardiac disease and not to become overinvested in this medicalization of life, particularly when we are well.

POSTWAR TECHNOLOGIES AND THE THRILL OF THE NEW

It was the "therapeutic explosion" following World War II that did away with any notion that medicine, that doctors, would remain mere "passive observers" of disease, writes physician William Silverman in his charming book of essays *Where's the Evidence? Debates in Modern Medicine.* The end of the war ushered in unprecedented changes, with the United States becoming a dominant world power, locked in a Cold War power struggle with the Soviet Union. In part as a result of this competition, massive changes were forged in science, research, and technology, which altered everything from agriculture (pesticides), aviation (commercial air and space travel), chemistry (plastics), and communications (radio, TV, telex) to everyday life (cars, suburbs) and, of course, medicine. The pace of change accelerated dramatically.

War has always been an excellent stimulus for medicine—the Napoleonic Wars improved surgery, notably amputation techniques, and led to the development of ambulances and the concept of triage (treating the sickest first). Anesthesia came into more common use with the American Civil War, which also created the first documentation on epidemiology and patient care, while the brutal wounds of World War I led to improvements in plastic surgery, burn techniques, and blood transfusions. It also was the first time that the psychological impact of war was noted, with the tremendous battle fatigue and posttraumatic stress experienced by soldiers of trench warfare.[34] World War II, of course, led to the widespread use of antibiotics. Even the Trojan War in ancient times had led to medical advances, mainly in analgesia (pain relief). But the twentieth century saw such extraordinary changes that it seemed for a time as though technology could solve *everything*. So prevalent was faith in technology's potential benefits, whether machines or processes (scientific, bureaucratic, medical, social), that by the 1990s, patients were being hurled down treatment trajectories that would have been unthinkable even a few decades earlier.[35] Ironically, the RCT now held up as *the* ultimate proof of truth in medicine was itself one of those promising postwar technologies, epitomizing the use of logic, mathematical algorithms, and progress.

The first drug to be systematically tested with an RCT was an antibiotic, streptomycin. Alexander Fleming had discovered the penicillin mold growing in a petri dish in 1938, but it was not until nearly a decade later that the compound was synthesized in a nontoxic form. (Gypsy women in eastern Europe had long used rotting cabbage leaves to dress wounds, but that was conveniently forgotten.) Supplies of these new drugs were scarce, which was why A. Bradford Hill, the first medical statistician on record (he had wanted to be a physician but poor health had prevented it), managed to convince Britain's Medical Research Council to agree to a "rigorously planned clinical investigation with concurrent controls"[36] to treat pulmonary tuberculosis and pave the way for a "scientific" medicine. And thus, in 1948, the RCT was born.

At heart, the RCT is blindingly simple: we assign patients to two groups, at random; we give one, the experimental group, the drug or therapy we are testing, and the second group gets nothing, or rather, a placebo, to see if our therapeutic intervention does what we want. The RCT is extraordinarily—and particularly—effective at demonstrating what interventions do *not* work.

In the case of streptomycin, the clinical trial did indeed prove the drug effective for tuberculosis: there were four deaths out of fifty-five patients in the drug group, versus fourteen deaths among the fifty-two patients treated with bed rest alone.* Interestingly, thirteen patients did get better on bed rest, suggesting that perhaps physiology and pathology were somewhat more complicated than laboratory chemistry.[37] Medical historian Marcia Meldrum writes,

> The RCT takes an essentially social problem—how do we treat disease—with complex epistemological aspects—what is disease? what is effective treatment? how do we know?—and structures it as a mathematical problem of probabilities to deal with the multiple unknown variables and the issue of subjectivity.[38]

By controlling for as many variables as we can (age, weight, diet, other medications), we keep the two groups as similar as possible. Then, all else being equal, any difference between the two groups over time can be attributed to the drug.

The time was right, and soon the RCT became the epitome of medical evidence, the gold standard, standing head and shoulders above observational studies, anecdotes or case studies, meta-analyses of observational studies, reviews, or anything else.† Various agencies, such as the FDA, began requiring clinical trials as proof of efficacy to approve drugs, and *evidence-based medicine* was on its way (although that, too, did not become a recognized term for a few more decades).

The discovery of antibiotics, the first drug to actually *do* something, had given medicine a huge lift, not just therapeutically and clinically, but in terms of prestige.

---

*Soon, the RCT evolved and became placebo-controlled (where, rather than the drug, an inert substance was given to patients) and blinded (where neither researcher nor subject knows who is given what).

†Meta-analyses of RCTs are now sometimes edging out the single RCT as a gold standard.

Then, with the RCT, came the cachet of having a scientific method. Medical institutions, such as the FDA, gained legitimacy and stature. When a handful of fledgling charity-type organizations joined under the funding banner of the National Institutes of Health (NIH), medical research became more streamlined and, ostensibly, more efficient—and soon, research and epidemiologic attention turned to finding different problems to solve, new frontiers to conquer, and unidentified diseases to describe (and cure). Scientific interest in the immune system and endocrinology, which had been at the center of medical efforts in earlier parts of the twentieth century, fell into disfavor; disease became of greater interest than physiology and its workings and soon it became the major subject of inquiry. The technological advances in medicine after World War II led to an "entrenched educational and research focus on the paradigm of 'curing' rather than 'caring,'"[39] which had been medicine's central tenet for centuries. In other words, focus moved *away* from the person and onto the disease.

FROM A MODEST PROPOSAL TO FRAMING RISK FACTORS

The belief that estrogen could prevent coronary artery disease (CAD), therefore, was not only seductive, but part and parcel of a major paradigm shift that had begun midcentury: an entirely new way of thinking about health and disease. Originally, hormones had been touted as replacements for those the body was unable to make, much as insulin replaced the failing pancreatic islets of diabetics or the estrogen supposedly made deficient by menopause. But now, attention (not to mention the marketing efforts of the drug companies) turned toward grander objectives and deadlier disease modalities. A whole new world of possibilities opened up, not least because of a longitudinal, population-based study begun in Framingham, Massachusetts, around the same time as the first clinical trial.

Initially conceived as a modest effort to test new cardiac diagnostic methods, such as the electrocardiogram, and perhaps discover what, if any, predisposing factors cardiovascular disease might have, this major epidemiological study in 1948 was a blend of efforts (and funding) between the Massachusetts Department of Health, the U.S. Public Health Service, and Harvard's Department of Preventive Medicine. The incidence of cardiac disease (and heart attacks) had been steadily increasing since World War I and had been largely attributed, during the first half of the twentieth century, to the hurly-burly and stress of modern life. But now the cardiology establishment was keen to understand how and why CAD developed. Plus, the advisory board of the newly established National Heart Institute needed a focus for fundraising (not to mention a catchy study that could provide them with suitable gravitas), and public health officials were looking for something new to focus on, because vaccines and antibiotics had largely done away with major public health problems such as epidemics of smallpox, polio, and tuberculosis. So researchers enrolled more than five thousand Framingham residents, free of CAD, to trace the course of heart disease in a study that continues to the present. Methodically following the Framingham residents, examining them, and interviewing them in person every two years would, over time, provide that new way of approaching disease that medical institutions were seeking.[40]

The first use of the term *risk factor* was coined in a 1961 report by the Framingham investigators, which means that the concept literally grew out of this one small town outside Boston and researchers' analysis of the associations they happened to notice and thought might be important. By the 1960s, however, screening for multiple risk factors had become the norm. A number of concurrent studies took up this approach, and within a few short years, CAD went from being a poorly understood, individual condition to one that was said to result from a handful of risks we could control. Where there had only been one or two (not terribly effective) drugs to lower blood pressure, drug companies, who had done very well from the war, raced to introduce newer and better ones. Their research and development grew, as did marketing and advertising budgets. By the 1980s, the face of medicine had altered so completely that not many people even remembered that the term *risk factor* had merely been a linguistic shortcut used in a report. (And, in all fairness to the Framingham researchers, they really had not intended their findings to be used in this reductionist fashion; on the contrary, their approach was broadly holistic.)

Research and therapeutic attention, which had once focused on the person, the patient, and his or her life and circumstances, shifted to biomarkers and surrogate end points, which were believed to predict the course of disease and lie on the causal pathway—never mind that nobody understood how disease evolved or why some people became sick and others did not. In fact, Framingham Study investigators themselves later found it difficult to explain the decline in cardiac disease mortality (from 1950 on throughout the West) via reduced risk factors.[41] Nevertheless, tests, scans, and so-called objective results soon began to trump individual perceptions because a person could be *at risk* and feel perfectly fine— just as what the person felt could be discounted through those same objective tests. For instance, a woman might feel a tightness in her chest and pain on the left side and be convinced that she was having a heart attack, but if, on admission to the emergency room, her heart was shown not to conform to previously agreed-on definitions of what constituted cardiac pathology (e.g., abnormal cardiogram or cardiac enzymes), well, she was out of luck. She would be sent on her way and told she had gas or that it was all in her head, a particularly devastating label that not only implied malingering and hypochondria but also suggested that a person's own subjective sense of ill health simply did not matter.

The term *psychosomatic* grew to have an ugly ring—yet all it means is that the source of the pain or the symptoms is not something that can be traced (with the existing technology) to a physical cause. So the source of the pain is the mind, the psyche (*soma* meaning "body" in Greek). But pain is pain, no matter what the source, and you can feel just as much pain whether the cause is your body or your mind. Such nuanced considerations, however, no longer are central to medicine.

HORMONES AND CARDIAC DISEASE

Ironically, the Framingham Study, which brought risk factors and the at-risk notion to the forefront of American medicine, did *not* find that estrogen prevented heart disease in older women, but the idea had already taken hold. Plus, in the early 1950s, a handful of animal studies mentioned in the journal *Circulation* had found a connection between a form of estrogen (estradiol benzoate) and a vague reduction in atherosclerotic lesions in the coronary arteries of "cholesterol-fed" chicks (your guess is as good as ours as to what that feed was). A handful of studies with rabbits had also found a connection between estrogen and lipids.[42] At the time, nobody really knew what to make of these results, but with the development of the risk factor argument (and the conviction, still prevalent today, that heart disease was a "man's disease" until a woman hits menopause), the consensus grew that what protected women had to be estrogen. Roughly a decade after menopause, a women's risk of cardiac disease, it was said, reached or even exceeded that of men (even though women's risk for CAD *never* equals that of men)—so what else could it be?

As an article in the journal *Cardiovascular Research*, which reviewed the cardiac evidence as recently as the early 2000s, adamantly wrote,

> There is strong evidence from both human and nonhuman primate studies support-
> ing the conclusion that *estrogen deficiency* [italics added] increases the progression of
> atherosclerosis. . . . [and] estrogen treatment of younger postmenopausal *women or*
> *monkeys* [italics added] in the early stages of atherosclerosis progression has marked
> beneficial effects.[43]

One does not need to be an expert in communications to see the blatant bias and sexism in this small excerpt (even if we ignore the near-comical tone in which the authors equate women and monkeys). The authors go on to add, with some alarm, that this was a public health issue of "major importance" because the average life span of the "rapidly increasing numbers of postmenopausal women" would mean that most women would live "about 35 years beyond *normal ovarian function* [italics added]."[44] Of course, precisely how "normal ovarian function" came to be defined as those thirty-five to forty years of menstruation versus the rest of a woman's natural life remains a mystery, as is how a normal transition in every woman's life can be dysfunctional. But as the reader will have noticed, the history of hormones is littered with contradictory messages, and this one is no exception.

The insistence on estrogen—or hormone "replacement" therapy—being a benefit to the heart received a major boost with the jauntily titled PEPI trial (or the Postmenopausal Estrogen/Progestin Interventions), the study that definitively demonstrated that unopposed estrogen caused endometrial cancer. Here the data hinted that a particular estrogen-progestin regimen might be related to a reduction in lipids (cholesterol levels).* The primary objective of the PEPI trial had been to assess the differences between unopposed estrogen, placebo, and each of three estrogen-progestin or estrogen-progesterone dosages and schedules to determine which one most affected four heart disease risk factors: high-density lipoprotein cholesterol (HDL), systolic blood pressure, or serum insulin and fibrinogen (a protein involved in the blood clotting process).[45] Some 875 healthy, postmenopausal women between the ages of forty-five and sixty-four were randomly assigned to the four groups in a multicenter, three-year study.

None of the hormone regimens differed substantively—all of them showed no change in systolic blood pressure, and postchallenge insulin levels decreased, as did LDL cholesterol. Placebo increased fibrinogen more than any active treatment but in quantities that were meaningless. Mean (average) levels of triglycerides were *increased* in all the estrogen-containing treatment groups. Nevertheless the conclusion drawn was that "estrogen alone or in combination with a progestin improves lipoproteins and lowers fibrinogen levels without detectable effects on insulin or blood pressure."[46]

The belief in the efficacy of estrogen in preventing heart disease was so staunch that some years earlier,[†] five thousand older *men* who had previously had a heart attack were randomized to receive two different regimens of high-dose estrogen (Premarin 5.0 or 2.5 mg) or placebo. The results were disastrous: the 5-mg dose *increased* heart attacks, and both doses led to higher mortality from cancer, pulmonary embolism, and heart attacks. Additionally, the men had terrible side effects: they became impotent and suffered from sore breasts, shrunken testicles, and decreased libido.[47] These spectacularly negative results, however, barely saw the light of day—the excuse was that the estrogen dose just must have been a little high.

Throughout the late 1970s and 1980s, the major impetus for the benefits of estrogen in preventing heart disease was from the Nurses' Health Study Cohort, a questionnaire-based study of 121,700 female, married nurses begun in 1976 at Harvard by epidemiologist Frank Speizer.[48] Speizer wanted to "study the

---

*One suspects that communications people, drug company PR staff, and/or adjunct personnel spend copious hours coming up with cool-sounding acronyms for studies. Those relating to heart disease (where the rewards, in terms of drugs sold, can be prodigious) are particularly cute: here we have PEPI, but also, later, HOPE (Heart Outcome Prevention Trial), CASS (Coronary Artery Surgery Study), HERS (Heart and Estrogen/Progestin Replacement Study), and more.

†Because there is a fairly major time lag between a study being undertaken and its results being published, it is sometimes difficult to create a proper chronology here, but the general timeline is right.

long-term effects of oral contraceptives," and the study was later expanded to include "postmenopausal estrogen therapy because both treatments involved long-term hormone use by millions of women," the consequences of which were totally unknown.[49] Questionnaire-based, longitudinal studies were all the rage at the time, and never more so than when their conclusions reinforced the researchers' own convictions: "More than 30 epidemiological studies have found that postmenopausal women who use estrogen are at lower risk for coronary disease," authoritatively stated *The New England Journal of Medicine* (*NEJM*) when summarizing the Nurse's Health Study data:

> We examined the relation between cardiovascular disease and postmenopausal hormone therapy during up to 16 years of follow-up in 59,337 women from the Nurse's Health Study, who were 30 to 55 years of age at base line. Information on hormone use was ascertained with biennial questionnaires. From 1976 to 1992, we documented 770 cases of myocardial infarction or death from coronary disease in this group and 572 strokes. . . . We observed a marked decrease in the risk of major coronary heart disease among women who took estrogen with progestin, as compared with the risk among women who did not.[50]

Researchers had been casting about for years trying to find something for estrogen to treat, much as those early Dutch researchers in the early 1900s had done,[51] and they had finally found it.

It is where we search and what we look for, however, that determines what we find, and not vice versa, as the respected Dutch epidemiologist Jan Vandenbroucke pointed out in a 1998 lecture to the Royal Society in London (later published in *The Lancet*). In other words, as Vandenbroucke wrote, "We believe or disbelieve the trial results because we believe or disbelieve the theory." Even RCTs show a "willingness to please the people who set them up."[52]

RESULTS SECONDARY TO BELIEF

Hormone researchers naturally already had exquisite faith in their own hypothesis, namely, that taking estrogen translated into a net cardiac benefit. By bringing in lipids and fibrinogen to test (as they tried to figure out how the process might work), they were merely coming up with an explanation that made sense *for the time*, which is the cornerstone of medicine. We come up with reasons to believe the things we believe, explains Vandenbroucke:

> What is the interplay between fact and theory? [Perhaps without theory] completely empirical knowledge could not exist; it would be a collection of facts like a pile of grains of sand, without any structure or purpose. The theory will vary over time. If 50 years ago, you had asked a doctor why he used salicylates [aspirin] for fever, he would have answered, "because it has antipyretic effect," which is saying in Latin

and Greek that it lowers fever, a trick at which medicine is so apt. If you had asked me 25 years ago, when I received my medical training, I would have answered that salicylates reset the body's temperature clock in the hypothalamus. Today, students will tell you about endorphins, prostaglandins, and, especially, cytokines. The theory changes and becomes more and more detailed, which is not important. The important observation is that we need a framework of explanatory stories to order the facts.[53]

It is not stories and narrative that we associate with medicine, however; we consider medical science to be objective, based on genuine knowledge and an understanding of physiology and pathology, disease and health. We *believe* screening technologies to be definitive (no matter what the error or false positive rates) and predictive of disease; we *believe* medical advice and medical science to be essentially trustworthy. Most important, we believe that it is better to do something than simply sit back and wait. After all, why else would all those magazines, television shows, and Web sites so confidently tell us to have our colons checked or have our mammograms and eat more of this or that type of food (antioxidants, fiber) to achieve optimal health? Why else would all those nice people be running marathons and doing all those amazing things to raise money for hospitals and cancer research? Do we *not* understand the basics of health—how the heart functions, for instance, or how various and sundry diseases and conditions evolve? Well, the short answer is, no. We do not.

Unfortunately for the women being prescribed hormones to protect their hearts, what was glossed over in the euphoria over the lipid reduction was the *increase* in triglycerides and blood clots. After all, what is a coronary artery thrombus but a clot in the heart's blood supply? (Never mind that the cholesterol-cardiac connection remains unproven, particularly as primary prevention.[54]) But, as with all things hormone related, none of it seemed to matter, any more than the earlier Framingham data, which had found that noncontraceptive use of estrogen increased the risk of CAD,[55] or that estrogen increased breast cancer. The pro-estrogen epidemiologists and researchers deplored this breast cancer "bias" as they pushed hormones as a means of lowering CAD. Here they were, smart academics and statisticians, explaining risk to us—and we, the lay public (sometimes supported by our primary care physicians), simply ignored them because we were scared of breast cancer.

Two such pro-estrogen researchers, the late epidemiologist Trudy Bush and physician Elizabeth Barrett-Conner (who has considerably softened her stance on hormones since then), were involved in the Lipid Research Clinics Program Follow-up Study, funded by the National Heart, Lung, and Blood Institute (for some reason, this study didn't get a cute name), that also had found an inverse association between estrogen and cardiovascular disease, at least in a group of 2,270 white women between the ages of forty and sixty-nine. The women were sent questionnaires for some eight and a half years.[56] The researchers did concede that "estrogen users* were better educated and thinner" (both known to reduce illness risk); nevertheless, their conclusion was that estrogen was cardioprotective, even if the women smoked and had high cholesterol. Later, Bush gushed that the benefits of estrogen affirmed "the old concept of feminine forever."[57] Given the tenuous level of the association and complete lack of causal evidence, the researchers did reluctantly concede that "some factor, as yet unidentified, is associated with both estrogen use and cardiovascular death" given the magnitude of difference: twenty-two deaths from ischemic heart disease (as per what was reported on the death certificate) in the nonusers of estrogen versus two in the estrogen users. In total, the contrast was striking—forty-four deaths versus six— but no ages or cause of death determinations were provided, so we have no idea if what was recorded on the death certificates bore any resemblance to the real cause of death.

DEATH FROM ILLOGIC

Here we come to an important point and one that tends to be ignored in both lay and medical writing: the accuracy of those "cause of death" labels. Often, the official cause of death is not the actual cause (if that can even be determined), and in the absence of an autopsy, never confirmed. Today, cardiac disease is often the de facto cause of death, the ubiquity and lethality of heart disease being so central to us culturally and medically. But, as communications professors Susan Leigh Star and Geoffrey Bowker write in their comprehensive book *Sorting Things Out: Classification and Its Consequences*, there has been a "secular change in the form that death takes." In 1900, the "overriding causes of death were the great epidemic diseases: tuberculosis, pneumonia, smallpox and influenza." Today, with antibiotics and ameliorated socioeconomic conditions, in the West at least, people tend to live longer and "break down more slowly." It is therefore difficult to "boil down a complex series of conditions to a single cause of death." Interpretation and opinion begins with the form itself—from the restrictions it imposes, for example, the insistence on a *single* cause of death when often death results from a "complex of diseases." What wins out is often more closely allied to the sociocultural landscape and what is deemed important than any so-called objective cause.[58] Additionally, there are major cultural differences in assigning cause of death—even in the West. One WHO study found that even when shown identical information from the same death certificates,

---

*The data were gathered between 1972 and 1976, when it was still not realized that unopposed estrogen could lead to endometrial cancer.

doctors in different countries came to different conclusions on cause of death.[59]

All descriptions or classifications of disease (of therapy, of death) make implicit theoretical and social assumptions, often specific to time and place, and as readers of history can attest, the future can be a harsh critic. We mock earlier generations, just as later ones will mock us. Not so long ago, most people died at home, of natural causes, unlike today, when the vast majority of us live in cities and die in hospitals. Even if we die at home, the cause of death is rarely listed as old age. Like birth, death is also filed, listed, and put away, and more often than not, the cause, when unknown, is listed as "cardiac." But as Hadler writes, not without irony, we all have to die of *something*:

> Terms such as myocardial infarction or heart attack, stroke or cerebral vascular accident, and atherosclerosis or hardening of the arteries are the darlings of the lay medical press. Pharmaceutical and hospital marketing budgets conspire to hang coronary artery disease like a curse, an imprecation, over North America. Pills, diets, and all manner of regimens are purveyed to ensure that blood continues to flow through the coronary arteries to keep the heart attack at bay. Failing all that, there's a technological solution—modern cardiovascular surgery and interventional cardiology (in which estrogen played its part for many years). The practitioners of these crafts are heroes . . . saving us from the scourge of our time. . . . [But] coronary artery disease is no scourge.[60]

Today, our risk of heart disease has actually decreased; our chance of dying of a heart attack at age sixty is about half that of our parents' risk, our survival rate after a heart attack is higher even without doing anything at all, but by taking a diuretic (an old, cheap drug) daily, we reduce even that risk considerably. The incidence of heart disease deaths, furthermore, has steadily declined over the last half-century. Suddenly the picture is not so gloomy—particularly when we look at the statistics and realize that heart disease went into decline long before we instigated the risk factor argument or had any major drugs or surgeries to deal with it. A controversial theory even suggests that cardiovascular disease is following a path much like that of an infectious disease because, when graphed, CAD incidence is moving from west to east. And the decline began long before there were drugs, surgeries, or prevention strategies of any kind in place.[61]

At the start of the twentieth century, angina was simply a form of chronic chest pain that some people had, one that often appeared to resolve on its own. (In fact, angina is simply exertion- or exercise-induced pain in the chest due to inadequate blood flow to a portion of the heart muscle.) But there was little point in considering angina pectoris anything other than a subjective symptom of chest pain at a time when there were no tests or scans to identify it, no underlying hypotheses to define it, no organization like the American Heart Association to publicize it, and no drugs to treat it. Once these emerged, however, it became possible to create objective boundaries (occluded arteries, plaque disease), come up with a label and disease classification, and shade in the borders. To what extent these will stand the test of time is simply not clear at this stage, but during the 1980s focus increasingly shifted toward disease prevention and away from the earlier approach of dealing with clinical phenomena (such as a urinary tract infection or a sore throat) and symptoms (how the person *felt*, in other words): what the late Yale physician Alvan Feinstein disapprovingly referred to as disease management. This meant that treatment was said to lie along a critical pathway that is assumed to lead to disease. So, because high blood pressure and cholesterol have been deemed part of the pathway toward cardiac health (by guideline writers, consensus conferences, and other group-think activities), treating and researching blood pressure or cholesterol takes precedence over the broader picture of the person's health, cardiac or otherwise.[62]

THE MYTH OF MENOPAUSE AND CARDIAC DISEASE

Women have long been said to have a ten-year window of freedom from cardiac disease: "Researchers have determined that women develop CAD approximately 10 years later than men," report cardiologists, around age sixty in other words. The reason was assumed to be "significant levels of circulating estrogens."[63] Given that women's estrogen levels fall at menopause, around age fifty, why this protection operates on a ten-year lag was never clear. The explanation proffered was that there is a "latent period" between menopause and "menopause-related disorders."[64] (Well, except for vasomotor symptoms, which appear early and are also allegedly caused by low estrogen—but for some reason, these seem to keep to a different schedule.) The underlying assumption is that while the ovaries are still active, women's hearts are protected, but once that estrogen-deficiency thing kicks in, cardiovascular disease follows close behind. A "natural menopause has an unfavorable effect on lipid metabolism," according to the *NEJM*,[65] hence replacing that estrogen—lamentably having to add some of that nasty progestin to the mix to prevent endometrial cancer—would naturally and obviously keep women's cardiac risk low.

There is a fundamental fallacy in this argument, however. The fact is that women's risk of cardiac disease *never* equals that of men. No matter how old women become, age- and survival-adjusted data suggest that a woman's heart disease risk simply does not rise as high as a man's—ever. As Hugh Tunstall-Pedoe of the Cardiovascular Epidemiology Unit in Dundee, Scotland, writes in *The Lancet*,

> It is unarguable that risk of myocardial infarction [heart attack] and coronary death is lower in women than in men in middle age. However, there is a myth that risk

Table 5.1

This table shows epidemiological data comparing deaths from coronary heart disease by age and gender. Reproduced with permission from Elsevier and Tunstall-Pedoe, H., "Myth and Paradox of Coronary Risk and the Menopause," *The Lancet 35*(9113), May 9, 1998, p. 1425.

Age Group	Population In thousands		CHD deaths (number)		CHD death rates per million	
	Men	Women	Men	Women	Men	Women
15–19	1681	1591	2.0	1.0	1.2	0.6
20–24	2008	1928	9.2	2.8	4.6	1.5
25–29	2123	2063	36	6.6	17	3.2
30–34	1888	1852	96	24	51	13
35–39	1696	1688	329	50	194	30
40–44	1795	1791	819	137	456	76
45–49	1603	1596	1588	265	991	166
50–54	1370	1371	2752	558	2008	407
55–59	1288	1307	4716	1258	3663	963
60–64	1234	1315	7878	2851	6386	2168
65–69	1157	1335	12075	5580	10438	4179
70–74	876	1148	13965	8518	15934	7417
75–79	639	996	15025	12381	23498	12426
80–84	381	748	12432	14982	32630	20024
85–89	158	421	6719	12486	42528	29629
90–94	na	na	2077	6306	na	na
95+	na	na	424	1899	na	na
90+	47	191	2501	8205	52764	42913
All ages 15+	19944	21343	80942	67305	4058	3153

CHD = coronary heart disease; na = not available.

in women is held low until the menopause, around age 50 years, when it rebounds, equaling, and later surpassing that in men. Although *challenged over 30 years by different mortality data and in reviews this myth persists* [italics added] . . . [pandering] to major commercial, professional and research lobbies.[66]

There is no blip in the heart disease data starting at menopause and never has been, but as Tunstall-Pedoe dryly points out, "Myths exist to explain everyday experiences."[67]

Coronary deaths are rare below age fifty in women, which means they are outside the experience of most medical practitioners; WHO statistics show that five times as many men under age fifty (2,900) as women (500) will die of coronary causes. But the only time cardiac deaths in women exceed that of men is over age eighty, and if one takes one's estrogen blinkers off for a second, it becomes blindingly obvious that this is because more women than men live past the age of eighty (Table 5.1). Longevity statistics from all developed countries show that women simply live longer; average life expectancy in 2005, according to the Centers for Disease Control and Prevention, for a woman in the United States was 80.4; for a man, 75.2 years. As for cardiovascular disease, a prospective epidemiology study showed that men whose cholesterol levels were at the lowest quintile (less than 5.0 mmol/L) had a higher cardiac death rate than those women in the highest cholesterol quintile (over 7.2), a finding that remained true after menopause.[68] Even a follow-up on the Framingham Study found that "between ages 35 to 84 years, men have about twice the total incidence of morbidity and mortality of women" in coronary heart disease.[69]

Furthermore, as Tunstall-Pedoe calmly points out, those who consider menopause "a catastrophic organ failure accompanying biological uselessness" would also suggest that it "implies major changes in mortality."[70] After all, if one is pushing the idea that being a woman equals being fertile—which equals estrogen—then it is useful to have cardiac mortality figures to back that up. Circumstantial evidence for this myth is found in studies of surgical menopause (hysterectomy) because these women were found to be at greater coronary risk than menstruating women of the same age. There is, however, a fundamental flaw in using such data, aside from the obvious, because anyone who has had surgery will not have the same risk profile as someone who has not, regardless of the type of surgery. Logically, those women who had hysterectomies were also the ones experiencing a difficult perimenopause; the majority of hysterectomies are done on women in their mid-forties, when women are perimenopausal, with the primary reason cited for surgery being excessive bleeding, with or without fibroids.

We know that women with heavy bleeding in midlife, at perimenopause, have higher estrogen levels.[71] These women, as discussed in a previous chapter, also have the lowest levels of progesterone to balance out the high estrogen. At a population level, this will translate into increased blood pressure and an increase in weight, waist circumference, body mass index, and lipids, which makes it highly likely that women who have had a hysterectomy already had *high* estrogen, which we now definitively know (from the Women's Health Initiative) causes cardiovascular disease. A Finnish study did, in fact, link cardiovascular risk factors, such as high blood pressure and a higher body mass index (being heavy, in other words), with women who had had a hysterectomy when compared to women who had not had surgery.[72] And although the study was small and did not note any difference in heart attacks or angina, it did indicate that the cardiac risk of the women who had hysterectomies was higher. More solid evidence comes from strokes: between the ages of forty-five and fifty-four, women's risk of stroke is higher than that of men, and because this is precisely the time women tend to be perimenopausal, the indirect implication is that it is high estrogen that causes heart disease, blood clots, and strokes.[73]

LOOKING FOR HEALTH IN ALL THE WRONG PLACES

If all we are doing is examining the higher incidence of cardiovascular disease in postmenopausal women (without comparing women to men because women's risk never reaches that of men), why could the reverse not be true? In other words, why does the lack of estrogen have to be at the root of CAD; why is it inconceivable that lower estrogen could be the effect, rather than the cause, of heart disease? Researchers at the University of Utrecht in the Netherlands and Boston University School of Medicine, working with data from the Framingham Study, came to precisely that conclusion in 2006, noting that women with an early menopause were at an increased risk of CAD. Ovaries, as Helen Kok and her colleagues point out in the *Journal of the American College of Cardiology*, are highly vascularized organs, so perhaps what was considered a consequence of menopause could actually be the cause.

These researchers examined the records of 695 women who had not reached menopause at the start of the study but did so later. What they found was that higher total cholesterol was linked with an earlier age at menopause, as were increases in blood pressure. A decrease in any of these risk factors was associated with a later menopause:

> Current views on the relationship between menopause and cardiovascular risk assume estrogen depletion to be a causal factor in the increase of cardiovascular risk. Conversely, however, menopause may not induce a change in cardiovascular risk profile, but a women's atherosclerotic status may influence age at onset of menopause.[74]

In other words, it might be that it is not the lack of estrogen that leads to CAD, but CAD that leads to the subsequent lowering of estrogen at menopause (bearing in mind that this is merely a theory and that one study does not constitute proof). The researchers also found that in those women whose risks for heart disease were high, the age of menopause went down. We bring this up not to say that an early menopause could lead to CAD, but rather, to point to the assumptions that have been made in trying to find heart benefits for estrogen.

Earlier, we described various women whose symptoms during their forties (much like the authors') seemed to reflect the higher cardiac risk associated with estrogen. During perimenopause, women feel fat, they sleep poorly, they are stressed, and often—if tested—their blood pressure is higher than they are used to. Women with a family history of diabetes found themselves thrown into the medical establishment's guideline-driven therapeutics at this time and were told they were at high risk—and there is some evidence that it was perimenopause that created this risk.[75] An Australian study of 2,540 women between the ages of thirty-five and seventy-nine, attempting to delineate the reasons for hormone therapy in menopausal women (with and without hysterectomy), found that women who were not taking hormones and who had had a hysterectomy had higher blood pressure (both systolic and diastolic), a higher waist-to-hip ratio, higher body mass index, and more bad cholesterol than women who had not had a hysterectomy, which suggests that the effects of the higher estrogen levels during perimenopause might persist in subsequent heart attack risk.[76]

Studies on menopause and heart disease, moreover, blithely tend to ignore the fact that estrogen is a risk for blood clots, whether it is endogenous estrogen (created by the body, as it is during perimenopause) or exogenous (primarily if ingested rather than pasted or rubbed on the skin). We have known this for years from the birth control pill as well as from the higher levels of estrogen during pregnancy; pregnant women are more prone than other women their own age to gestational diabetes and blood clots. Ironically, as we saw earlier, estrogen was implicated in heart disease in men more than thirty years ago; men given estrogen had more blood clots and heart attacks.[77] Estrogen also caused cancer, a risk that persisted even after the estrogen was stopped.[78] As early as 1992, one of the authors of this book (J.C.P.), in a letter to the *NEJM*, firmly predicted that estrogen would be found to increase heart disease risks.[79] Not that anybody listened.

All of us—women and men alike—lose some elasticity in our blood vessels and arteries as we age. Like our joints, the vessels through which blood flows in and out of the heart become slightly stiff, and as we hit our fifties (more or less, individual variability being what it is), systolic blood pressure (although not diastolic) goes up.* In the elderly, the highest cardiovascular risk is a decreased diastolic pressure combined with a higher systolic pressure.[80] (So it is best if your grandmother's blood pressure is not 210/55.) These blood pressure changes happen to all of us as we age, regardless of estrogen, but so besotted were researchers with the estrogen connection that all else was pushed to the side or ignored altogether, and gynecology and cardiology continued to insist throughout the 1980s and 1990s that the estrogen-progestin combination simply *had* to be good for the heart.

STOPPING THE MADNESS

Even at the height of the estrogen-is-good-for-your-heart craze, a few critical voices did urge caution; unfortunately, their voices were drowned out in the in the clamor of hype and hope and hysteria. California epidemiologist Diana Petitti, writing in *JAMA* in 1998, pointed to the "limitations of observational research"

---

*Systolic blood pressure (the higher number) is created by the heart muscle contracting and diastolic pressure (the lower number), is caused by the relaxation between heartbeats. So if your blood pressure is 128/76, the 128 is the systolic blood pressure and the 76 is the diastolic. It is the 128 number that is affected by age. High blood pressure is also known as hypertension.

and the "incompleteness" of the current understanding of the "mechanisms of vascular disease," not to mention the risks of extrapolating from a handful of studies.[81] No matter how convincing they might seem, another *JAMA* editorial warned, observational studies cannot "establish causality."[82] The point was repeatedly made that not only were these observational studies prone to the healthy user bias, but the nurses and other questionnaire-filling subjects were clearly also compliant with therapy. They took the drugs, listened to advice, and did as they were asked, all of which has been shown to make a difference: in two different randomized trials of coronary heart disease, "the subjects who faithfully took their *placebo* [italics added] had a lower risk of CHD [coronary heart disease]" than the ones noncompliant with therapy.[83]

In 1997, Elina Hemminki, a Finnish research professor, and Klim McPherson, a British public health professor, published a meta-analysis of existing observational studies in the *British Medical Journal*, pooling results from twenty-two trials and 4,124 women. Their conclusion was that the data in favor of estrogen were not compelling: "The results of these pooled data *do not support* [italics added] the notion that postmenopausal hormone therapy prevents cardiovascular events," they wrote.[84] But the tenor of the times was clearly obvious in the tone of subsequent letters—vitriolic, albeit icily polite. Mostly written by gynecologists, the writers heaped scorn on the researchers, nitpicked their methodology, and expressed outrage that articles such as this could "deprive women of the potential benefit of hormone replacement therapy."[85] Belief in the efficacy of estrogen ran so deep that dissent simply could not be tolerated—even though doubt is the basis for all scientific inquiry. (Note that none of the cautious voices said that estrogen wouldn't work; merely urged caution, pointing out that the evidence was not in.)

Faith in the cardioprotective powers of estrogen ought to have eroded, once and for all, in the late 1990s with the HERS trial; unfortunately, nothing seemed to make a dent in America's faith in hormones. In a randomized, double-blind study undertaken between January 1993 and September 1994, twenty HERS clinical centers enrolled 2,763 women with "established coronary disease" (but who were not sick); 1,380 received hormones (a single pill containing 0.625 mg equine estrogen and 2.5 mg medroxyprogesterone acetate), and 1,383 were given a placebo. HERS, standing for Heart and Estrogen/Progestin Replacement Study, was funded by Wyeth-Ayerst to obtain FDA approval to label their drug as cardioprotective, and everyone fully expected the results to be positive. But on the contrary, after approximately four years, the HERS results found that not only did hormones "not reduce the overall rate of CHD events," but that the treatment group experienced "net *harm*."[86] Undaunted, the researchers pushed on with HERS II. They just knew in their *bones* that there might be a "decreased risk of CHD during years 3 to 5" (versus those first three years). Tenaciously, they followed 2,321 of these extraordinary women (93% of the HERS survivors) for another 2.7 years. Randomly assigning 1,250 women to hormones and 1,260 to placebo, again they found that "hormone therapy did not reduce risk of cardiovascular events."[87] (The trial was stopped early; it had been scheduled to run for four years.) Was anyone listening? Not so you'd notice: by 2001, some 15 million women in the United States were filling prescriptions for hormones annually, perhaps one-third solely to prevent heart disease.[88] Despite the calls for "well-designed clinical trials" to establish the cardioprotective effect of hormones at menopause,[89] nobody wanted to hear about negative results.

Finally, a year later, in 2002, when the largest randomized clinical hormone trial in history, the Women's Health Initiative (WHI), was stopped early because the risk-benefit quotient simply did not compute, people listened—at least for five minutes. The WHI was simply too big to ignore. It had taken twenty-five years and billions of dollars in estrogen sales (and who knows how many unnecessary deaths), but this necessary randomized trial finally had reached a conclusion.

THE WOMEN'S HEALTH INITIATIVE

A massive, $625 million, fourteen-year study, the WHI had enrolled some 160,000 postmenopausal women between the ages of fifty and seventy-nine into the largest trial ever funded by the NIH. (It was probably no coincidence that a woman, Bernadine Healy, a cardiologist, was the director of the NIH at the time.) This long-awaited study ("When the WHI is finished" was a throwaway line common throughout the 1990s in any discussion on hormones) was designed between 1991 and 1992. Based on what was hopefully (and, as it turned out, erroneously) called "the accumulated evidence at that time," the WHI focused on "defining the risks and benefits of strategies that could potentially reduce the incidence of heart disease, breast and colorectal cancer, and fractures in postmenopausal women."[90] The study had several arms, a number of them interventional, and one observational, to study various and sundry aspects of women's health such as a low-fat diet and the efficacy of calcium/vitamin D in preventing fractures. There were high hopes for cardiac prevention, based on what were considered "supportive data on lipid levels" and from primate studies—not to mention all those terrific observational studies everyone kept quoting.[91]

But then the unthinkable happened. The trial was stopped early, at the end of May 2002, after an average follow-up of 5.2 years—when, to their horror, proponents of "HRT" discovered that not only did the women taking the estrogen-progestin hormone cocktail have a far higher incidence of major cardiovascular events, but that the incidence of breast cancer was "excessive" or, in more statistical terms, the "test statistic for invasive breast cancer exceeded the stopping boundary."[92] In other words, even though the researchers had expected the incidence of breast cancer to rise somewhat, they were horrified to realize just how much estrogen could increase that risk. Hormone therapy simply could not be said to be beneficial in reducing a healthy menopausal woman's risk of future disease.

For once, the media did not ignore the results, and while "millions of women and their physicians wondered what to do next, the scientific community wondered what went wrong."[93] Of course, what the scientific community *should* have been wondering is how they could have been so wrong, so unscientific, so biased, and so stubbornly sure of estrogen, given their lack of evidence and the fact that the entire basis for science as a form of inquiry is *doubt*. As geneticist Marion Namenworth writes in a segment of the book *Feminist Approaches to Science*, such "authoritative" pronouncements are "antithetical to the nature of science," which, by definition, is supposed to be a dynamic, fluid process and not carved in stone.[94]

Be that as it may, shock and consternation was the order of the day. The stopping of the WHI was medical history in the making: the miniscule decrease in the incidence of colon cancer (a infinitesimal risk to begin with) and the clear but small decrease in hip fractures was simply no match for the increases seen in breast cancer, heart disease, blood clots, stroke, and gallbladder disease.

For years, epidemiologists had been scornful of women for worrying about breast cancer when their risk of dying from cardiovascular disease was so much higher; as it turned out, women were smarter than they were. We have all known women, sisters, mothers, friends, with breast cancer, some of whom never made it out alive. And we did get that heart disease might be numerically more impressive—but we also understood that CAD was unlikely to be a problem until down the road, when we were older. And, as Hadler says, we all have to die of something. Plus, hormones simply did not *feel* right: we got migraines; we felt bloated, anxious, and fat. Our breasts became sore. (Even the WHI allowed some "flexibility" in the dosage to accommodate various side effects.[95]) So in the end, it was epidemiologists who had not understood that an abstract risk is not quite the same thing as the very real threat of a breast tumor that could easily kill you—and even if the tumor didn't, the treatment could. (The writer Calvin Trillin wrote a moving, extended farewell to his wife, who had had breast cancer in the 1960s but died in the late 1990s because the radiation treatment had irrevocably damaged her heart muscle.) Our subjective reality finally managed to trump their objective one, and, for once; science backed us up. The strident voices insisting hormones *had* to be good were silenced—for a nanosecond.

Then, as difficult as it might be for the rational mind to believe, given the huge impact the stopping of the WHI had had, the excuses, justifications, and but-maybe arguments began to stream in. "But was the WHI really a primary cardio-vascular prevention study?" asked a group of vehemently pro-estrogen researchers, unable (or unwilling) to give up their pet theory. After all, the women taking the hormones were older, with an average age of sixty-three, compared with those of the observational studies.[96] (Actually, in subsequent subgroup analyses, age was a "nonsignificant" factor.[97]) Estrogen proponents felt sure that their earlier "hypothesis that early initiation of hormone therapy, in women who are at the inception of their menopause" would "delay the onset of subclinical cardiovascular disease" had to be right—or, at least, remain an "open question" requiring further "rigorous testing."[98]

NEVER GIVE UP, NEVER SURRENDER

When a hypothesis, an idea, like that of estrogen being fundamentally positive, refuses to die—as social scientists and cross-cultural observers have noted—the reason has nothing to do with science and everything to do with culture. Any evidence, no matter how sound, that does not fit in with prevailing social mores or cultural beliefs of what *ought* to work is, inevitably, said to require "more proof," as Lynn Payer pointed out in her comprehensive book *Medicine and Culture*.* The United States had whole-heartedly embraced the hormone—or at least estrogen—thesis for nearly a century; even the DES debacle had not convinced the medical establishment that estrogen (particularly by itself) was simply not the answer and would cause harm. And in the United States, once the rationale for a specific idea has taken hold—particularly if that idea is one of *doing* something, versus sitting back and allowing nature to take its course—the national character (unlike that of other countries such as Britain or France) is tenacious. Perhaps this was inevitable in a country painstakingly built on and through the gradual colonization of an unfriendly frontier. Other Western countries, such as England, do not tend to extrapolate beyond the specific, as Payer describes, but America does. To illustrate the point, she uses the American penchant for giving adjuvant (additional) chemotherapy to remove the potential spread beyond lymph nodes in patients with breast cancer, as a prominent British professor dryly explains:

> I can understand as well as any oncologist why it *should* work. The arguments are very persuasive. But because it ought to work doesn't mean it does. I ought to be rich, I can produce the most compelling arguments why I should be rich, yet I seem to be poor. The data are more important than the hypothesis.[99]

Therein lies the rub. Just because it *ought* to work—and the theory explaining why it should is an excellent one—does not mean that it does. But a culture that valorizes advance, progress, and speed; a country where medicine is characterized in military terms and revolves around the notion that we must *do* something; a country that considers aging an enemy to be conquered is a country where

---

*For more, see Notes.

giving up is not an option,[100] particularly if what is being given up is a hormone, estrogen, whose essence has been considered fundamental to the concept of women's health for nearly a century.

"Bravo, bravo, bravo," wrote I. Kerber and R. Turner (a vet) in response to the article suggesting it was not hormone therapy that was at fault (in the WHI results) but the age of the women involved, and the timing. To start "estrogen in newly menopausal women before endothelial damage has occurred" made perfect sense, they enthusiastically agreed, since "it makes little biological sense for estrogen receptors to *lie fallow* [italics added] for one-third of a woman's life."[101] Yet again, another phase of denial seems about to begin, as the media now also seem to have picked up on the timing hypothesis and has begun to insist that there is still a discussion to be had because we "just don't know." *Yes, we do.*

Estrogen has not been beneficial in reducing cardiac disease. That ship has sailed. Women need to understand that. Estrogen causes strokes, heart attacks, and breast cancer. It did not prevent dementia, heart disease, or any of the other terrible things it was supposed to be good for. During perimenopause, when some women experience onerous symptoms, their risk of cardiac disease (and hysterectomy) rises along with their estrogen levels. During that time, taking progesterone to balance out their wildly spiking estrogen might well serve as a physiologic anchor and prevent some of the potential risks of this stormy transition into menopause. After that, normal, healthy, well women have no reason to consider taking hormones. Estrogen was not and is not useful in preventing disease and has, in fact, been shown to cause harm.

In the next chapter, we continue to examine the myths surrounding estrogen and other epidemiologic justifications of these ostensibly pro-active preventive treatments, notably with respect to osteoporosis and breast cancer. We will continue our analysis of modern medicine and its history as well as its estrogen infatuation, where, as always, we return to the obvious: that it is the *balance* of hormones—estrogen and progesterone—that matters.

6

THE BASICS OF BONE

The organizers of Australia's "healthy bones week" have come under fire for making exaggerated and misleading claims about the dangers of osteoporosis—the loss of bone density that raises the risk of fracture with age. "Fact 1" on the poster sent to Australian general practitioners last week read: "More Australian women die from osteoporosis than all female cancers combined." There was no reference to back up the statement. . . . Sydney general practitioner Mark Donohoe, a government adviser of false health claims whose surgery was sent the poster, described the claim as "patent rubbish" and a "bald faced lie." . . . Osteoporosis is not listed in the top 12 causes of death. . . . The false claim . . . was being promoted by Osteoporosis Australia.

—Ray Moynihan[1]

Osteoporosis. A word that few of us had heard when we were young and certainly our grandmothers knew little of, although they did know about the "dowager's hump" (a forward bending of the upper back) caused by vertebral compression-type fractures. Over the last decades, however, we have heard nothing but bad news about our bones—how they are hollowing out, becoming frail and fragile; putting us at risk of falling and not being able to get up. Advertisements on television remind us of the alarming statistics: once we reach fifty our bones are on the brink of disaster, "one in four" of us is at risk of osteoporosis. Yet again, we are told that we must be proactive, involved; stay on top of it lest we shrink away and, who knows, maybe disappear altogether. (Perhaps this is a not-so-hidden metaphor for the way aging women vanish—in films, ads, or as role models throughout the culture.) Recommendations for scans and screening programs pour in thick and fast, as do the exhortations to take drugs and supplements to ward off this skeletal disaster, "bolstered by advocacy groups, professional societies, educational programs."[2] Hormones naturally have also had their role. In fact, the common term for osteoporosis in women is "postmenopausal osteoporosis," because the current thought process goes something like this: menopause causes "estrogen deficiency" which, in turn, causes rapid bone loss; therefore women have fractures after menopause—lack of estrogen must be to blame. Although dropping estrogen levels do cause bone loss, this perspective is not only narrow and myopic, but just plain wrong.

Osteoporosis was first called a disease by Fuller Albright in a 1940 paper in which he said it occurred after menopause and in women, not men, so "estin" (what he called estrogen therapy) might help.[3] But, the reality is that, taking the life-cycle view, as we have throughout this book, there are multiple factors involved in whether or not a woman will have fractures at an older age: maintaining a healthy weight with a high enough intake of calcium; having reasonably regular cycles that become ovulatory ones during the teen years (all of which contribute to a high peak bone mass),[4] and preventing bone loss by menstruating and ovulating normally through the premenopausal years.[5] Also important is that rapid bone loss can occur in perimenopause when cycles become irregular (and despite still high average estrogen levels) although we don't know why.[6] All these aspects of later fracture risk occur *before* menopause, when estrogen levels are usually normal. Therefore to focus solely on older women and their supposed "estrogen deficiency" is shortsighted and unhelpful.

Quoting one of his teachers, the vociferously pro-hormone head of the International Menopause Society disapprovingly wrote in 1990: "Why do we accept it as inevitable that grandmothers should always be short?"[7] (Subtext: If more women took hormones at menopause this would not happen.) Except, of course, by menopause, bone is already low for the majority of those women who will end up having a fracture. It is also unclear whether five years of estrogen therapy (hopefully with progesterone to stimulate bone formation) will be sufficient to restore fragile bone to normal. And of course, hormones or no, not all grandmothers *are* short, merely shorter than they were, as are grandfathers.*

We all lose height as we age: the disks in our spines compress, in men and women alike; in fact, few people over sixty-five have not lost some disk spacing in their spine.[8] What women picture with the threat of osteoporosis, however, is not this slow, natural process but breakage and that kyphosis, or forward bend of the spine that we occasionally see on an older person, which results from a series of small, often painless (although about one-third of them may be very painful) vertebral fractures that some people are prone to, men and women alike. So there

---

*My own grandmother was short, but she was short all her life, not just when she became a grandmother. As it happens (and for the record), I am also short (S.B.); whereas J.C.P. is not.

is a prejudicial slant in ascribing this simply to women.* The stalwart Benjamin Franklin developed this condition. The question then becomes whether these spine fractures, also called *compression fractures*, which some radiologists refer to as genuine "clinical markers of established osteoporosis" that frequently "go undiagnosed,"[9] should be a major public health concern. What we do know is that those who have these silent spine fractures are somewhat more likely to break a wrist or a hip over the next ten years and that, even when unaware of such fractures, at least in a population-based cohort of women, quality of life was significantly lower.[10] (Although we don't know what else was going on in these women's lives; quality of life figures are notoriously vague.)

What this does *not* mean is that most of us will end up breaking bones in our backs as we get older. In a large Canadian study, a group of (16,505) women over the age of fifty were followed over a four-year period (through a retrospective examination of hospital records, in the province of Manitoba). Only 208 had a clinical spine fracture (meaning that sudden back pain, commonly between the shoulder blades and under the bra in women, made them seek medical help). Most were at least sixty-five, with the majority of cases occurring over age seventy-five. Put another way, what this study showed was that out of one hundred women over the age of fifty, not even one (0.7) under age sixty-five would have a spinal fracture. Over age sixty-five, the incidence rose to somewhere between one and two (1.2) women.[11] True, once that initial fracture happens, there are other studies that show that the risk for a second one does go up about 20 percent.[12] But what the alarmists don't tell you is that clinical vertebral fractures are vanishingly rare and that they primarily tend to occur in the elderly (in the absence of some precipitating disease or drug, e.g., prednisone), in particular, among the frail, *institutionalized* elderly or people nearing eighty. But it is not that older group that garners the media attention and who are the focus of the television advertisements and brochures highlighting the need for mass screening programs and wider access to drug therapies. On the contrary, these messages are almost always aimed at *younger* women (between ages fifty and sixty-five) who have not yet had a fracture.

PERIMENOPAUSE, EARLY MENOPAUSE, AND BREAKAGE

What most of us associate with the term *osteoporosis* is broken bones: having a fracture for no obvious reason. These commonly are important clinically and in terms of public health because fractures do seem to be associated with higher mortality—about one year after a fracture, the risk of dying rises 20 percent—plus loss of functional state, even having to enter long-term care.[13] As alarming as these

---

*And as we saw before, women simply live longer, so there are more older women than older men.

statistics sound, however, yet again, it is important to put these figures in context and appreciate that they do not routinely mention age, and, inevitably, it is being older that is the most important risk factor for, and predictor of, osteoporosis.[14] (Of course, being older is also a risk for all manner of other conditions, from CAD to Parkinson's disease.) So, contrary to the hype, it is not her fiftieth birthday (and menopause) that a normal, healthy midlife woman should be concerned about, but (if she insists on being concerned) her eightieth, because the frequency of osteoporosis rises to *approximately* 25 percent of women by age eighty or ninety. That is where that scary phrase "one in four women will develop osteoporosis" comes from.

The emotive tone notwithstanding, it is also important to stress that statistics, by definition, are phrased in general, rounded-out terms and subject to error and misrepresentation. (As Mark Twain said, "There are lies, damn lies and then there are statistics.") And much as we would like to lump all older people together, the reality is that as we age, the more different we become. As an article in *The Lancet* succinctly explains, physiologically, aging is simply a "progressive constriction of each organ system's capacity to maintain homeostasis in the face of challenge" and is "influenced by diet, environment, and personal habits as well as by genetic factors." As a result, *individuals become more dissimilar as they age,* making generalizations increasingly difficult the older we get.[15] The authors add that to speak of a "healthy old age" is not a paradox. As such, the numbers on osteoporosis or any other threat(s) of old age should be put in context.

This is not the kind of language we tend to hear, however. More common is the advice to have tests, scans, or screenings of one sort or another, ranging from colonoscopies and having one's cholesterol checked to mammograms and, for osteoporosis, bone density scans. But are these strategies truly preventive, and are they useful? In terms of bone density scans, it can get tricky because the evidence connecting bone densitometry or bone density scans to fracture is often contradictory, and perhaps unsurprisingly, those studies finding the strongest link between bone density and fractures are either funded by, or strongly associated with, pharmaceutical companies.[16] For instance, when a group of researchers affiliated with Merck* (three of whom were employed by the drug company) studied a group of white, female nursing home residents in Maryland over the age of sixty-five, what they concluded was that low bone mineral density (BMD) and "independence in transfer" (mobility) were "significant predictors of osteoporotic fractures."[17] Yet the large Canadian study, cited previously, of more than sixteen thousand women concluded that "most of the postmenopausal women with osteoporotic fractures had *nonosteoporotic* [italics added] bone mineral density values."[18] That is because the risks for falling increase as we get older, and we are more likely to fall awkwardly

---

*Merck manufactures one of the most popular drugs for osteoporosis, Alendronate.

and thus sustain a fracture. Because, again—although bone density is what we talk about—it is falls that are more germane.

In the same vein, a meta-analysis of some ninety thousand person years, published in the *British Medical Journal* (*BMJ*), found that although bone density measurements *might* predict some fracture risk, they "cannot identify *individuals* [italics added] who will have a fracture." In other words, the predictive value of BMD is fair-to-middling useless, unless that BMD is coupled with other important information like age, sex, having taken prednisone (a drug used for some autoimmune diseases that causes bone loss and also paralyzes bone gain), or, most important, having a history of a low trauma fracture or a strong family history of fracture.*

Nevertheless, those women whose menopause is early or who experience a difficult perimenopause, which, as we saw in an earlier chapter, is often a sign of fluctuating (often wildly) estrogen levels and low progesterone, may indeed lose bone mass during this transition. Every woman loses bone mass fairly rapidly during late perimenopause when her cycles become irregular; one meta-analysis suggests that the rate of loss averages 1.8 percent a year.[19] So if bone mass was low to begin with (plus there was bone loss during the premenopausal years), this could tip one into the fracture risk early. This small subgroup may indeed need medical help. One such woman was Reka, a forty-seven-year-old executive, who caught her toe and fell in a step class, breaking her wrist:

> Reka has never been pregnant and says she was healthy as a young woman, except that she had rather severe weight loss around age twelve. But she reports that she has always been thin. Her periods began at thirteen and a half, and she has no family history of osteoporosis. Until she was forty-five, her periods were regular (she didn't really keep track), and then they suddenly stopped when she was forty-six. She has recently experienced night sweats, several times a week, that wake her during the night. After she broke her wrist, she read up on bones and has begun drinking calcium-fortified soy milk and taking a 1,000-mg calcium carbonate pill at bedtime. She asked that her family doctor send her for a bone density scan. She is diagnosed with osteoporosis (a spine T-score of –2.9 and a hip T-score of –2.3) and sees an osteoporosis specialist, who starts her on a once-a-week dose of biphosphonate, Fosamax (alendronate).
>
> Although she takes it as directed—staying up and moving around after she takes it, waiting two hours before eating breakfast, and so on—she begins having heartburn that worsens with time. One evening, she is too nauseated to eat and wakes in the night vomiting blood. She goes to the emergency room and is told to stop the drug and is treated with acid-blocking drugs. She returns to her family doctor greatly distressed—and is referred to Dr. Prior.
>
> A detailed history and physical exam reveals that Reka probably never ovulated (she never knew when her period was coming plus her breasts are immature, like a

---

*See note 55, D. Marshall et al., 1254.

girl who has just started her period). Her extreme thinness as a youth suggests she might have had an eating disorder, perhaps anorexia, which, along with other stresses, prevented the brain, pituitary, and ovary from learning how to ovulate normally.

The connection between *ovulatory* periods—not merely a regular menstrual cycle, which can occur in the absence of ovulation—throughout our adult lives and bone *strength* seems to be important, although we are not sure precisely what the mechanism is. We suspect that there is a link with progesterone, the forgotten hormone in the hormone discourse, and its ability to enhance bone formation.[20] This bone loss, which seems to be caused by disturbances related to the hypothalamus, occurs in women like Reka with chronic anovulatory cycles. Progesterone (as Provera) given in a "luteal phase replacement pattern" (through the second half of the cycle, mimicking the body's natural balance), in conjunction with other strategies, such as stress reduction and restoration of normal body weight, not only appears to prevent bone loss, but is associated with bone gain.[21] Progesterone appears to stimulate osteoblasts to increase their ability in making the osteoid, protein substance of bone, and to increase the number of osteoblasts[22]:

> Reka was not keen on the idea of gaining weight: she insisted that she was happy the way she was and felt "fat" if she weighed any more. Dr. Prior suggested she at least take 1,400 IU/day of vitamin D₃ and have about 500 mg of elemental calcium (one or more servings of dairy, fortified soy, rice, or other beverage) with each meal and at bedtime. She also started Reka on 300 mg of bioidentical progesterone (Prometrium) at bedtime and encouraged her to keep up her step classes and yoga and to keep using the rowing machine. Dr. Prior also gave Reka a lower-dose estrogen (Estragel, which is a clear jelly spread on as wide an area of soft skin as possible), half a pump a day on days one to twenty-five of the month. This is a natural way for Reka, who is menopausal, to decrease bone loss (and prevent the rapid bone loss that normally occurs during the first few years of menopause). This regimen can be revisited in five years, when estrogen should be stopped and a bone-loss stopping drug substituted.

Estrogen as well as progesterone has a role in this case because Reka has both severe night sweats (that would need hormone therapy) and osteoporosis. It is quite clear that dropping estrogen levels, or swinging ones, as in perimenopause, cause bone loss,[23] and estrogen is approved by the FDA for the prevention (although not the treatment) of osteoporosis.[24] In this instance, the estrogen will not increase Reka's risk of breast cancer because her risk is already lower than average due to her early menopause; plus, estrogen therapy for five years, even in women with a higher age at menopause, does not seem to increase breast cancer risk.[25] A study from France, furthermore, showed that oral micronized progesterone (but not progestin) actually prevents breast cancer from developing when one takes estrogen.[26]

Reka's resistance to the idea of gaining weight suggests that she, like many women today, practices eating restraint—in other words, she is vigilant about what she eats. This might not seem like a problem, except that continually worrying or thinking about what you eat is inevitably stressful, which in turn leads to higher cortisol levels, a stress hormone that is linked to not ovulating or having sufficient progesterone. These two risk factors were recently found to differ significantly between twenty-four young women with osteoporosis and seventy-two similarly aged women with normal bone density randomly picked from the local population. Plus, Reka's weight has always been low, and the smaller one is, the higher one's risk of having fragile bones. Other risks are a family history of fragility fractures, being physically inactive (or having small muscles), a history of skipping more than three periods, excessive worry about weight gain (dietary restraint), chronically low calcium and vitamin D intake, smoking, and various diseases (bowel, kidney, thyroid). Additionally, there are several medications, such as the steroids used in inflammatory conditions and oral contraceptives,[27] that appear to negatively affect bone. Of course, having any of these does not mean one has, or will ever have, osteoporosis, and it is vital to keep that in mind. Statistics and general conclusions, even when they are based on excellent research, do not predict anything for any individual person.

DEM BONES, DEM BONES

In women, osteoporosis—"bone fractures that are not secondary to trauma"—increases with age, which obviously refers to the time after menopause.[28] Similar to CAD, women said to be at risk were often told that taking hormones was the answer, even though the evidence was never compelling: "Although HRT has been used for over 60 years to treat osteoporosis," wrote the authors of the 2002 Canadian guidelines for osteoporosis dryly, the "evidence for its efficacy has been suboptimal."[29]

The estrogen-progestin arm of the Women's Health Initiative (WHI), as we saw earlier, was stopped early due to the elevated risk of cardiac disease, stroke, and so on, but it did demonstrate that the regimen reduced the risk of fractures, including hip fractures. Similar prevention of fracture was also shown with estrogen alone.[30] Nevertheless, the risks inherent to taking estrogen meant that it could not be recommended to healthy women as an osteoporosis safeguard or preventative. As a commentary in the *Canadian Medical Association Journal* by physician Anna Day pointed out, the WHI results "elegantly demonstrate" that the "scientific validity of ideas that appear to be intuitively correct"—such as the one that had us believe it was our "deficiency" of hormones after menopause that was to blame for all manner of diseases years later—need good evidence to back them up.[31] Intuition and faith in the inherent goodness of your theory is not enough. She goes on:

> the results of the WHI should make us evaluate whether we are targeting and funding primary prevention efforts appropriately. If the risks of hormone replacement

outweigh the benefits, what are the options for women who hope to avoid the fractures associated with osteoporosis? Recent studies demonstrate that the risk of osteoporosis is related to the peak bone mass achieved in the teens and twenties. Primary prevention of osteoporosis could therefore consist of ensuring that teenagers and young adults maximize their bone mass with appropriate exercise and diet.

In terms of midlife women, however, because we cannot go back in time and change what we did when we were sixteen, what we need to consider is that the accelerated phase of bone loss begins with the irregular flow of perimenopause, and not after menopause as we are continually warned.[32] Although we have no good studies, it seems likely that the higher social and physiological stress of perimenopause (like night sweats and insomnia), fluctuating estrogen levels, and insufficient or absent progesterone might be the culprits in rapid bone loss.[33] And as we noted earlier, progesterone seems to have a positive impact on bone.[34]

OSTEOPOROSIS (SORT OF, ALMOST, MAYBE) DEFINED

It is important to stress that the processes through which various biochemical mechanisms—including hormones—exert their effects on bone are complex, and our understanding of how it all works remains piecemeal and incomplete.[35] Bone is an extraordinary biological material, a living organ. Contrary to what most of us believe, it is neither static nor unchanging, but dynamic. The composition of bone is site-specific; for instance, the bones of the spine and vertebrae differ from the femur (thighbone) or the skull. It appears that long bones and vertebrae respond to the "habitual application of physical forces by compensatory changes in architecture," for obvious reasons.[36] They need to. This explains why some bones will shatter more quickly than others, even in a youth or child; they simply are not, by nature, equipped to deal with the sudden trauma of an awkward fall.

Bones continually renew themselves through a sophisticated process of de- and re-mineralization. In simple terms, the collagen that makes up the bone is first reduced down (resorption) by substances known as *osteoclasts*, then rebuilt (accretion) by *osteoblasts*, a process known as remodeling. Soon after puberty, all our bones finish growing in size, even though they continue the remodeling or renovating throughout our lives. This *peak bone mass* we achieve in our early years is affected by heredity, childhood activity, overall nutrition and calcium intake, and in women, menstruation and ovulation.[37]

Interestingly, in women, progesterone (the presence of the luteal phase during our menstrual cycle) also plays a part in that maximum or peak bone mass we achieve; for instance, in the Michigan Bone Health Study, premenopausal women with the lowest progesterone levels seemed to have the lowest peak bone mass.[38] In other words, normal ovulatory cycles seem to have an impact on how well our bones form. Until we reach midlife, the bone remodeling tends to be even; there is neither a net gain or loss, but once we reach a certain point in our adult lives (usually around age thirty, but in this, as in anything else, there is enormous individual variability), both men and women experience gradual bone loss, at a rate of about 0.5 percent every year.[39]

The term *osteoporosis* originated in France circa 1820 to describe a deteriorated, porous human bone—and osteoporotic fractures have been identified in skeletons dating as far back as the third century.[40] By the late nineteenth century, women were said to suffer from the condition more than men, which was attributed to them "tripping over their long skirts." Today, osteoporosis has been labeled the "disease of the twenty-first century," even though it remains a controversial designation. Much of what we currently read or hear about osteoporosis (and its apparent precursor, low bone mass, or *osteopenia*) puts the major emphasis on recognition and prevention, rather than treatment; it also stresses the value of bone density screening. Recommendations with respect to osteoporosis often stress this BMD number as well as various therapeutic and lifestyle interventions that are believed to slow this seemingly inevitable decline of menopausal, weak, brittle, or hollow bones. Reasons for bone loss include thinness, smoking, low levels of vitamin D and calcium, and being of Asian or white ancestry.

The language used to describe and treat osteoporosis is permeated with those Western military metaphors of which we are so fond (might is right, after all), and we often hear of treatments that *combat* the declining bone mass to make it *strong* and able to withstand any kind of *onslaught* or *attack* (like an icy sidewalk, perhaps). Again, as with cardiac disease, the discourse is one that moves us toward the new "morality of public health where the individual has control over her health through self-governance" and prevention strategies of one sort or another.[41]

In many ways, "osteoporosis and bone measurements have each become a focus for different world views," writes Canadian radiologist Brian Lentle. On one hand, it is argued that losing bone mass is simply a natural part of aging, and overemphasizing the matter consists of "medicalizing the menopause." Conversely:

> Others are afraid that bone measurements will cause undue concern in people found to have low bone mass. Such people may paradoxically avoid exercise for fear of fracture. Another perspective is the impending time when, because of changing demographics, far too many hospital beds will be occupied by people undergoing surgery for osteoporotic fractures of the proximal femur—either spontaneous or resulting from trivial trauma—unless preventive measures are taken.[42]

The problem in terms of diagnosis is that osteoporosis has no symptoms and, until the early 1990s, before bone measurement technologies and methods were developed, providing a more convenient label, osteoporosis was simply a diagnosis made after the fact, after someone had suffered a broken bone—what is known as a fragility fracture, In other words, when someone had suffered a broken bone without having had a previous trauma of major sort, such as a fall down the stairs.[43]

Then, in 1994, a Working Group of the World Health Organization (WHO) on osteoporosis created a set of diagnostic bone density criteria—which they clearly defined as intended for *epidemiological* purposes, not as interventional thresholds. According to these WHO values, "normal" was defined as within 1 standard deviation* of the "young adult reference mean" and osteoporosis as 2.5 standard deviations or more below the young adult mean, with "severe" or established osteoporosis also including one or more fragility fractures. (In the preceding clinical vignette, Reka's spine score was –2.9.) In effect, this definition used young adults as the norm and considered anything too far removed from that as aberrant or potentially diseased.[44]

The inherent problem with this comparison is obvious—we all know that things change with the years. Whether this is abnormal (given that it happens to everyone) is open to question. Also open to question is precisely how objective that WHO meeting really was, given that the drug industry contributed to its funding, notably Sandoz Pharmaceuticals and Smith Kline Beecham (both of which have since merged with other drug companies that manufacture bone agents).[45]

DISEASEMONGERING OR GENUINE PROBLEM?

Osteoporosis is authoritatively presented to us at present as a "silent but deadly epidemic," one that is a sad fact of life for "tens of millions of postmenopausal women," the risk of which increases rapidly once women reach midlife.[46] As the many TV advertisements and pamphlets drive home, that magical cutoff point is somewhere around age fifty (menopause), after which osteoporosis begins to take its toll. There is only one problem with this narrative: the bulk of the data are from women who are sixty and over, and even then, the risk is small—not that that fact ever stopped anyone with an interest in the subject.

An article in the weighty *New England Journal of Medicine* (*NEJM*) states that women over age fifty have a "40 percent lifetime risk of an osteoporotic fracture," which sounds absolutely terrible. But if we take a deep breath and translate this into normal human terms, what it means is that four out of ten American women over the age of fifty *might* have a fracture of the hip, wrist, or some other bone at some point during the remainder of their (projected) lives. Or not. The *NEJM* article goes on to say that one woman in three and one man in nine "older than 80 years of age" will end up sustaining a "hip fracture at

---

*A standard deviation is the number calculated from subtracting each score from the mean (the average—or all the scores added up and divided by the number of scores) and then getting the mean (average) of that. For more on how to calculate statistics, see Notes.

some point" and, worse, some "15 to 20 percent of these patients will die" from "attendant complications."[47] Again, this sounds completely horrifying, until one is reminded that average life expectancy in the United States is seventy-seven,* which already makes these eighty-year-olds long-lived, actuarial anomalies.[48] In any event, compared to what? Expressing numbers in terms of probability (what is called relative risk) makes it fair-to-middling meaningless, particularly because the *reference group* is unclear.†

As health economist Gerd Gigerenzer explains in his illuminating book *Calculated Risks*, the way risk values are usually presented—as percentages, or relative risk—can make even a small difference seem much larger than it is.[49] In normal human terms, it makes far more sense to consider risk in terms of frequencies. So, if we deconstruct the numbers the *NEJM* gave us, what they mean is that out of one hundred American men and women over the age of eighty, forty-four will be at risk of having a hip fracture. Of these forty-four, six to nine could die. Up to seven times that number, thirty-three to thirty-eight people, will be just fine even after that hypothetical fracture (because only 15 to 20% are at risk of death). In this already hardy group, the majority, or well over half (fifty-six), will have no fractures at all—hardly stop-the-presses news. Furthermore, it stands to reason that among those eighty- and ninety-year-olds who end up in hospital for any reason, there will be some deaths. Ultimately, it makes no difference how many conditions or diseases are vying for the cause of death; what matters is that one's life, leading up to that age, was a good one.[50] Perhaps the near-hysterical tones of the *NEJM* article had more to do with the fact that its author and his work were "sponsored by Merck" labs, which makes one of the most widely prescribed osteoporosis drugs on the market.[51]

"Disease mongering" is what critics call the tone and slant of articles such as this one in the *NEJM*, where "a risk factor"—or a bone density value lower than 2.5 standard deviations below that of robust youth—has been "transformed into a medical disease in order to sell tests and drugs to relatively healthy women." This not only expands the size of the "osteoporosis market" but pushes us into the arena of the dubious idea of "pre"-osteoporosis—or women "apparently at risk of being at risk."[52]

As we saw earlier, both men and women lose bone mass as they age, after achieving their highest, or peak, bone mass somewhere between ages twenty and thirty. It has recently become obvious that that original peak, that ultimate bone mass we reach when we are young, is significant, which makes perfect sense since going downhill means something very different depending on how high you were when you started going down. In fact, some observers have noted that

---

*Or 76.9, if one is opting for what some statisticians call spurious accuracy.

†Readers interested in knowing how to calculate relative risk, absolute risk, and so on will find information in the Notes.

because what appears to matter most in terms of later life is bone mass when we are teenagers and young adults, public health efforts should be far more concerned with ensuring that young people have healthy diets, get enough bone-building calcium and vitamin D, do not smoke, and engage in enough exercise to build up that peak bone mass to begin with, not scaring fiftyish women into having their bone densitometry measured.[53] This is particularly true given that *osteopenia,* the gray zone in that WHO scheme, defined as between normal and whatever magical number that is said to define osteoporosis, is a description, not a disease.

As a comprehensive "Clinical Crossroads" article in the *JAMA* flatly says,

> "Osteopenia" is not a disease. Before the advent of bone densitometry, "osteopenia" was used by radiologists to describe bones that seemed more translucent than normal, and "osteoporosis" was defined by the occurrence of vertebral fracture. The widespread use of densitometry changed these terms.

The WHO delineations further cemented this "unsettling" term, which is often presented to patients as though it is a diagnosis—and which most patients interpret as meaning they have a disease, leading to stress and "persistent anxiety."[54]

MAKING THE INVISIBLE BODY VISIBLE

For midlife women, retrospective regrets about their dieting, less healthy younger selves is neither useful nor productive. To stay well, or so we are told, we should instead focus on making sure that we get our bone density scans (the "to do" list keeps growing: check blood pressure, cholesterol, and glucose; have mammograms and colonoscopies; the list goes on and on). But as Deborah Marshall and her colleagues at the Swedish Council on Technology Assessment wrote in the *BMJ*, "using bone density measurements alone to predict fractures is analogous to using blood pressure to predict stroke and serum cholesterol concentrations to predict coronary heart disease."[55] It is simply not possible. We cannot use correlations reflected in large, epidemiological studies that are the result of large numbers and statistics to predict what will happen to an individual. Ever. Although it is true that high blood pressure does seem to be connected to stroke in some people, in many more people, it is not. Similarly, many people who have heart attacks have cholesterol levels that fall within the low-normal range.

Our ability to predict disease is nowhere near as piercingly accurate as we are led to believe—much like our analysis and understanding of the genome, which is similarly presented as meticulous and exact, when it is nothing of the kind.*

---

*Terms such as *splicing* the gene add to this confusion, when the reality is that we wildly bombard chromosomes, hoping to hit something. (For more, see *Genetic Engineering* by Mae Wan Ho [2000] or *The Triple Helix* by R.C. Lewontin [2000].)

Yet taking hormones or drugs to lower blood pressure or having various and sundry screening tests and scans is presented as empowering for the person and predisposes both women and doctors "to view their current health status in terms of their risk of *future* [italics added] ill health"[56]—a perspective that not only encourages "medicalization of the future," but squarely puts the onus and responsibility for staying well on the individual.

Medically, screening is presented as neutral; it is promoted as part of a sensible program of prevention. Having a bone density scan is considered simple and painless. Yet the consequences of being told one's bones may be on the verge of becoming brittle—or, worse, being labeled as having "osteopenia"—are complicated and often *dis*empowering, as a group of Scandinavian researchers found, for not only did such knowledge produce "new symptom interpretations" and affect how women perceived themselves, but it resulted in a "reconstruction of the body self as weak" and being of "reduced" capacity. Writing in the journal *Social Science & Medicine*, they go on to say:

> Modern medicine works by making the body's invisible parts visible, and the culturally established confirmation of the primacy of the visual also extends to medical technology [linking] the imperatives of "objectivity" and the establishment of visual modes of representations as instruments of knowledge and "truth." . . . The bone scan focuses on the difference between normal and low bone mass (the abnormal). . . . The question is, what implications does a bone scan have for each individual's bodily experience and self perception?[57]

Knowledge is said to equal power, yet the reality, as even this small study starkly demonstrated, falls a long way short of that ideal.

In interviews with sixteen Danish women between the ages of sixty-one and sixty-three, what these researchers found was that women took the bone density scan very literally: as proof of an underlying truth about themselves. Where they once might have discounted a slight backache or fatigue as the result of having done too much, now, post scan, the women felt themselves and their bodies as being diminished. Having been advised that they might be at risk not only did *not* make them feel powerful, but it led to hypervigilance and an overawareness of physical symptoms. Yet as the medical doctor on the research team pointed out,

> From a biomedical viewpoint, osteoporosis is . . . a progressive systemic disease characterized by low bone density and micro-architectural deterioration of the bone tissue, with a consequent increase in bone fragility and susceptibility to fractures. Most frequent are fractures in the wrist, the hip and the backbone, with hip fractures as the most important, because of the association with medical complications and disability and the costs of hospitalisation. However, fractures of the backbone have great significance for women as they may cause . . . a stooped appearance. Among 60-year-old women, the 10-year incidence of a hip fracture is 2.3%. If they have osteoporosis [low bone density; *t*-score below –2.5 SD compared with the average of young healthy adults] the incidence is 7.8%. Hence, *nearly 8 out of 100 women*

with osteoporosis will have a hip fracture within a time frame of 10 years, while 92 will not [italics added].[58]

The women interviewed did not see it that way.* Their reactions ranged from the stoic to the despondent, but all of them were affected, and all of them expressed enormous faith in the technology—with osteopenia, reduced bone mass, and a possible tendency toward osteoporosis all being interpreted as being the same thing as *having* osteoporosis. And many women reporting that they could almost feel the "calcium oozing away from the bones." This complicated the medical advice to stay active (because exercise, particularly weight-bearing exercise such as walking, strengthens bone); many of the women expressed uncertainty as to how much their "osteoporotic bones" could stand—even though none of them were told they actually had osteoporosis. They felt newly fragile, helpless. The scan had created a new self-image. So much for bone density scans being quick and painless or screening being a simple, empowering way of staying on top of your health.

THE TROUBLE WITH OBJECTIVE RESULTS

These women, like most of us, had accepted their so-called diagnosis as having expressed a fundamental truth about themselves. They believed the results of the technology. Yet, as Harvard hematologist Jerome Groopman explains in his popular book *How Doctors Think*, radiological and other results—bone scans, lab results, mammograms, and all the various and sundry types of screening we undergo over time—are the highly subjective distillation of expert opinion. It is a *person*, a human being, who looks at the X-ray or scan or mammogram or blood test and decides whether it is normal or not.

Primary care physicians regularly look to radiologists to confirm or deny a diagnosis, but the process is broken down into two processes: perception and cognition. So, not only must the person reading the scan analyze what she sees, but he must evaluate what it means for the patient. "This dual process is repeated second by second, minute by minute, hour after hour," writes Groopman. A contour, a blur, a variation: any of these could mean something—or nothing. Some screenings result in hundreds of images and "radiologists are expected to look at and analyze images very quickly." Between the speed and the magnitude of the job, it is inevitable that there will be disagreements, not only between different analyses, but even if the same person is shown the same picture at a different time. In one study of one hundred certified radiologists in which some sixty chest X-rays were examined, the same person disagreed with himself or herself an average of 20 percent of the time.[59] As for disagreements between

---

*This type of thinking is reflected in other types of screening; for instance, women who had had a mammogram that had found an anomaly believed they were already suffering from breast cancer.

different doctors, depending on the type and complexity of the test in question, that number can be as high as 80 percent.[60]

Yet medicine—and we—tend to gloss over the frequency of errors (never mind the accuracy of what constitutes "normal"). Depending on the test, the expertise of the person analyzing the results, the care with which the lab handles results, and individual patients and their physiology, different screening procedures can result in false-positive or negative results in ranges anywhere from 74 percent to 96 percent of the time for mammograms, to 75 percent of the time in colorectal screening.[61] These are people we are talking about reading tests, people who get tired, who have bad days, who react with and at their lives. A radiologist who has been sued, for instance, will err on the side of caution—leading to an excess of false positives. Even reading the results of an ultrasound, bone density scan, or an old-fashioned X-ray depends on the skill (and bias) of the radiologist, but in our zeal for medical and linguistic mastery of this scourge we call illness, we set aside doubt and believe in the experts.[62]

So here is a test that purports to make our bones visible, that is said to empower us and allow us to face our future with impunity, allow us to make good decisions about how to cope with impending osteoporosis (which, we are assured, faces a great many of us), based on a group comparison that was never intended for this purpose—a comparison, furthermore, that compares our bones to a statistical average of our younger selves (so to speak) and is increasingly being touted as part of good, preventive care.

For years, we were told that hormone "replacement" therapy at menopause was the solution; then, in 2002, it turned out that the risks of long-term hormones outweighed the benefits. So now we are told to have our bone density measured and to take drugs if our diagnosis warrants it. All this for a disease whose severity appears to have appeared on the scene with alarming rapidity. How did this happen?

Many things happened, of course, but three of them stand out and were particularly important. First, we moved from an acute model of health care, in which medicine was there when we got sick to one that emphasized risk factors and comparisons to an ideal of some sort. Second, there were advances in various technologies, such as bone density scanners, which had both medical and commercial possibilities (and a lot of people interested in both). And finally, because no preventive strategy can have any coherence unless it also includes some kind of intervention or treatment, a new class of drugs appeared on the scene, and these, the biphosphonates, truly made osteoporosis a household word.

FROM SOAP TO NUTS

In the 1960s, the chemists at Proctor & Gamble, the giant corporation that today brings us everything from Crest toothpaste to Mr. Clean, managed to solve a problem that had been plaguing all soap manufacturers for a long time: how to keep their pipes clean. Saponification, or the process of making soap, was a simple business, but the process inevitably produced a type of effluent, a by-product, that was rich in calcium salts and stuck to the plumbing. These salts coated the pipes and had to be cleaned, shutting down production and generally being a pain. Proctor & Gamble engineers, in testing various solutions, came across a class of calcium-binding molecules, the biphosphonates, that seemed to work extraordinarily well at keeping the pipes clear of calcium. Nobody really considered using these as a pharmaceutical, but one day, years before there were too many FDA or legal consequences for creative drug use, a well-read clinician, possibly with a background in biochemistry, wondered if these biphosphonates might be useful in treating a particularly nasty (and rare) disease, myositis ossificans, that causes muscle to harden and turn into bone.

Unfortunately for the patients with this horrible disease, biphosphonates were not therapeutic for the condition. The lone clinician did, nevertheless, publish his observations on this "promising" compound as a clinical anecdote somewhere. This, in turn, caught the attention of the pharmaceutical division of Proctor & Gamble, which set them to thinking: what if these compounds had the potential to do more than just clean pipes? They were not intrinsically toxic, and were conceivably useable, so perhaps these biphosphonates could be used for some other pharmaceutical purpose.[63] After some trial and error, it was found that biphosphonates did not behave in humans as they did in those calcium-clogged pipes; they did not bind to the calcium in the body, but they did, nevertheless, seem to have an effect on the cells, preventing them from removing calcium from the bone. And a new class of drugs was born.

These new drugs were marketed aggressively: their benefits, exaggerated and their side effects, downplayed. Yet these drugs are known for causing (sometimes severe) abdominal side effects and diarrhea, and there is even "concern over an increased risk of vascular, neurological, and laboratory abnormalities" in people who take them.[64] In addition, their cost has been of concern to national health care systems and HMOs, given that the cost/benefit ratio (where health economists determine, numerically and in terms of cold, hard cash, how much needs to be spent to prevent an undesirable result such as a fracture) is low. This overwhelming emphasis on bone density scans and medication, furthermore, has reduced any conceptualization of fracture risk in the frail or institutionalized elderly (which is where the real risk lies) outside these narrow medical limits. Yet, as Finnish researchers writing in the *BMJ* point out (it is interesting that the majority of critical voices seem to originate outside North America),

Numerous studies show that among older people falling, not osteoporosis, is the strongest risk factor for fracture. When a person falls, the type and severity of the fall (including fall height, energy, and direction) largely determine whether a fracture occurs. . . . These fall induced fracture risks are "strong" associations—comparable to those between smoking and lung cancer. Thus, preventing falls is a logical approach to preventing fracture.[65]

Preventing falls would involve various strategies, ranging from exercise (to improve mobility, balance, and muscle strength) to altering the physical environment, such as keeping nursing homes and other sites free of loose bits of carpet or other hazards over which someone might trip. An additional, important, preventive (medical) step would be to ensure that people at risk for falls can see as well as possible (that their glasses fit and are of the right strength, that there is sufficient and good lighting) and that they are not taking medication that makes them dizzy or otherwise impaired and prone to falling. This last step would be significant on many levels because the elderly are notoriously overmedicated. Indeed, a recent U.S. retrospective cohort study of 765,423 patient records from patients over age sixty-five expressed concern for the "common use of potentially inappropriate drugs."[66]

LEAPS OF LOGIC

Prior to the biphosphonates, of course, were hormones and the "estrogen-deficiency disease" paradigm of menopause. As with cardiac disease, proponents did not seem to notice that there was a rather large time lag between menopause and the onset of these conditions; they merely called it a *latent period* that occurred postmenopause, and before symptoms actually developed. (Amazing how one can twist reality to fit one's theory if one sets one's mind to it.) Of course, this time lag could just as easily have been interpreted to mean that the two were not connected.[67] In fact, to suggest that menopause was the "cause" of various age-related ailments always seemed like a stretch, at least to any logical mind.

In medicine, the study of causal relationships is fundamental.[68] First formulated by the immunologist and Nobel laureate Robert Koch in the late nineteenth century (Koch died in 1910), Koch's postulates, as they came to be known, were originally used to describe the bacterial basis (*mycobacterium tuberculosis*) of tuberculosis, with causality expressed as the presence of the bacterium in the organism for the disease to occur. Koch's postulates, later updated by Bradford Hill, the originator of the RCT, added that the *temporal* (or time) relationship between cause and effect also mattered.* But even in infectious disease, where the cause is a virus, bacterium, or fungus, causality is never quite that simple. Unlike what happens in the physical sciences (e.g., in a chemistry laboratory, with the behavior of gases when heated, which always respond in exactly the same way), in a living

---

*For more on causal relationships in medicine, see Notes.

host, the microbe is a *necessary* component but is not *sufficient* in causing disease: poor, immune-suppressed, malnourished, stressed individuals are generally far more prone to illness than their healthy, wealthy, well-nourished counterparts. Even today, when there is an outbreak of some kind—*E. coli* is found in packaged lettuce, for instance—it is always the elderly, immune-compromised, or otherwise weak or ill who are at higher risk; most healthy individuals can weather an extra microbial load.

The nuances and complexities inherent in determining causality medically, however, did not seem to particularly concern the proponents of estrogen. It had been decided, practically since the discovery of sex hormones, that "normal" for a woman translated into those years when she was fertile and menstruating. Anything after that was simply aberrant, wrong, or diseased, and from there, it was an easy, albeit unsound, jump to the notion that it was menopause and the putative lack of estrogen that caused anything that came with age, even though men experienced age-related conditions as well, up to and including in a bone disorder that might or might not occur. This was particularly true with the publication of that famous (or infamous) book, *Feminine Forever*, which cemented the idea that estrogen was marvelous and all women past a certain age needed to take it. This clicked with the time and the technological bent of the time not to mention the American cultural psyche, and estrogen, for many years, was considered *the* most potent force against aging, one that kept the desiccation and wrinkling of time at bay and prevented fractures.

In the previous chapter, we touched on how a confluence of factors after World War II converged during the 1950s and 1960s to change the face of medicine; everything from the discovery of antibiotics (the first drugs that could actually *do* something) to the development and growth of various institutions that could approve drugs (like the FDA) and fund studies (e.g., the National Institutes of Health), as well as single-disease institutions such as the American Heart Association (now the Heart and Stroke Foundation), which dealt solely with cardiovascular disease.

Pharmaceutical companies also gained prestige, power, and influence during this time, moreover, even as new technologies were developed and made their way into practice and common use—in medicine, as in communications, travel, and every other aspect of life. Medical education and the focus of primary medicine shifted from the simple and clinical toward a more generic, prevention-based model. Of course, trauma and acute care also developed in leaps and bounds, not least because the twentieth century had its fair share of wars, and, over time, emergency care, neurosurgery, plastic surgery, and other techniques to repair a wounded and traumatized patient emerged. Today, the wars in Iraq and Afghanistan are fast advancing trauma techniques even as improvements in protective gear create new types of neurological and orthopedic injuries. (When the torso is protected, it is the nether regions that suffer; with better helmets, injuries to the head no longer kill, but as an anonymous army doctor once described, instead, they "scramble" the brain, often leading to vicious, impossible-to-treat, closed-head injuries.)

The RCT, also developed in the late 1940s, provided a means of testing medical interventions, and with the rise of insurance companies and HMOs in the United States, and national health care systems in Canada and Europe, new funding systems and policies came into play. The concept of medical necessity, or what medicine *ought* to be, came to occupy a much larger place than it had before, and health economists and administrators soon became involved as well, to do cost/benefit analyses and analyze risk. In opposition to these groups attempting to restrict care, lobbyists and activists worked the opposite side of the street, trying to sway public and political opinion toward more and more accessible medical care—and succeeded in areas such as AIDS and breast cancer, even as various and sundry chronic conditions and diseases (Parkinson's, Alzheimer's, arthritis, osteoporosis) gained attention and a somewhat larger slice of the health care pie.

Drug companies refined their marketing and promotional efforts, as did non-governmental organizations and not-for-profit and charitable groups, to the point where it seems that every other week now some relay, run, marathon, bake sale, or other worthy fundraising effort is attempting to raise money and increase awareness of one condition or another. Today, as we write this book, the front page of the newspaper is of two pink-wigged women finishing the race "to end breast cancer." Ribbons of all colors, teddy bears, bracelets, brooches, and pins compete for our attention and charitable donations.

Such efforts, although commendable and no doubt important to those who participate (and which have had some success, at least at the start, at bringing orphan diseases like cystic fibrosis or amyotrophic lateral sclerosis—Lou Gehrig's disease—to the public's attention), unfortunately also have the paradoxical effect of shifting attention, money, and individual concern toward particular diseases and distracting us from other important issues, for instance, the fact that more people die from motor vehicle accidents every day than from AIDS, that poverty is actually a greater risk than secondhand smoke, or that lung cancer kills more women than breast cancer. This idea, that some diseases are more worthy than others, raises an interesting point with respect to values and how we rate a disease as being good or bad—not to mention our lamentable tendency to stress our individual contribution to disease and undervalue social, economic, and environmental factors.

Which brings us to back to osteoporosis. Once a little known condition diagnosed retrospectively after a person broke a bone for no apparent reason (in medical parlance, called a fragility fracture)—without a big fall or being in a car accident or what have you—today, osteoporosis has become such a major part of the lexicon and sociocultural landscape that Web popups or TV ads for supplements containing calcium and vitamin D casually use the term, aware that their intended audience knows exactly what they are talking about. In one ad, a group of fifty-something women celebrating a birthday ominously tell the birthday girl that now that she has hit fifty her bones are at risk (as though physiology can tell time and knows your birthday). Our risk of osteoporosis, as we are repeatedly told, is "one in four," a phrase nearly as ubiquitous as the "one woman in nine" who apparently will get breast cancer. A risk that is linked medically, culturally, and socially to menopause and its supposed subtext of estrogen "deficiency."

EMPOWERMENT?

Does anyone actually understand what that phrase "one in four women will get osteoporosis" means (or "one in nine" with respect to breast cancer)? That is unlikely, for although it could be argued that the phrase is technically true (as long as one has total faith in statistics, information gathering, classification systems, and everything else that goes into determining those statistics in the first place), what it translates into is that women's *lifetime* risks of osteoporosis and breast cancer are, respectively, one in four and one in nine. What it does *not* mean is that one woman in four will be diagnosed with osteoporosis; that if there are four women playing bridge one of them will end up with a fragility fracture.

Lifetime risk means throughout a woman's life span, calculated in actuarial terms (which are the tables insurance companies use to determine your risk of living or dying within a certain length of time). In the West, where the average life span is somewhere around eighty or eighty-five depending on where one lives,* the chance of developing osteoporosis is probably one in four. In other words, if a woman lives past eighty, she has a 25 percent chance of getting osteoporosis. She also has a 75 percent chance of *not* getting it. At earlier ages our risk of having osteoporosis or breast cancer is miniscule. By way of comparison with that "one in nine" figure, between the age of thirty and thirty-nine, in a cohort of one thousand women, three were diagnosed with breast cancer and none, *zero*, died of breast cancer. In that age group, there were five deaths, all from "other" causes (which in women of that age probably, unfortunately, meant accident, suicide, or murder). During one's forties, the figures are similar: there were thirteen diagnoses of breast cancer and three deaths. In fact, out of those 1,000 women, even over the age of eighty-five, 434 were still alive.[69] So how did statistics turn from a dry, numeric form of describing the world (versus art, music, or literature) and turn into the boogeyman, the monster under the bed, used to frighten us and convince

---

*For instance, a woman in Japan has an average life expectancy of about 85.2; a woman in Canada, 82.6; an American woman, 80.6.

us to have ourselves "checked" continually for one disease or another and take medication—what some observers call "selling sickness" or "diseasemongering?"

We all need to take a deep breath and relax. There is little we can do by the time we hit midlife with respect to how we lived life as teenagers, which is the single biggest predictor of bone health later in life. Neither can we change our heredity. However, we can take commonsense measures to strengthen our bones such as becoming more active and building strong muscles that help prevent falls (and absorb energy if we do fall). This, incidentally, would be a good idea whether or not we are at risk for osteoporosis. Elemental calcium, a building block for bones, is necessary—and available in dairy (like milk and yogurt) or in pill form—as is vitamin D_3. (It is significant that northern countries, such as Norway and Canada, where sunshine is limited for half the year, often seem to have higher rates of osteoporosis than sunnier climes.[70]) Finally, it is always a good idea to reduce stress, which tends to make any physical condition worse. We could also encourage our daughters to be active, to eat well, maintain a healthy weight (in the hope that they will ovulate normally and maintain optimal health), as well as not overfocus on the negative, as so much medical advice currently seems to do.

In the next, and final, chapter, we cover one last condition that may well be related to healthy ovulation and sufficient progesterone, a disease that scares women terribly—breast cancer—and attempt to put it in a wider context of hormones, culture, the risk factor argument, and life.

BREASTS, BREAST CANCER, AND OVERCOMING OUR FEARS

Although the causal link hasn't been conclusively established, US researchers say there's been a remarkable decline in breast cancer rates since fewer women began taking hormone replacement therapy (HRT) to alleviate the symptoms of menopause. The overall incidence of breast cancer in the US declined 7% between 2002 and 2003, while the number of women aged 50–69 diagnosed with estrogen receptor positive (ER-positive) breast cancer declined 12% over the same period, when millions of women stopped taking HRT after the release of a July 2002 Women's Health Initiative study indicating HRT bore more risks than benefits.

—Wayne Kondro[1]

In the Song of Solomon, the breasts of a woman are compared to "twin fawns" that "feed among the lilies," baby deer on wobbly legs—a fanciful phrase suggesting that even two thousand years ago, women's breasts were the archetypal symbol of attraction, desire, femininity, and womanhood. Today, in North American culture especially, breasts retain their iconic status (unlike more nonchalant cultures where going topless is no big deal), and often a young boy's first foray into manhood is his furtive glance at the *Playboy* centerfold and the model's breasts. As the actress Halle Berry wryly remarked, "The truest cliché about Hollywood is that women have boobs and everybody wants to see them."

The tragedy for adult women (especially at midlife) is that even the most beautiful breasts have the potential to generate fear and the ghastly onslaught of oncology into her life, which makes maintaining breast health and avoiding breast cancer—a disease women fear more than any other—more pertinent than any other topic having to do with their breasts. Breast cancer is a terrifying thing: all of us have known someone with the disease, shared the pain at what is euphemistically called "therapy," and, for many of us, the disease has also meant loss: of a dear friend, sister, mother. Breast cancer is a disease that "seldom countenances dispassionate or objective treatment,"[2] writes professor of medicine Nortin Hadler; the topic "roils" with gender issues and is fraught with a vast, emotive layer of bad medicine and iatrogenesis.* This has had particular resonance in recent years as women realized that the hormones so casually prescribed—estrogen, in particular—were a major factor in the increased rates of breast cancer.

Estrogen is necessary for breasts to grow, as we described in an earlier chapter, but we need *progesterone* for breast maturation—not only in terms of shape and size but to develop the milk ducts beneath. As with all other aspects of women's physiology, therefore, breasts also require the balance, the complementary roles, of these two primary hormones for development and, as it turns out, optimal health.[3] In fact, we believe that regular menstrual cycles with consistently normal ovulation (and progesterone) can potentially prevent fractures and osteoporosis, breast cancer, and heart disease. Yet inevitably, as with virtually every other aspect of women's endocrinology throughout the twentieth century, the centrality of estrogen persists, even as evidence steadily mounts as to its harms.[4]

HORMONE "REPLACEMENT" AND BREAST CANCER

The possible association "between the use of estrogen replacement therapy or combined estrogen-progestin replacement therapy and the incidence of breast cancer" has been evaluated, assessed, analyzed, noted, commented on, and clearly proven in nearly thirty studies, dispassionately observed Seattle public health researcher Chi-Leng Chen in 2002 (and there have been many more studies since then). The incidence of breast cancer, this *JAMA* article adds, for "all histological types combined," increased between 60 and 85 percent in those women who were long-term users of HRT.[5] The evidence linking hormone use with breast cancer had, in fact, been steadily rising for nearly a quarter century; for, although breast cancer has been around since time immemorial, its incidence increased exponentially throughout the twentieth century, specifically with the synthetic estrogen DES, which was given to pregnant women in the 1940s. In particular, the estrogen receptor–positive kind of breast cancer (meaning that the tumor is "fed" by estrogen) has skyrocketed. Throughout most of those years,

---

*Iatrogenesis, from the Greek *iatros,* or "physician," plus *genesis,* "originating in," refers to disease or dysfunction caused by medical examination or treatment. The term usually refers to errors of commission, although many people also include errors of omission.

even as women were being prescribed hormones (well, estrogen), they were falsely assured (and reassured) that although hormone "therapy" might increase their odds of getting breast cancer, it really was nothing to worry about—the cancers connected to estrogen were of a "favorable" type that "did not result in increased mortality."[6] In other words, even though you might find a lump and be diagnosed with breast cancer, the chances were good that the disease would not actually kill you. Cold comfort to a woman who had taken hormones for her health and then found a lump in her breast, even as her mind flew to every worst-case scenario, with all the terrifying implications that the term *breast cancer* has within our breast-obsessed culture.

In fact, "a history of HRT use had only beneficial, and no discernible adverse, effects on breast cancer," soothingly concluded surgical oncologist Julie Cheek, Judith Lacy, and colleagues in the *Archives of Surgery* in 2002, in an article so convoluted it verges on the surreal. Particularly because their primary argument, prior to their bizarre conclusion that HRT had "only beneficial" effects, was that because taking hormones creates denser breast tissue, it made it more difficult for a mammogram to detect a lump. So, tumors were more likely to be found through palpitation (touch), which meant they were "statistically larger" and node-positive. This clearly implied, they wrote, that "women who receive HRT and then develop breast cancer would likely have a *worse prognosis* [italics added]."[7] Pardon? How did a *worse* prognosis manage to morph into a *benefit* in the abstract (summary) at the beginning of the article, probably the most important part because it is the one most people read? And how did this blatant error get by the peer reviewers of this medical journal? The mind boggles. But if this defense of hormone "therapy" seems extreme and irrational, try the one that came up in the spring of 2008.

At this time, the lawyers for the pharmaceutical firm Wyeth (who make Premarin, the most popular estrogen tablet on the planet) asked the judge hearing a class-action suit against "HRT" at the Arkansas Supreme Court to rule that there were no grounds to the argument that estrogen had anything to do with breast cancer. Now that's chutzpah, as our Jewish friends would say (along the lines of the man who murdered his parents throwing himself on the mercy of the court because he was an orphan). As you recall, in 2002, the Women's Health Initiative (WHI) had been stopped early because not only did the estrogen-progestin regimen not decrease cardiac risk, but it *raised* breast cancer rates to an unacceptably high level.[8] Furthermore, the longer women took hormones, the higher the risk.[9] The Wyeth legal team based their preposterous request on the fact that the WHI estrogen-only trial arm did not show any increase in breast cancer, whereas the estrogen-progestin one did. Hence, it *had to be* the smidgeon of progestin, the synthetic progesterone added to prevent the endometrial hyperplasia and cancer that unopposed estrogen could cause in the women who had not had a hysterectomy, that caused the increase in breast cancer.

The estrogen-only arm, of course, was entirely made up of women who had had a hysterectomy. Yet, as Chen and colleagues had clearly found in 705 post-menopausal women in Puget Sound; as the Iowa Women's Health Study had found (although not really admitted);[10] and as a host of articles in prestigious journals such as the *NEJM*, *JAMA*, and *Cancer* had explained; in women from Canada to Greece, there was, as Chen and colleagues wrote, "an elevated risk of invasive breast cancer among postmenopausal women who were long-term, recent users of oral estrogen, either alone or in combination with progestin."[11] No matter how much generations of believers and experts had consistently insisted that estrogen could not *possibly* be implicated in anything so nasty as breast cancer, finally, an analysis with combined data from fifty-one trials and more than 52,000 women (with almost 110,000 controls) convincingly documented that there was a much higher incidence of breast cancer in those women who had taken estrogen.[12] Even more damning were the clear results of the Million Women Study, showing that for every one thousand women taking hormones over ten years, there were five new breast cancers in women on estrogen alone and nineteen new breast cancers for women taking estrogen-progestin.[13] These studies, however, were observational, although prospective, and, as we have learned from the heart disease–estrogen story, observational studies can only show associations. This was something the Wyeth legal team used to their advantage, using the results of the WHI to suggest that breast cancer only increased in the estrogen-progestin arm.[14] (They also omitted to mention that previously, women who had taken only estrogen had an increased risk of ovarian cancer.[15]) Moreover, many researchers also suspect that the estrogen-only arm of the WHI was insufficiently powered (had too few people, in other words) to be convincing.

ESTROGEN AND BREAST CANCER

In terms of the WHI, the reasons for the disparity in breast cancer incidence between the two arms (estrogen alone versus estrogen-progestin) are logical, albeit complex—so bear with us. First off, the dosing: the Premarin used in the trial was 100 percent of a young woman's estrogen, whereas the medroxyprogesterone was a mere 25 percent. The progestin dose simply wasn't strong enough. Second, the women on estrogen-progestin had not had a hysterectomy, and a hysterectomy, which cuts off ovarian blood supply, decreases breast cancer risk significantly, by at least 25 percent.[16] (Interestingly, *any* pelvic surgery reduces the risk of breast cancer, perhaps because the surgery decreases ovarian testosterone and interferes with ovarian blood supply.) Therefore, the women with the higher risk received the combination regimen, whereas the women whose risk was already lower were given estrogen. Additionally, the estrogen-only study enrolled more than five thousand fewer women than the estrogen-progestin one, although it did run longer. Finally, and most important, progestin (medroxyprogesterone) is *not* progesterone. This last difference is crucial, as a French study effectively demonstrated in a massive, prospective observational study of one hundred thousand women, called the E3N, from a health insurance program. What this study found was that menopausal women taking estrogen (in patch or gel form, as is the custom in France) had about 30 percent more breast cancer (similar to the British Million Women Study), and that estrogen with progestin increased breast cancer by 70 percent—but that estrogen plus *progesterone* was not associated with any increase at all.[17] This suggests that it is prudent to use natural progesterone, as we have consistently recommended throughout this book. In France, where dosages of common medications are lower than those of the United States,[18] women were given 100 to 200 mg of progesterone at bedtime rather than progestin (or medroxyprogesterone). Why the synthetic form of progesterone is so different from the bioidentical, oral micronized form remains unknown, although it stands to reason that a bioidentical form of a hormone will be better than a synthetic version.

In terms of estrogen and breast cancer, moreover, as we all know, breast cancer is a disease largely specific to women—men do not tend to develop breast tumors (although it does happen). The ratio of women to men in breast cancer is more than five thousand to one. Furthermore, drugs such as tamoxifen[19] and raloxifene,[20] which are specifically made to antagonize the action of estrogen in the breast, have been shown to prevent breast cancer. That is why they are used. That estrogen is part of the genesis of breast cancer has been demonstrated so often and in so many different ways that it is as close to a fact as we ever have had in medicine. The more estrogen a woman is exposed to throughout her life, therefore, whether it is endogenous or exogenous, the higher her risk for the disease. For instance, a woman whose first period, or menarche, was early, which appears to carry with it higher estrogen levels (and also seems to mean she will be heavier as she grows up), or a woman who has higher than average levels of the male hormone testosterone, possibly because testosterone readily converts into estrogen, has a slightly higher risk of breast cancer. In fact, an incidental finding in a study of older women with osteoporosis (who should have a lower risk of breast cancer than average) noted that those women who were in the highest range for estrogen and testosterone, compared with those in the lowest, had over six times the risk of developing breast cancer.[21]

Additionally, we have also known for a long time that women who, for one reason or another, do not have their first child until they are thirty have a much higher risk of breast cancer. Whether that is primarily in those who are *unable* to have children (of whom about one-third will likely not ovulate normally) or in those who took the Pill for many years is not clear. Weight (fat) and higher levels of estrogen also go hand in hand (as endogenous estrogen levels rise, the more one weighs); women who gained the most weight between their twenties and menopause appear to have a higher breast cancer risk than women who gained the least. In this latter context, it seems that having an apple shape (being rounder, in other words, and carrying the extra weight in the midriff) is more of a risk than being pear-shaped (with a smaller waist but larger hips). In the Nurse's Health Study, furthermore, there was a link between breast cancer and the women who drank alcohol (which increases estrogen levels in the tissues—how we are not exactly sure) versus those who did not drink at all.

What does this gloomy litany imply for those of us who are a bit heavy, like to have the occasional drink, or never managed to have our first child before we hit thirty? Nothing really, because risks, as we discussed earlier, are simply known connections gleaned from populations—epidemiological studies—and statistical analyses of large groups of people. They imply absolutely nothing for the individual. All that any of these associations demonstrate is that virtually any aspect of our lives, any factor, that enhances estrogen appears to promote breast cancer in those susceptible to the disease. Having said that, one of the most consistent risks for breast cancer, one that was noted in the era prior to reliable contraception and in vitro fertilization, is never having been pregnant. In most cases, except for nuns and otherwise celibate groups, this in all likelihood meant that the woman was not ovulating (and therefore did not have sufficient levels of progesterone in her endocrine system to counterbalance what were quite possibly normal estrogen levels). In other words, a lack of progesterone (ovulation) could well be implicated in the how cancerous tissue develops in the breast.[22]

However, as we have repeatedly seen, throughout modern times, anything negative that might be due to estrogen has inevitably been blamed on progesterone. So as the Wyeth lawyers, protesting the innocence of Premarin, their best-selling estrogen pill, insisted, it was not the estrogen that could be at fault; it had to be the progestin—which is quite a stretch. Happily, in the face of the wide array of estrogen–breast cancer associations we have just discussed, the judge declined to accept Wyeth's version of events and the company lost their case.

COULD PROGESTERONE PROTECT THE BREAST?

Estrogen has an important role in enlarging the breasts (and other reproductive organs) at puberty; in addition, estrogen stimulates the proliferation of every tissue in the body. For a long time, scientists believed that progesterone was the same; this was based on examinations of cells in culture exposed to estrogen or progesterone, and on clinical biopsies or by examining the tissues of (menstruating) women having breast reduction surgery (not quite ordinary women). Some of these women were on the Pill or in the second half of their monthly cycle—and there was no way of knowing whether they ovulated or achieved optimum levels of progesterone during each cycle. What these researchers did find was that there was breast cell proliferation, meaning that new cells were being created. Aha, they said. Progestin or progesterone *ought* to be here; the tissue shows proliferation (which, in excess, is a risk for cancer), so it must be progesterone that causes this and therefore breast cancer[23]—the same leap in logic that led the WHI doubters to insist that it was not estrogen, but progestin, that caused the increase in breast cancer. As the alert reader will quickly have noticed, however, this contradicts everything we already know about the basic endocrinology of the menstrual cycle, during which it is the rise of estrogen, prior to ovulation, that causes the endometrial cells to proliferate and the progesterone during the second half of the cycle that transforms and reduces that overgrowth. So why would progesterone suddenly completely change its character as it changed site? It simply makes no sense that it would.

Admittedly, it is difficult to separate the effects of estrogen and progesterone in the latter half of the cycle because estrogen must reach a peak and must have been increasing for about ten days before it becomes possible for the body to even begin to make progesterone. However, two rather good studies—in women (not mice or rats, who have completely different ovarian cycles than humans and whose baseline progesterone is higher)—have cleverly teased out the separate effects of estrogen and progesterone in breast cells. An unlikely collaboration of scientists from Singapore and France* recruited a group of premenopausal women, all of whom had found a worrying breast lump needing surgical removal.[24] They gave each woman an unusual, *local* hormone therapy in the form of a gel, which they applied to the breast that was to be biopsied, starting on the first day of the women's periods. (It is interesting that outside of North America, researchers are far more prone to including women's natural menstrual cycles within their scientific thinking instead of just ignoring them.) This regimen continued for eleven days, up to the day surgery was scheduled.

The women were randomized to receive a gel containing either alcohol alone, natural estrogen (estradiol, in mid-cycle doses), natural progesterone (in luteal peak doses), or both estrogen and progesterone. When these women went into surgery, the surgeon also removed a minute piece of normal tissue about an inch away from the lump to later examine and analyze for hormone levels. The alcohol gel, which was the placebo, predictably showed that estrogen levels were moderate (because the women were eleven days into their cycles). But in the tissue that had had the estrogen gel applied, not only were there high levels of estrogen, but one-fifth of the cells were turning over rapidly (growing/proliferating). The progesterone gel, gratifyingly, overcame the rising estrogen effects so that only a miniscule number of cells (1%) were proliferating. Even with the high-dose estrogen, progesterone sizably decreased cell growth, which is clear evidence that in breast cells (as well as the uterine lining), progesterone seems to *calm* tissue

---

*Although the French have long had a presence in Indochina.

growth—just as it does within the normal menstrual cycle. In other words, progesterone appears to complement estrogen.

If it is indeed true, as we have been saying all along, that progesterone is fundamental to the natural maturation of the breast, that progesterone decreases estrogen's tendency to make cells proliferate, and that having enough progesterone translates into ovulating every month during the menstrual years, then does it also mean that sufficient levels of progesterone lower our risk of breast cancer? Well, that is entirely possible except here there is a problem.

THE TIME ELEMENT

Breast cancer is not an acute illness: the development of a tumor in the breast takes many years—decades. Studying human ovulation, therefore, to see if progesterone could protect against breast cancer would take a long time and be excruciatingly complicated, particularly because it is next to impossible to retrospectively know for certain whether or not a woman has ovulated throughout her life. The only exception is a woman who has persistently been unable to conceive yet has a fertile partner and no blockage in her fallopian tubes, which strongly suggests that she is probably not ovulating normally. Fortuitously, we do have a study along those lines.

From the mid-1940s on, one thousand infertile women were studied for about nineteen years. The objective was to better understand the development of breast cancer, and because this study took place largely before the 1960s, the Pill did not confound the results. One-third of the women were presumed not to ovulate (they were anovulatory), which meant that their infertility was therefore related to "progesterone deficiency." In this group, the risk of *premenopausal* breast cancer was increased five hundred times,* compared to those women who were determined to be infertile due to male-factor or tubal insterility.[25] A second, similar study of breast cancer and ovulation was conducted at the Mayo Clinic in the 1950s and 1960s. Here, thirteen hundred women with polycystic ovary syndrome (better called anovulatory androgen excess, or AAE) who menstruated infrequently and were also obese were compared to a complement of women of similar age in order to track the development of breast cancer over a ten-year period. What they found was that the women who had AAE (characterized by obesity, facial hair, and anovulation) had a risk that was 360 times higher† for *menopausal* breast cancer.[26] So here we have two studies, which may be old but are nevertheless detailed and well conducted, suggesting that not ovulating regularly increases the risk of breast cancer: that estrogen left unchecked, without sufficient

---

*Actual details: risk ratio 5.4, 95 percent confidence interval (CI), 1.1–49.
†Relative risk 3.6, 95 percent; CI, 1.2–8.3.

progesterone to balance it out, can lead to excessive tissue growth in breast cells. This makes intuitive sense as well, for as we have seen throughout this book, it is when our hormones are in balance that we are most likely to be healthy reproductively and endocrinologically.

The time element—and the years that it takes for a breast cancer to develop—creates a different kind of problem, though, one that ties in with our present infatuation for screening, risk factors, preventive health, and staying proactive in our search to root out the cause of all disease. We saw this happen with cardiac disease and osteoporosis; we heard it in the exuberant recommendations for women to take hormones to ward off future disease, without any evidence or logic behind it, and we continue to be subjected to the arrogant advice of prevention gurus, what one ethicist has called the rise of "risk factorology." Yet, if the WHI has taught us nothing, it should at least remind us to pause, take stock, and be cautious, not least at the sheer presumption of so much of this advice.[27]

THE FEAR OF BREAST CANCER

Breast cancer is a frightening illness, and women wrongly believe it is the most common cause of death, which is in fact not true. Even women with breast cancer often die of other causes, as physician Kerry-Ann Phillips and her colleagues demonstrated using data from a cohort of one thousand Ontario girls. Their work, published in the prestigious *NEJM*, found that even women as young as thirty-five who had breast cancer often died from other causes—notably accidents and cardiovascular disease.[28] In fact, the older the woman with breast cancer, the lower her risk of dying from it (see Table 7.1). This mirrors what we know of other cancers; for instance, an older man is far more likely to die *with* prostate cancer than *of* it. Breast cancer, however, is not one illness, and it appears that women with one or other particular genetic mutations (*BRCA 1* and *2*) seem to have a higher risk of the disease. These are the women whose family trees contain long lists of women who have died from the disease (and other linked cancers such as ovarian cancer): aunts, cousins, sisters, grandmothers. And for these women, it is often a frightening race against time:

Jill* was forty when she found a tiny lump in her breast. This was before the genetic link had been identified, but Jill already knew her family history: two aunts, a cousin, her sister, and various distant relatives had all had breast cancer, and some had died of it. Jill had regular mammograms from the time she was in her late thirties. She had a mammogram in April and it showed no cancer. Four months later, she felt that lump. It was cancer; a virulent, fast-growing tumor. Over the following months

---

*This is the only patient narrative where the name was not changed. Jill would not have minded. S.B.

Table 7.1

This table shows 1995 population data from Ontario, Canada looking at the incidence of breast cancer by age, and comparing deaths from breast cancers, cardiovascular diseases, and other causes in a life table for a birth cohort of one thousand women according to five-year age intervals. Reproduced with permission from Phillips, K. A., "Putting the Risk of Breast Cancer in its Place," *New England Journal of Medicine 340*(2), January 14, 1999, pp. 141–144. Copyright 1998 Massachusetts Medical Society. All rights reserved.

Age (yr)	No. Alive at Beginning of Interval	No. of Incident Breast Cancers	No. of Deaths from Breast Cancer	No. of Deaths from Cardiovascular Causes†	No. of Deaths from Other Causes
0–4	1000	0	0	0	6
5–9	994	0	0	0	1
10–14	993	0	0	0	1
15–19	992	0	0	0	1
20–24	991	0	0	0	1
25–29	990	0	0	0	2
30–34	988	1	0	0	2
35–39	986	3	0	0	3
40–44	983	5	1	1	4
45–49	977	8	2	1	6
50–54	968	11	3	2	11
55–59	952	12	3	5	15
60–64	929	12	3	9	25
65–69	892	14	4	16	36
70–74	836	13	5	28	51
75–79	752	11	6	52	70
80–84	624	9	6	89	95
≥85	434	5	7	224	203

*The data were based on the 1995 incidence and mortality rates in the Ontario Cancer Registry.
†This category includes deaths from cerebrovascular causes.

and years, Jill had a mastectomy in the left breast, then had the right one removed prophylactically. After a few years, she had both breasts reconstructed and implants put in.

A petite, blue-eyed dynamo with a huge mass of curly blonde hair, Jill had a small, successful PR firm with five employees. She knew a lot of people and everyone adored her, for what she had in droves was charm. When her friends came to see her in the hospital after that first surgery, she was surrounded by flowers, candy, and every conceivable stuffed toy known to humankind. "I couldn't meet a man when I had two breasts," she complained. "I'll never meet one now, with only one." But she did. Cancer had taught her to take risks, and she knew her time was short. She met Bob, a quiet, humorous man a few years her junior, who adored her. They had two dogs, three cats, and a bird—and Jill rescued every stray animal she met.

For nearly two years, her cancer was in remission. She traveled, grew her business, and worked long hours, trying to cram as much living into the time she had left as possible. Perhaps it was stress and overwork, or perhaps the cancer was simply going to return regardless, but the disease came back. Jill consulted alternative medicine practitioners, healers, anyone she thought could help, while never giving up on the so-called traditional therapies—many of which left her sick, weak, and too ill to move. But Jill was a feisty, fiery fighter, and she kept going. She planned a huge, amazing wedding, a spectacle, starting in a church and ending up in a marina on a hot August day. In Edwardian lace (her late mother's) and a vintage car, she looked like a princess—a very thin princess. She served organic vegetables and dip—she had changed her diet completely and wouldn't even go near anything packaged. She read every book, listened to every bit of advice. She became so focused on doing all the right things that one day, when she realized that she was becoming frantic because she hadn't experienced "joy" in her life that day (as all the self-help books said was necessary), or laughed, she did laugh—at herself. Again, the cancer went into remission.

New tumors grew just as fast as the chemo and radiation could push them back. Her doctors and nurses had her dead and buried and on palliative doses of morphine years before the fact; each time she weaned herself off, refusing to die before she was good and ready. She attended one group therapy session for breast cancer survivors and left halfway through; they depressed her. "They only want to talk about dying," she said. Because her cancer was node-positive for estrogen (and it had just been realized this was significant), she was given the new drug, tamoxifen. She hated it but took it anyway. The hospitalizations became more frequent, but she took her work in with her, along with her cell phone (driving hospital staff wild).

Seven years after that first lump, her body gave out. The oncologist, looking as though he would cry, told her there was nothing more he could do. She went home. Two days later, she slipped into a coma, surrounded by tall trees, her garden, her pets, and all the friends and family who had gathered to tell "Jill stories" and raise a glass of wine to her. The nurse said she could probably hear us. Five days later, she died.

We have all known someone like Jill—which is why breast cancer scares us so much. But the takeaway message from Jill's story is not what you think. It is to demonstrate how futile mammograms are as a proper screening tool, for finding cancer while it is in its early stages as we are so often told it does by everyone from women's groups to random brochures scattered in pharmacies or doctors' offices.

THE MAMMOGRAPHY QUESTION

Mammograms are said to pinpoint abnormal tissue, to find those miniscule lumps we cannot feel, to catch them before they are a problem, except that with those virulent tumors like the one Jill had—the ones you *want* found early— they are almost always useless, their accuracy, negligible. What mammograms do find are noninvasive lumps that, when tested, may indeed prove to have some cancerous (or, increasingly, "pre" cancerous) tissue, which is not going to kill a woman throughout her life.[29] Furthermore, as physician and Dartmouth professor of community health Gilbert Welch points out, there is an enormous amount of disagreement as to what, exactly, constitutes an "abnormal" piece of tissue, particularly in terms of how it will behave in the future.[30] One study that asked ten radiologists to read the same 150 mammograms over again found that they detected cancer correctly (as later confirmed by biopsy results) between 74 and 96 percent of the time. But (wait for it), when it came to *noncancerous* lumps, their errors ranged from 11 to 65 percent.[31] In other words, up to sixty-five women out of one hundred, or two-thirds, could have a false positive and would undergo the strain, stress, and sheer terror of a biopsy, not to mention the physiologic trauma of a surgery (which could, in addition, create scar tissue that could confound or impede future screening). Such surgeries, rooting out a possible cancer that may or may not exist, are neither neutral nor benign—and could bode badly for the health of the breast. There is some suggestion that surgery itself—merely disturbing or traumatizing the tissue (as surgery inevitably does)—could in and of itself stimulate the proliferation of cancer cells by creating new blood vessels (angiogenesis) that "feed" the tumor.[32]

The proponents of early detection, nevertheless, insist that finding these small lumps early and treating them (with surgery, followed by radiation) translates into cancer-free longevity, and they have statistics to back them up—just as the proponents of estrogen, for so many years, had reams of numeric results from observational studies to back up their contention that estrogen saved lives. Yet the evidence that we can cure metastatic cancer is anything but compelling, as is the claim that we can prolong life. In fact, a recent, well-designed study from Norway published in the *Archives of Internal Medicine*, that compared cumulative breast cancer rates in age-matched women residing in four different counties, even makes the revolutionary suggestion that "some breast cancers detected by repeated mammographic screening would not persist" after six years, and could "spontaneously regress" on their own. So by following the recommendations to have regular mammograms we may be subjecting ourselves to the trauma of an unnecessary diagnosis as well as surgery, chemotherapy, and more.[33]

"Improvements are more likely to be apparent than real," writes physician and critic Nortin Hadler. Plus, "much of the 'advance' can be ascribed to 'lead-time bias,' as our ability to detect metastases has steadily increased."[34] In other words, because we are finding lumps that are smaller and smaller, and identifying these women as cancer survivors, which we then throw into the statistical mix, what actually happens is that we are adding time at the beginning of the process, not the end. In other words, it is not that women are living longer, merely that they are living longer with the diagnosis of cancer—a cancer that is unlikely to have caused them any problems throughout their lives, with or without that diagnosis[35]—a diagnosis, furthermore, that is not neutral and can have fundamental consequences, as does the label "in remission."[36]

Previously, we thought of the world in terms of sick or well. Today, we have this peculiar "at risk" category—or "presick" label—that pushes us into the diseased camp even when we feel well. These classifications and characterizations change and evolve, furthermore, and are not always for the best. For instance, small lesions (about the size of the head of a pin) referred to as ductal carcinoma in situ (DCIS), are controversial as to whether they are a cancer at all—ten years ago, they were not, but today, they are, leading to aggressive treatment. What changed? The classification, that's all. There is little evidence that DCIS goes on to become invasive breast cancer.[37]

A perhaps controversial option for a woman given this precancer diagnosis of DCIS is to consider taking progesterone—in a slightly higher dose (400 mg Prometrium at bedtime).[38] This would be a safer, noninvasive first step rather than surgery or estrogen-antagonist drugs (such as tamoxifen*) or some of the newer high-tech, gene-specific therapies. Surgery and radiation are still possible in the future if they are needed. Progesterone is a safer estrogen-antagonist than any drug, particularly because there is some suggestion that estrogen could even "block" the immune system from destroying tumor cells.[39]

CONFOUNDING FACTORS

As with osteoporosis and heart disease, however, influences other than the medical have converged on this emotive subject and how we define "normal." Physiologic issues appear to be the least of our concerns too much of time, even as rules and guidelines dictating the form and structure of medical practice take over. These are often less than objective, as the majority of the experts convened at the consensus conferences at which such determinations are made have been found to have connections to pharmaceutical and medical technology companies, all of whom have a serious vested interest in the subject.[40] Who else would buy their high-tech machines, their drugs, their surgical paraphernalia?[41] Politicians have also become involved in the discussion; after all, what better way to profess support for women, without really having to do anything substantive (such as improving the environment, supporting child care, reducing estrogenic additives and compounds or raising living standards and wages for women)? The U.S. Senate even became involved at one point, passing a resolution that demanded guidelines be changed in favor of mammograms.

Three large, excellent, RCTs, one Canadian and two Swedish, disputed the veracity and value of mammograms as a useful screening tool. In the Canadian

---

*There has been some suggestion that tamoxifen could backfire—by mimicking estrogen—and actually help some breast cancers to grow, according to a molecular scientist at the University of California (see http://www.newscientist.com).

study, widely considered the best, 50,000 women between the ages of forty and forty-nine and 39,000 women between fifty and fifty-nine were randomized into two groups and followed for up to sixteen years. One group had their usual medical care, and the other also had mammograms. In the group that had started out in their forties, 213 women had died after eleven to sixteen years: half the deaths were in the mammogram group, half in the other. After thirteen years, of the roughly 40,000 women who were in their fifties at the beginning of the trial, 622 invasive and 71 in situ cancers (i.e., cancers that had not spread) were found in the mammography group, compared to 610 and 16 in the other. There were 107 deaths in the mammography group, and 105 in the unscreened group. No difference, in other words.[42]

Several august panels have backed down from their authoritative recommendations for all women over forty to have mammograms but many have not, and today many other groups have entered the discussion, from ostensibly charitable organizations to grassroots women's groups (who could, for all we know, be funded by the makers of tamoxifen or one of the newer estrogen-antagonist drugs, because many such groups are, and unless we dig deep, we have no way of knowing whether a group developed organically or was organized as a PR maneuver). It has become politically incorrect to say one does not have mammograms, tantamount to admitting to some heinous crime (or at least a felony), as one of the authors of this book (S.B.) has found out. Mammograms, as someone ironically said, constitute our god-given right to radiation. And that is another issue we tend to forget: namely, that mammograms are radioactive and that radioactivity can *cause* cancer. This is not to say that they inevitably will, but in a vulnerable host, repeated doses of radiation could be carcinogenic. Unfortunately, science is no match for advocacy and PR.[43]

The two other large mammography trials, both Swedish, were also comprehensive, although not as detailed as the Canadian one. Both these studies—one in the city of Malmo and the other in Stockholm—had similar results and conclusions.* In terms of evidence, the Cochrane Database, the repository for the best available studies, considers the Canadian and Malmo studies as the only ones of "sufficient quality" to include in their list. In short, it appears that we are asking more of this particular imaging technology, the mammogram, than it can possibly deliver.[44]

This is not to say that no woman should ever have a mammogram; rather, it is a plea for moderation and less either/or thinking. There is no reason for all women to be shamed or pressured into having a mammogram; no reason for funds that could be used more effectively against breast cancer to be sunk into more mammography machines. Nevertheless, if a woman is genuinely frightened

---

*The Malmo study (of mammography) enrolled forty-two thousand residents aged forty-five to seventy between 1976 and 1978. The Stockholm trials enrolled sixty thousand residents in 1981. Both monitored subjects for at least eleven years. There was little suggestion that mammography saved lives.

of breast cancer—to the point where it is keeping her up at night—and a mammogram would give her peace of mind, fair enough. Or, if there is a family history fraught with stories about the disease, and, for some reason, you would genuinely feel better knowing you had tried to be proactive (especially if given a clean bill of health), then, by all means, seek one out. Just be aware that the process is considerably more ambiguous, more uncertain, and less accurate than it has been presented—like so much else in medicine generally and women's health specifically.

WOMEN AND MEDICINE

Women have not been well served by medicine generally, throughout the modern era especially, and nowhere is this more obvious than in the history of hormones or in the diagnosis and treatment of breast cancer. Initially, breast cancer surgery was a mutilating, horrific process during which surgeons removed not only the tumor and surrounding breast, but every bit of muscle and tissue, practically scraping the chest cavity. Surgeons drained the lymph nodes in the armpit (not to mention the neck, chest wall and cavity, and every conceivable orifice that might harbor a bit of cancer), and the story of this procedure, radical mastectomy, remains one of the more cautionary tales. This surgery was considered right and proper, undertaken ostensibly to protect the woman, because the scalpel was considered the instrument of cure.[45] (As surgeons still sometimes say, nothing heals like clean steel.) Radical mastectomy was the standard of practice for far, far longer than it should have been because that is how it was done and how it had always been done.

This type of thinking, also known as heuristics, has been the driver for most medical practice throughout the years, as the estrogen debacle aptly demonstrates. The rules of thumb and common practices that medical heuristics involve were passed down through the years, repeated over and over, and contrary to what many people believe, medicine has not had to face up to the harsh reality that many, if not the majority, of its practices have been—not to put too fine a point on it—just plain wrong.[46] As physician Clement McDonald writes, the "conceit" of medicine has long been that it is broadly scientific and empiric, yet nothing could be further from the truth—particularly today, as medicine has grown in size and scope, increasingly driven by abstract rules and statistical precepts, even as treatment thresholds are set progressively lower. He adds:

> As a resident I was often chided to "treat the patient, not the numbers." . . . [Today] most of the arguments about "treating the numbers" in the case of asymptomatic patients have been won by the "numbers treaters." . . . The medical community has always been prone to assume that it knows most of what there is to know. This is a

common mistake in science. During the 18th century, physicists decided that their real work was done; the only thing left was to grind out solutions to the Newtonian equations. . . . Then along came quantum mechanics.

Women's health care, in particular, has, for too long, been blighted by this shortsighted arrogance, as various feminist writers have forcefully pointed out. Women rarely had the power or status to contradict the authority of medicine, and much of the time they also had no idea of (and were not told) the risks or the downside so they didn't know to speak out against mutilating or harmful practices.

A professor of surgery in Massachusetts during the late 1960s, Oliver Cope was a physician who did not believe radical mastectomies were necessary. Not only did they not improve survival compared to historical controls (earlier generations of women who had not had the extensive surgery had the same 50% survival rate), but the process was a horrific one, with drastic side effects. Yet no medical journal would publish Cope's observations, and his work was rejected over and over again, never making it past the peer-review process (compare this to the gobbledygook published about hormones not causing invasive breast cancer earlier in this chapter). Cope eventually gave up on the medical journals and wrote a piece in a women's magazine.[47] Women, thankfully, read it, and what revolution there was began with women patients demanding that the procedure be done less harshly. Women surgeons like Susan Love (author of *Dr. Susan Love's Breast Cancer Book*) also made an impact, and, eventually, lumpectomies (taking out the lump and leaving in the surrounding tissue) became the norm.

In the 1970s, Cope's perspective led to renewed interest in mastectomy surgery, and Bernard Fisher, in the United States, and Umberto Veronesi, in Italy, undertook RCTs of the various surgical approaches to treat breast cancer, discovering that ancillary lymph node removal made no difference.* This finally turned the heuristics of radical mastectomy upside down, but alas, medicine continues to be as slow as it ever was in terms of changing its practices, beliefs, and firmly held convictions—the belief in the power of hormones to fix all manner of problems being a case in point.

Patients, doctors themselves, and researchers often truly believe that medicine is founded on objective science, yet this "quantitative research paradigm" represents only a small fraction of medicine and "confined access" to clinical knowledge, suggests Norwegian physician Kristi Malterud. And the difficulty for medicine is not that such problems occur but that medicine lacks strategies for integrating interpretive and dynamic strategies into medical practice, in effect threatening to "expunge its primary subject," the living, breathing person who is the patient.[48] Doctors such as Cope, who challenge accepted practice, are shunted aside, their

---

*The removal of the lymph nodes goes on, however, causing disabling edema and other symptoms. Those of us with an interest in the immune system also wonder how removing the immune cells closest to the affected site could possibly help the woman recover in the long term.

observations ignored, in favor of the tried and the so-called true, without any real understanding of the underlying physiologic processes involved or the convoluted pathways through which clinical decisions are made. As patients, in our quest for certainty, our desire to believe in the inherent truth of what we are told about our health, we are often complicit in this, seeking out certainties and rejecting any mention of ambiguity or doubt. It is important, therefore, that we remind ourselves that medicine, like all other human activities, involves what Malterud calls "living bodies of human beings in their sociocultural environments" that are subject to all manner of biases, prejudices, false beliefs, and magical thinking. This means that as individuals, as patients, we not only need to be vigilant, but we should take much of what we are told with a large grain of salt. We need to realize that there is—and need to be prepared to live with—a measure of uncertainty. There is always ambiguity in individual physiology, in medicine, in therapeutics, and always will be.

INTEGRATING TOWARD A HEALTHY FUTURE

In this book, we hope to have given the reader much to think about, not only about hormones and the complexities of physiology and endocrinology, but also about the broader context—the time, place, and even position—within which our knowledge, of medicine, as of anything else, is portrayed, presented, and explained.

Perhaps you had never thought terribly hard about what menopause means; conversely, you could be one of the millions of women who had internalized the notion of "estrogen deficiency." Certainly it is a common enough phrase. Perhaps you had never heard of perimenopause—on the other hand, perhaps you are one of those women, like us, who are having or have had enormous difficulties concentrating, sleeping, or maintaining any thermal regularity, making it nearly impossible for you to function with any degree of normalcy. Yet your cycles are still regular and your doctor assures you that you are too "young for menopause." It seems unlikely that you are that familiar with the fundamentals of perimenopause, however, particularly because—contrary to the assurances we have been given about hormones for so long—not only is this time not a "deficiency" of estrogen, but an *excess*, a transition period during which estrogen levels veer out of control, often fluctuating wildly. It is progesterone, the forgotten hormone, whose levels are low and not present in sufficient quantities to create that essential balance of hormones we need to function normally.

Most important, what we hope to have helped you realize is that there is no such thing as a "good" or a "bad" hormone—unlike the rhetoric that proponents of estrogen have been so quick to promulgate, even as they vilified progesterone and raised estrogen on a pedestal so high it was bound to fall off and hurt something.

As it did. Hundreds of thousands, millions, even tens of millions of women, if we go back to the earlier part of the twentieth century, were told to take estrogen, and sadly, too many of these women suffered the consequences of this blind faith that there was only one hormone, estrogen, worth bothering about. Who knows how many women died or were disabled permanently from the breast cancers, heart disease, strokes, blood clots, and more that this imbalance of hormones created for them. With this book, we have simply tried to put estrogen in its place, where it belongs, next to and alongside progesterone—waxing and waning over time and as our bodies change, from puberty and young womanhood through to adulthood, pregnancy, midlife, menopause, and beyond. And it is in their essential *balance* that these two hormones, estrogen and progesterone, need to be conceptualized.

Physiology is what it is. Disease and dysfunction are what they are. There is no point in directing negative emotions or angry language, using those military metaphors of which we are so fond, insisting that we are going to *kill* the cancer or *destroy* the tumor; to insist that we are going to *fight* this all the way with whatever *weapons* or drugs are on hand, as though there are ever winners and losers in a game where the goal is just to live as well, as healthily, as fully as we can.

It is not possible to understand the workings of progesterone or estrogen or any other aspect of health or illness outside the context of society and culture and the world in which we live, any more than we can taste something by simply reading its ingredients out loud. The air we breathe, the food we eat; our lives, the stresses in our lives, and how we fit into the society at large: all of these affect us physiologically as well as psychologically, socially, domestically, personally, and more. In terms of medicine and endocrinology, however, the real world—from pop culture to social norms and patterns, beliefs, values, politics, economics, and commerce—has a far greater impact on us than we sometimes appreciate, not only in terms of how we feel, but what we determine as being health or sickness. For instance, our world, our culture, casually creates estrogen excess through everything from the plastics and other compounds we are exposed to on a daily basis to the food we eat—in the hormones that factory animals are fed to make them grow faster, in the additives and colorings that make things look and taste nice, even though all they are designed to do is give these products a longer shelf life.*

As for other aspects of health, such as staying slender or maintaining good bones, our highway- and car-obsessed culture does not encourage walking (a terrific, weight-bearing exercise that is good for bones as well as weight). Often,

---

*We also tend to use soy as an additive in everything from chocolate bars to frozen pizza. Soy, a crop that did not exist on this continent until recently, contains phytoestrogens, which may well be beneficial in small quantities, but for those of us who have migraines, for instance, it can add up and cause symptoms. Eastern cultures use soy sparingly, not in the amounts we do.

there are no sidewalks next to roads, and you take your life in your hands if you try to walk or ride a bicycle to pick up a loaf of bread at the store, so we end up taking the car—and we gain weight and lose bone density. Then, with increasing stress and weight gain, our protective brain cuts back on energy and inhibits ovulation, for as we described earlier, it is the survival of the organism in its entirety that concerns the brain; reproduction can be put aside for a time. So, we have to contend with infertility or cysts on our ovaries or other such problems—which we now classify as medical even though their basis is, at least in part, social, cultural, and political. We medicalize life, menopause, hormones and easily describe any problems in our lives by using the idioms of physical distress. Yet it is *everything*—who we are, where we live, and what happens in our homes, our neighborhood, our city, our country, within the larger economy, and around the world. In short, everything is connected, and to suggest otherwise is simplistic and reductionist—the two types of thinking we have tried to steer clear of in this book.

ATTEMPTING TO TRANSCEND GENDER

The most cursory glance around us reveals just how persistent and regularly reinforced our notions of gender difference are. Commercials hone in on women's domestic and child-care roles, and even diapers come in gender-defined colors lest anyone forget that boys are the active ones and girls the pretty ones. A respected American author, immunologist, and political commentator, recalls that when her son was an infant, his hair was quite long and blonde. "Aren't you pretty," a waitress, mistaking him for a girl, cooed. On being told he was a boy, the waitress didn't skip a beat: "*Tough* little guy, eh?" No irony intended. We talk differently to babies, depending on whether they wear pink or blue, and encourage them to behave differently: boys are encouraged to explore and move (even when they're too young to) and girls are held, encircled, and toys are brought over to them.* Such immediate and continual conditioning cannot help but have an effect.

From the time they are tiny, boys learn that men are in charge, that men run the world, and real men don't clean (even their own barbecue); girls learn to be good, not to interrupt, and to model themselves on mommy, who does all the housework regardless of her work outside the home or the money she brings to the household. Yet human behavior is so variable that it is impossible to reduce differences between people down to a single factor, gender, and have it stand up

---

*This is based on a study that S.B. watched as an undergraduate. A small baby was dressed in pink or blue (nobody was told what the sex of the baby was) and reactions to the baby were filmed. The differences were striking.

to scrutiny. There is no question that boys and girls, men and women, behave differently, but, from the moment a child is born and the sex is determined, every child is treated differently depending on what sex the surrounding social group believes it is—right down to the color of the bib. The Nobel Prize–winning chemist Eric Kandel, among others, has demonstrated with enormous elegance that *how* we think and behave physically alters brain chemistry, which means that the neurological makeup of the brain is not set, but develops throughout our lives and is affected by what we do, how we think, and how we are treated.[49] So any differences we subsequently "see" in scans and tests (or autopsies) are not necessarily innate, as we assume them to be. Yet so convinced are we of the binary nature of sentient beings that even those barely mobile, asexual blobs of marine goo, algae, are assigned gender roles, as biologist Ruth Hubbard ironically describes a male ethologist doing, in her book *The Politics of Women's Biology:*

> Even among very simple organisms such as algae, which have threadlike rows of cells one behind the other, one can observe that during copulation the cells of one thread act as males with regard to the cells of a second thread, but as females with regard to the cells of a third thread. The mark of male behavior is that the cell actively crawls or swims over to the other; the female cells remain passive.[50]

Medicine is not immune from this deep gender bias. Take a recent (2004) edition of an endocrinology textbook,[51] which lists, in the section on infertility, among the causes for the inability of a couple to have children "ovulatory defects, pelvic disorders [and] male factors," without anyone having noticed that the blame is squarely placed on the sex organs of the woman, medically and linguistically.*

Or, as anthropologist Emily Martin describes in the introduction to the 1992 edition of her book, *The Woman in the Body*, a graduate student in biology had not even begun to realize how much our cultural assumptions had affected her scientific studies until she understood that she had so internalized the notion that sperm are "virile" and aggressive that when she first observed lobster sperm through the microscope she thought they were dead—because they didn't move as she assumed all sperm must (and lobster sperm do not).[52]

TAKING BACK OUR POWER

This book is our attempt—as women who experienced a difficult perimenopause, as scholars, as feminists, and authors†—to give women a new way of

---

*In communications science, this is referred to as the connotative meaning of a text, which is often invisible to the reader. A text such as this actively constructs the reality of which it speaks. Alas, this is not an area science and medicine understands or appreciates.

†Perhaps even as activists, although J.C.P. is far more an activist than S.B. could ever be.

thinking: about medicine, about their bodies, about hormones, and about their journey into midlife, menopause, and beyond. It is also our attempt to introduce some sanity into the discussion on women's hormones and remind medicine, remind women, that progesterone *matters*—perhaps more than anyone currently could imagine. Progesterone can treat perimenopausal symptoms, such as heavy flow,[53] and help with sleep problems and night sweats.[54] It can help with the mood swings[55] caused by high estrogen.[56] If, once into the calm of menopause, hot flushes and night sweats continue to interrupt sleep and drain energy, progesterone (or in this case, medroxyprogesterone) is just as effective as estrogen.[57] And it is likely, although the trial (by J.C.P.) is not yet finished, that oral micronized progesterone will be highly effective at treating night sweats and will protect against breast cancer[58] and help with sleep,[59] and may well also play a part in a healthy cardiovascular system.

Unfortunately, when the template for "normal" is that of a man (and often a young man at that), then women's physiology, particularly relating to hormones, which change throughout our lives, becomes somehow "wrong" and pathological. It was only in the mid-1980s—through intense lobbying on the part of feminists and women activists—that issues relating to women and research even began to be noticed and some political interest developed in the United States with respect to the dearth of women taking part in clinical trials. Until the early 1990s, in fact, FDA policy had actually prohibited women in their childbearing years from participating in drug trials, whether these were Phase I or Phase II trials (in which drug safety profiles were established), probably due to the lingering memory of the thalidomide disaster and the deformed babies. Eventually, politicians became involved (notably several congresswomen), and Congress directed the National Institutes of Health, on whose funding many researchers relied, to conduct research according to the standards they themselves had set up some years earlier (in 1986), requiring researchers to specify whether women were included in a study and, if not, why not. The change in policy, undertaken under duress and pressure from feminists and politicians, was in response to growing criticisms that women's health was being ignored. The reason that had been cited, of course, was that women might become pregnant—but even women who were not going to become pregnant (because they used birth control, were abstaining from sex for some reason, or had partners who had had vasectomies or were sterile, for instance) were not allowed in.[60]

If that were not bad enough, the cutoff date for entry into clinical trials was and continues to be either sixty (usually) or sixty-four, which means that as we age we have no idea whether the drugs we take actually will work for us. This has created numerous problems with pharmacotherapy because once a drug is approved, it is prescribed to both men and women, young and old, with the assumption always being that everyone will react in the same way—like the young men on whom they tested the drugs. Naturally, older women were also excluded in case they took hormones or had had a hysterectomy, which might affect the efficacy of the trial drugs.[61] What this translates to is that women of a certain age often have no way of predicting whether the drugs they are prescribed are safe or appropriate for them.[62] It is therefore important that we, as individuals, not take evidence—even good evidence—to necessarily mean "truth" and approach such therapeutic options with some caution. It is also important to remember that clinical trials, by their very nature, are an artificial slice of life that can only be extrapolated to the general population with extreme caution—as the Hawthorne effect shows.

OF GOLD STANDARDS AND CLINICAL TRIALS

In 1927, at the Hawthorne Works of the Western Electric Company in Chicago, a group of the company's engineers wanted to better understand productivity and what could be done to improve it. With a representative from the U.S. National Research Council, these men set out to "determine the effects of different levels of illumination on workers' performance." So, they turned the lights up in one section of the company (where the workers, all women, were experienced at "winding induction coils on a wooden spool") and left the light of another group (the controls) alone. Much to their amazement, the productivity of both groups went up identically.[63]

Puzzled, they then decreased the light. Productivity still went up for both groups. Despite the difficulties inherent in working in next to no light, the women worked faster and better. Thinking it might be some kind of group effect, they then tested just two workers; just as before, productivity and speed increased. At one point, "the light was reduced to .06 of a foot-candle," which is about the same as a moonlit night, and the women still maintained their efficiency. They reported no eyestrain and even said they found it less tiring to work with less light. What was going on?

These surprising results caught the attention of researchers at Harvard Business School, who trekked over to Chicago to investigate, and, over the next five years, they tried manipulating anything and everything they could think of. They changed rest periods and breaks, altered the duration of the working day, and any other external factor that came to mind. Productivity just kept going up and up. Finally, the researchers realized that it was not *what* they did; rather, it was the fact that they were doing anything at all. As retired physician and essayist Robert Silverman writes,

> Interviews with the workers suggested that the mental attitude of the group of test workers had undergone a definite change during the protracted experimentation. The women felt they received special recognition as participants in the study and, as a consequence, were responding more to prestige gained than to any specified change

in working conditions. These classic studies of the work output of Western Electric Company workers established the Hawthorne Effect as a distinct and important influence in studies of industrial relations: The effect (usually positive or beneficial) of being under study upon the persons being studied; their knowledge of the study often influences their behaviour.[64]

In other words, the women had responded to the attention. Here they were, factory workers, women, not terribly important in the grand scheme of things, especially in the 1920s and 1930s, and these grand people from Harvard had come down to see their work. The women blossomed. We all do when we feel good, when we feel valued, when we feel as though our work, our lives, *matter*.

So in the end, it is this that we need to hold on to. Once we know and have the courage to face what is real in ourselves, regardless of what anyone else thinks, when we can think for ourselves and trust our own judgment—especially with respect to our health, our bodies, and ourselves—then we will be less likely to believe the myths or the statistics, the misinformation and half-truths, whatever the subject. In this book the focus has been perimenopause, menopause and hormones, and progesterone especially, but the basics hold true in all manner of areas. If we are able to accept ambiguity and vanquish fear, we can accept our bodies and their changes, hormonal and otherwise. As Eleanor Roosevelt said, "You gain strength, courage and confidence by every experience in which you really stop to look fear in the face." Or as her husband said, there is nothing to fear but fear itself.

Afterword: The Estrogen Conspiracy

Jerilynn C. Prior, MD

If we are to raise young women to be confident about knowing how their bodies work . . . we would have to start teaching them body-management as schoolgirls. We would soon discover that we had no answers to the most obvious questions about how healthy women function. Three hundred years of male professionals' lancing women's bodies as if they were abscesses is not easily undone.

—*Germaine Greer*[1]

my heart is moved by all I cannot save;
so much has been destroyed,
I have cast my lot with those
who age after age, perversely
with no extraordinary power
reconstitute the world.

—*Adrienne Rich*[2]

Susan Baxter and I have covered a lot of territory—historic, scientific, medical, and cultural—in this book so far. This chapter is my chance to provide a personal perspective on how "the estrogen errors" look from my vantage point as a woman, physician, researcher, and teacher who has struggled to make a factual understanding of women's reproduction—including progesterone as well as estrogen—part of our whole health as women.

To say I feel there is an estrogen conspiracy sounds overly dramatic—I'll admit that it even seems paranoid—in the vein of cures "they" don't want you to know about. However, I feel like the medical or hormonal conflicts in which I have been unwittingly embroiled for more than thirty years are more than a passing error or mere controversy; this is not just about differing points of view. The concept that Estrogen is Good and embodies all that is alluring, sexy, and accommodating about womanliness—coupled with the notion that Progesterone is Evil and related to all that is fickle, bitchy, and bad about being female is so pervasive as to be carefully crafted and equally meticulously maintained.

Clearly, there is more here than debate about "scientific truth." Most thoughtful people agree on certain ways of doing research—there is no gender gap in research methodology and philosophy. Well-designed studies lead to reliable and accurate information that is usually accepted, or at least accommodated until proven false. The most dependable research boils down to a synthesis of results of randomized double-blind, placebo-controlled trials asking the same or similar questions but performed in different places and populations. Ideally, this meta-analysis should lead to a robust, true result. However, there is much more to scientific endeavor than that simple and clear idea. There are many steps in the process of doing science into which culture, the dominant theories of the day, and the most powerful thought leaders of the era have potentially crippling input: what questions are allowed, what kinds of hypotheses can be funded (by various granting bodies), what studies people (women, in this case) will participate in, what experts can say, what medical students can be taught and what results are ultimately publishable.

Thus, there are many issues in this so-called estrogen conspiracy story, but the one that has recently been front and center for me relates to the treatment of night sweats and hot flushes. In 2007, after almost thirteen years of repeated (I think totaling twenty-six) rejections, I finally got data from a randomized, double-blind, one-year comparative trial published.[3] These data are unique: no other randomized and blinded study of women following premenopausal surgical menopause (meaning a menstruating woman who had both the uterus and the ovaries removed) has made a head-to-head comparison of any form of estrogen to a progestin (progesterone-like drug) for the treatment of hot flushes and night sweats. This study directly compared conjugated equine estrogen (Premarin), the largest-selling estrogen preparation, especially in the United States, with medroxyprogesterone acetate (Provera), the most commonly prescribed synthetic version of progesterone (progestin, or progestogen) in North America. It is a unique study because women participants were enrolled immediately as they left the hospital following their surgery—thus all were experiencing the same major hormonal disruption of moving from premenopausal to menopausal with a figurative scalpel stroke.

The multiple rejections of this paper bring us back to my feeling that there is an estrogen conspiracy. I believe the key reason that this study was repeatedly rejected, despite the uniqueness and clarity of its design, is in the results. The reason is that the data showed something unthinkable in this estrogen-centric culture—namely, that medroxyprogesterone is as effective as estrogen at treating hot flushes.[4] Meanwhile, during the thirteen long years I was trying in vain to put into the public domain the important new information that medroxyprogesterone was an effective alternative to estrogen for treatment of severe night sweats, three large, well-publicized, RCTs were published showing that conjugated equine estrogen (the same estrogen I studied) caused strokes and blood clots and did not (as was fervently hoped) prevent heart attacks.[5] In response, millions of menopausal women who had been taking hormonal therapy wanted to, and tried to, stop.[6] Because stopping estrogen commonly makes hot flushes, night sweats, and general misery worse (much like withdrawal from heroin), many were forced to restart the estrogen therapy despite their justifiable fears. Estrogen was the only thing (i.e., about which their physicians knew) strong enough to treat severe sleep-disturbing hot flushes for which herbs, soy supplements, clonidine (a lower dose of an older blood pressure pill), newer antidepressants in the Prozac family, or antiseizure/pain medicines (like gabapentin) were unable to offer adequate relief.

When I designed that study in the early 1990s—which, incidentally, had a primary bone physiology outcome—I suspected that the progestin would be as good or better than the estrogen for severe hot flushes based on the published results of six randomized, placebo-controlled trials of medroxyprogesterone. As a woman who had experienced severe night sweats in perimenopause/menopause, I knew an effective therapy was essential. I also felt strongly that an effective alternative to estrogen was important for women's health, having predicted the disastrously negative results of those big hormone trials.[7] For all of those reasons, I was determined to get our positive, helpful, and scientific results published. Instead, they were repeatedly rejected. So I spent almost half the years of my academic career sending this paper out, getting a rejection, revising it, reanalyzing the data, asking for more advice from statisticians and other researchers, sending it out, getting yet further rejections, and sending it out again.

Why should it be controversial that progestin was as effective as estrogen for menopausal hot flushes? Why should I have to work that hard to get this well-designed and well-executed study published? That's the rub. Everyone—physician and woman alike—knows that estrogen is the gold standard for treating hot flushes.[8] Estrogen is the gold standard not just for hot flushes, but for all of women's health—it will take a lot more than shockingly negative results in randomized, double-blind, placebo-controlled trials in more than thirty thousand women to change our minds on that. Gynecologists and obstetricians, as a medical specialty, appear to consider that their acquired personal wisdom trumps any experimental design[9] or the results of any NIH–supported trial.[10]

What is so controversial about the notion that medroxyprogesterone is effective for severe night sweats and hot flushes? I feel that these data are controversial because of the conspiracy to keep estrogen atop its eighty-five-year-old pedestal.* I believe that this exalted position for estrogen is intimately related to the inferiority of women in this culture. Estrogen occupies this position because it can be used by experts to fix women. That fixable-with-estrogen idea is based on the beliefs of a lot of scientists and physicians, and with support from billions of pharmaceutical company dollars. Wyeth is the main drug company (formerly Ayerst, then Wyeth-Ayerst) for it is the brilliant inventor of two all-pervasive myths: (1) menopause as an estrogen-deficiency disease and (2) hormone *replacement* therapy. There is nothing in the world to compare with estrogen. Estrogen is the bee's knees for the treatment of women—no data can possibly challenge that truth.

I believe that were the rational, the logical, even (dare I say it) the scientific view prevailing in women's health, no woman would take estrogen therapy for hot flushes and night sweats. Furthermore, no physician would prescribe it (for fear of losing his medical license, being blackballed in the medical community, or being sued by her patients). The only justification for estrogen therapy for hot flushes is an early menopause (before age forty). A woman with early menopause has come up short of the thirty-five to forty years of her normal life cycle in which estrogen and progesterone are cyclically high. For early menopause, the physician should prescribe a human form of progesterone daily, in second-half-of-the-cycle (luteal phase) doses, plus transdermal (through the skin as a patch, gel, or cream) 17-βestradiol, the estrogen that is natural for humans. It is important that estrogen be prescribed in a form absorbed through the skin because our best evidence indicates that oral estrogen is four times more likely to cause blood clots than transdermal estrogen.[11] Progesterone (the kind that is identical to what our ovaries can make) is available as a pharmaceutical little round capsule—three of them (300 mg) at bedtime keep the blood level of progesterone in the luteal phase range for twenty-four hours.[12]

If a woman has severe hot flushes, why not give her the *choice* between medroxy-progesterone and a transdermal estrogen? (Obviously remembering that she needs progesterone with estrogen to prevent endometrial cancer if she still has her uterus.) With appropriate dissemination of the available information, including that medroxyprogesterone is similarly effective as estrogen—and that there is no solid evidence that it, without estrogen, causes blood clots, heart attacks, or strokes—I believe few women would be so foolhardy as to want estrogen therapy. In a better world, I believe all menopausal women with sleep-disturbing

---

*Most recently, after the initial draft of this book was submitted, *The New York Times* broke a story that Wyeth, maker of Premarin, had paid ghostwriters for favorable articles and editorials about estrogen (http://www.nytimes.com/2008/12/12/business/13wyeth.html).

hot flushes would be treated with a progestin (or better yet, oral micronized progesterone).*

However, there is another side to the deification of estrogen in women's health—since the 1930s, everything negative about estrogen, or being a woman, or feeling bad premenstrually has been blamed on *progesterone*. Medroxyprogesterone is repeatedly blamed for every side effect during menopausal hormone therapy, despite the fact that two randomized, double-blind, placebo-controlled trials have shown that it does not cause premenstrual symptoms, depression, weight gain, or anything else seriously negative.[13]

Results of well-conducted scientific trials, however, do not matter—women and physicians have become convinced that progestin and progesterone are bad.

For every god, there is a corresponding devil. I give a recent example of the extent of this persistent bias against progesterone. I was attending the American Society for Bone and Mineral Research meeting in 2007, diligently reviewing posters. I went to look at one about treatment of osteoporosis in young women. I was curious why the authors had tried estrogen therapy (with a smidgeon of progestin) for these *pre*menopausal women with fractures. I spoke with the senior author, a prominent scientist and former president of the Society for Bone and Mineral Research, asking her why she had not studied cyclic oral micronized progesterone for these women (given that I had shown cyclic medroxyprogesterone to significantly increase bone in a similar population[14]). She retorted angrily, "Progesterone is an evil hormone!" Taken aback, I asked—trying to calm myself against her vehemence—why she thought that. "I know how I felt when I was on it," she spluttered.

"But weren't you also on estrogen?" I asked. Undoubtedly she, who was middle-aged like me, had been treated with estrogen. She turned away—end of discussion.

The forces that keep so-called hormone "replacement" therapy in the news and under doctors' prescribing pens have a power greater even than that of omniscient science in our culture. They have a power stronger than the trillions of pharmaceutical dollars vested in them. They have the power of women's centuries-old inferior status in our present culture. (I hold out faint hope because this gender power imbalance has not always been present.)[15] Since written history we, as women, are privileged only when acquiescing to men and, since the 1930s, taking the various forms of estrogen that rescue us from otherwise certain degradation.

---

*We are currently completing a randomized, double-blind placebo-controlled trial of oral micronized progesterone (marketed as Prometrium in North America) for severe hot flushes and night sweats in menopausal women. This trial is in women without any historical, physical, or laboratory evidence for heart disease so it will provide information on progesterone and weight, waist circumference, blood pressure, cholesterol and other lipids, inflammation, blood vessel function, and coagulation.

I feel that the estrogen conspiracy is against women who ask questions, against women who value normal life cycles and an accurate, observation-based understanding of their own hormonal mysteries. It is centered on the idea of estrogen as transforming us into acceptable members of the human race. And, when begrudgingly, as occurred with the estrogen-only arm of the WHI, harm is shown from estrogen, then quickly, the blame shifts to something else—women were too old or it had been too long since their last period at the time they started therapy (the so-called "timing hypothesis") for the estrogen to work, as it surely must, to prevent heart disease. Or every negative is because of that quarter-dose equivalent of progestin in combined therapy, for if estrogen rescues women from subhuman status, progesterone is the embodiment of all that makes women mysterious, defiant, and dangerous.

At this point, I should admit to having personal as well as scientific reasons for my skepticism about estrogen. As a medical student who was about to be married in 1967, I was desperate to avoid pregnancy. I obtained a sample oral contraceptive from the local Planned Parenthood. I took it only five days. Nausea, depression, fatigue, and swelling (I measured nine pounds of weight loss in hours after I took half a water pill I had begged off a friendly intern) and my first ever migraine headache forced me to stop. That Sequens pill I took, which was later discontinued because it was not effective contraception, contained only estrogen during the first fourteen days of the pack, and in a massive dose. I think you will forgive me if I have been dubious about all the positive estrogen messages I have heard since.

Throughout this book, I have contributed to our joint effort illustrating misogyny and the prejudice in the processes that we call science, the conventions and narrow, reductionist thinking that prevent scientists from even asking certain questions. To come back to my research and questions that could not be asked, I was motivated by my personal joy in running—and the feminist emancipation that long-distance races represented for women in the 1970s—to find out the truth about women's cycles and exercise training. At that time, everyone *knew* that *exercise causes amenorrhea*. This message was created as soon as women started participating in long-distance exercise—without any proof, it rapidly became Fact. Because everyone knows that exercise is for men—women who exercise will undoubtedly disadvantage themselves as women, their wombs will fall out, or they will lose their cycles—I had performed an unfunded, cross-sectional study with women runners similarly motivated as I was and observed that mature, healthy, and normal-weight women who were regularly running maintained perfectly regular cycles. Within this group, however, those who did longer training runs (who were thus ramping up the intensity of exercise) had short luteal phases (meaning that the time from release of an egg until the next flow was too short for fertility) or anovulation (no egg was released at all).[16] Around the same time, having devoured what was currently known about women's cycles and exercise, I postulated that all the missed periods being reported in runners were in women dealing, not only with exercise, but with *many* stressors—like obsessive worry about weight gain,[17] performance anxiety, dislocation to a strange environment, or being young and just past their first period. Those who fit within this over-stressed category were the ones who developed amenorrhea. In fact, I found a magazine picture of running women who were obviously pregnant, and I made a slide of it with the label "Athletic Amenorrhea" (my tongue firmly fixed in my cheek).

Thinking about women in context, not dissecting out the smallest bit, I marvel now when I look back—as a new part-time academic, shoved from nook to cranny in the hospital and university, a woman in a medical man's world, and just going through a divorce—at my confidence in holistically reviewing exercise-related menstrual cycle changes.[18] I postulated then, in the early 1980s, that women's reproduction could *adapt* to increasing exercise, just as our lungs and legs adapted to our running.

I had done my homework and was ready to test this reproductive adaptation notion in an observational study that lasted a year. I already knew that I would study women who were mature and healthy, at least ten years after their first period, of normal weight, nonsmokers, more than six months since they had used the Pill, and who were noncompulsive exercisers. I decided I also needed to prove initially that they were normally ovulatory. Toward this end, I designed the study so that, to be eligible to participate, women had to have two, consecutive, normal-length cycles that also had normal ovulation and luteal phases that were ten or more days long. I asked all participants to write their first morning temperature in a list at the bottom of a menstrual cycle diary I had devised when studying premenstrual changes with increasing exercise.[19] When applying for funds to study the menstrual cycle changes during increasing exercise aimed at running a marathon, I decided I needed women who were similar to the running women but normally active (a no-running and no-training control) and also that I needed women who were regularly running but not training (a running but nontraining control). I didn't dare write my postulate that the menstrual cycle *lengths* would not change (in that climate, even I didn't have the courage to postulate that amenorrhea wouldn't develop), but rather that whatever cycle-length changes might occur would also include decreases in the women's ovulation and progesterone production. At that time, I felt compelled to frame the hypothesis in terms of low estrogen or amenorrhea (no flow). Estrogen deficiency is what the world worried about. It was the ultimate in bad news for women. That grant was not funded.

Not daunted, and wanting to make my way in a very competitive (i.e., woman-unfriendly) academic world, I applied again with the same proposal, but this time with a high-tech outcome: quantitative computed tomography of bone. Although I was interested in bone and had done a few studies on the osteoporosis and fractures experienced by those in renal failure, I knew that a sexy and objective outcome—like applying the then exciting and new CT radiography to bone density—would help.

It did—the grant was funded. I also remember figuring that the women training for a marathon, but not the consistent runners, would develop short luteal phases and anovulation, but within regular menstrual cycles. I wondered whether progesterone was related to bone formation and whether less progesterone would cause bone loss. But I couldn't write that preposterous hypothesis—although it was already well supported by cell culture, animal, and other studies[20]—and expect to get funded. I was being prevented from postulating what was, already for me, a logical guess. (I reasoned that there were two hormones of women's reproduction. We knew that bone renews itself in an ideally balanced way, with some being lost and some being replaced all the time. We also knew that estrogen decreased bone loss. Why would progesterone not be a logical candidate to increase bone formation?)

Once I found, to my ecstasy, that my true (unmentionable) hypothesis was correct—those women who developed ovulation disturbances during the year-long study lost bone. Neither the marathon training nor regular running caused periods to go away, to differ from the cycles of normally active women, or even caused luteal phase lengths to shorten. But—I couldn't get it published. I tried for three years and endured, I think, six rejections before I got a revise-and-resubmit letter from the *NEJM* editor, who was retiring. The new editor assigned to my file changed every second word in my draft, in green ink. I made all the changes requested (if they didn't alter the facts or the meaning). I again got a request to revise the draft with every second word corrected, this time in brown ink. Again, I made the changes, noting (to myself, mind you) that now he was asking I change back to my original words. Finally, the paper, titled "Spinal Bone Loss and Ovulatory Disturbances," was accepted for publication.[21]

However, when I got the proofs, the title had been changed to "Spinal Bone Loss and Menstrual Cycle Disturbances," and the abstract had been similarly altered to talk about the menstrual cycle, rather than ovulatory, changes. I was crushed, then mad. Here I was, a junior person, having just achieved the lowest academic rank after years of working full time and being paid for half time, wanting so much for that paper to be published, for women to know that it was okay to run (just be well fed and happy and healthy while doing it), and the proofs were wrong. I now can better interpret the editor's resistance: "Menstrual cycle disturbances" to him meant problems with estrogen, which fit the existing notions about women and bone (after all, menopause and estrogen deficiency cause "postmenopausal osteoporosis"). However, what I had found, what was totally new, was evidence that *ovulation disturbances* (i.e., lower progesterone levels) were associated with bone loss and in a dose–response-like manner, depending on the luteal phase length—estrogen levels were fine, whether women were gaining, maintaining, or losing bone. That meant progesterone was important for women's bone, which was not a thinkable thought in those days.

I had the gall to object to those erroneous proofs. How I had the courage, I don't know. Perhaps because I *believe* in science—meaning, as it can and should be. What I was dealing with, this time in the publishing end of women's health research, was perversion of science to maintain the status quo. I called the journal long distance from a rustic lakeside Manitoba resort (ironically, at the time, I was at a Canadian sports medicine conference to deliver the keynote "The Myth of Athletic Amenorrhea"). I asserted on the telephone, and later by faxing the corrected proofs, that the title and the abstract had to be returned to what I had submitted (what they had accepted) or they did not have my permission to publish. I pulled their bluff: the paper was published as I wrote it.

I suspect, however, that many women in medicine and in basic science, with a less intense commitment to Science, or more of an I-want-to-fit-in-and-be-accepted motivation than I have, would have acquiesced, then or earlier, in the harassment stage that passed for editorial correction. I was raised in the wilderness in Alaska, where I had to be self-sufficient. I also—from the perspective of a poor girl in first grade in a Berkeley Hills school, a white girl in an aboriginal village, and later a medical student living on a quarter a day for food—had insight into class and race and other common prejudices.

Having come up with an idea (hypothesis) and having tested it in a prospective, observational study called the Prospective Ovulation Cohort, I decided it needed confirmation in an RCT. So, following the same protocol described previously, with funding from the Dairy Bureau of Canada, we enrolled healthy, normal-weight, exercising women with *abnormal* menstrual cycles or *abnormal* ovulation (those with regular cycles had to have two consecutive cycles with either short luteal phases or anovulation) and called it the Prospective Anovulation Cohort. The main randomized therapy was medroxyprogesterone (10 mg/day for ten days a month) or progestin placebo, and we also tested the effect of extra calcium (1,000 mg/day) or calcium placebo. The observational study had shown that ten to sixteen days of endogenous progesterone during the luteal phase of a normal menstrual cycle prevented bone loss in women with enough estrogen and regular cycles[22]—would it do so in women with amenorrhea or oligomenorrhea and sometimes low estrogen levels? The outcome for this study was also spinal bone density (this time with the now-conventional dual-energy X-ray absorptiometer machine that this grant funding allowed Vancouver General Hospital to purchase for the first time). When the results showed a highly significant, 2 percent annual bone gain in women on cyclic medroxyprogesterone versus a 2 percent loss in women on double placebos, I was beyond the moon. This was proof that progesterone *caused* a gain in bone.

Then came the nine rejections over three years—it was finally published in the *American Journal of Medicine* in 1994.[23] During those agonizingly long three years, I was applying for tenure. Because I could not get this paper published, I almost failed that ultimate academic challenge. That would have meant no further funded position at my university or uprooting my children and trying to make a fresh start at a new academic medical center—this is the power of what I feel is an estrogen conspiracy. I have no doubt, had I shown that *estrogen* increased bone density, that paper would have been published immediately. No worries, career secure.

I have described examples of what I believe are an estrogen conspiracy— from my research in women's health—preventing the formulation of new ideas, preventing the funding of studies to test these new hypotheses, and preventing the publication of results. Following that work, by now, into the early 1990s, I decided we needed information about the relationship of ovulation to bone in the whole population. In other words, we needed to know the epidemiology of ovulation. Using ways of recruitment that I had learned by being responsible for one center of the Canadian Multicentre Osteoporosis Study,[24] I applied to Canada's national medical funding agency and was rejected. Later, as I was learning from my own experience about the paradoxical increases in estrogen during perimenopause, I tried to get funding for an observational study of women's experiences and hormone levels in perimenopause. Multiple applications over about ten years were unsuccessful.

Some years later, having failed to *observe* perimenopause, I realized it was crucial to scientifically discover something that would effectively *treat* the miseries of midlife women. Estrogen is assumed to work fine for "menopausal symptoms" (it is ambiguous whether that term means symptoms in perimenopause or in menopause). It did not make sense to me, however, that women whose estrogen levels were too high, and whose brain–pituitary–ovary balance was defective, thus causing that high estrogen, would get better by giving them even *more* estrogen. The ineffectiveness of estrogen in perimenopause was confirmed (for me) by a large, well-performed, placebo-controlled trial that had already proven that low-dose oral contraceptives were not effective or acceptable therapy for heavy bleeding, hot flushes, or quality of life in symptomatic perimenopausal women.[25] I designed a randomized comparative trial of the Pill (standard therapy then, and still) versus cyclic oral micronized progesterone. The rejections, three years in a row, implied that I was an idiot because we already *had* effective therapy: the Pill worked charmingly—the paper was written cleverly enough by the drug company that funded the study so that the casual and estrogen-enchanted reader would think it a highly successful therapy. However, it was clear that from the small print that there was worsening of vaginal bleeding for three cycles before improvement, and that the Pill caused no significant decrease compared with placebo in hot flushes or overall improved quality of life.[26] The estrogen conspiracy allowed publication of the data that were so well spun that the true ineffectiveness of estrogen for perimenopause was buried. No further research was needed. We knew all we needed to about the treatment of symptomatic perimenopause—hysterectomy and antidepressants like serotonin reuptake inhibitors, if the Pill didn't work.

About this time, I was fed up with applying for the research grants that someone with my research and academic record should have had no trouble attaining. I had spent sixteen years of my career applying for funding for logical (to me) extensions of my previous work and not gotten any major grants. (The personal behind this statement is that each grant meant months of work; hours of tedium for long-suffering assistants; producing eighteen to twenty copies of the final grant, each of which was at least 4.2 cm thick; and considerable angst as well as anger.) By this time, it was the early 2000s, and I was increasingly convinced that there was an estrogen conspiracy. For several years, I had declared my office a grant-application-free zone. I had continued doing research but simply funded the studies myself, from my salary or honoraria for speaking, or from donations.

Then, I decided to apply to the Canadian medical granting agency to do an international collaborative, population-based study of ovulation (by measuring progesterone levels) within a whole-county study in Norway that was already re-cruiting young women and collecting blood. Still seeking to observe relationships between ovulation and bone, I also applied for funds to study a questionnaire method to document ovulation. For both grants, when asked to name review-ers I *didn't* want, I wrote, "Please don't ask any gynecologist to review this. I don't believe they will be able to scientifically or fairly evaluate it." Those are fighting words. I realized that this medical specialty's strong belief in estrogen might be preventing grant funding and decided to see if I could avoid it. Part of me felt, when I wrote that, like I wasn't playing fair. But another part said, hang it all, the *system* isn't fair. If this is what it takes to continue exploring the non-estrogen-based ideas I have for women's health, so be it.

I got both grants! To my mind, this was proof that gynecology—the medical specialty that is accepted socially as *the* experts in women's health—were squashing any research that didn't conform to the notion that "Estrogen's what makes a girl, a girl."

Not only does what I feel is an estrogen conspiracy prevent new ideas, impede funding, and deny research publication, but it also prevents free speech. There is (supposedly) no more sacred aspect of the Academy than free speech. I say I feel that the estrogen conspiracy prevents free expression based on many experiences, but one, in particular, that is explicative. I was invited to speak at a national program jointly organized by two not-for-profit (but pharmaceutically supported) Canadian organizations: the Osteoporosis Society and the Society for Obstetrics and Gynecology. I was to deliver a keynote at a menopause conference held in the historic Convocation Hall on the University of Toronto campus. About a month before the event, I was asked by the president of the Osteoporosis Society to provide an outline of my talk. I protested. He insisted. So I wrote that I would discuss the science-based and safe reasons why estrogen and progesterone should be used in menopausal therapy: early menopause, menopause with existing osteoporosis, or severe hot flushes that nothing else effectively treated. I also said I would talk about RCT evidence that estrogen *caused* heart attacks, blood clots, and low libido in *men*.[27]

Finally, I would outline the numerous ways women have for preventing heart attacks (namely, exercise, normal weight, not smoking, correcting abnormal blood sugar, and eating to prevent abnormal cholesterol). However, I was told—mind you, this time by an academic acquaintance, and endocrinology colleague—that I *had* to say that estrogen therapy prevented heart attacks. I said I couldn't. Finally, I reluctantly agreed that I would say, "Most physicians and experts *believe* that estrogen prevents heart disease."

A year or so later, in 1998, when the results of the HERS confirmed my beliefs about estrogen not preventing heart disease, I literally ran into him at a conference. I greeted him, and then punched him semiplayfully on the shoulder, telling him that I was right. Somewhat taken aback, he spluttered that he hadn't yet read the HERS results. He professed to have forgotten trying to make me say that estrogen prevented heart disease in women.

Finally, I feel that the estrogen conspiracy is limiting what I may teach the second-year medical students in their problem-based learning curriculum about bone and osteoporosis. I am responsible for the week on metabolic bone disease. Following is the case history the students are given: a 63-year-old woman stumbles and breaks her hip; she has no obvious hormonal or reproductive abnormalities— a normal menarche age, regular cycles during her premenopausal years, and she became menopausal at a normal age. However, the rub came when the case history expanded to include the fact that despite regular cycles, she was unable to get pregnant during the first fifteen years of her marriage. Then, when she was no longer trying, she got pregnant at age thirty-eight. I made a key issue in this case that enough estrogen without enough progesterone is a reason for important premenopausal bone loss. This idea is founded on the irrefutable basic science evidence that progesterone stimulates osteoblasts (the bone-forming cells) to increase their number and the amount of the osteoid (protein matrix of bone) they create thus stimulating new bone formation.[28] Most important, this is based on the evidence I know from three prospective human studies[29] and two proof-of-principle randomized, double-blind, placebo-controlled trials.[30] However, the notion that progesterone is important for bone formation still is not in the textbooks or the common reference sources that students usually use.

Repeatedly, I tried to make clear the ideas about progesterone complementing estrogen's important role in preventing bone loss. I explained that the falling estrogen levels before menstrual flow increase bone loss that needs progesterone's stimulation of increased formation to offset the loss. And year after year, each new crop of medical students grumbled. Their complaints were couched that they could not find reliable information to support that idea. I gave them two original papers; now they objected that it was extra work to read them. The tutors sympathized with the students; the administrators and, eventually, the head of the entire block on musculoskeletal health demanded that I "take progesterone out of the case."

I was shattered that my leader and colleague would make such a demand. I considered resigning from osteoporosis teaching. I tried hard to imagine teaching about bone balance without the notion of stopping bone loss (estrogen) and promoting bone gain (progesterone)—that was simply impossible for me to visualize. After a lot of thought, I decided to continue. I rewrote the case this year to have the woman in the clinical story investigated for infertility in her twenties and told that she had "trouble ovulating and her progesterone levels were too low." That should make her menstrual hormonal situation very clear. All of the references supporting the role of progesterone and bone were on reserve in all the academic libraries, and they were all listed for the tutors in the tutor guide. I was hopeful that things had improved and that the perpetual "progesterone problem" was solved.

The feedback session about my week this year began on a high note when one of the senior tutors said, "This week is a shining example of what PBL [problem-based learning] should be—it delved into the basic science aspects as expressed in an interesting clinical situation." Following that, however, the same fundamental problem reared its ugly head—only old women get osteoporosis, we know estrogen deficiency causes it, and that's that. One after one, the tutors said they did not like the week, that the "emphasis on progesterone" was a problem, and I was the only one who believed that progesterone was important for bone. One tutor even went so far as to say, "She is using the students to advance her own progesterone research agenda."

The only way that I can understand this response is in the context of what feels like an estrogen conspiracy. Although the undergraduate curriculum is supposed to be "evidence-based," most tutors and students are more comfortable with what is in textbooks and with the estrogen-centered osteoporosis dogma that everyone knows. I will continue to try to convey a physiology-based (meaning both estrogen and progesterone are important) approach to bone. The academic administration will have to fire me before I will quit teaching this week. I believe it is important for students to know about progesterone's role in bone formation because in the future, they will be trying to prevent and treat osteoporosis in their patients.

In summary, I have somehow, amazing still to me, clawed my way up through academic ranks to full professor despite my heretical notions. I have been able to establish a poorly funded but highly productive Centre for Menstrual Cycle and Ovulation Research within my university and to initiate and maintain a vibrant and contemporary Web site (http://www.cemcor.ubc.ca). I am excited at the opportunity this book has provided to share my insights with you. I am also sure that what we relate about how progesterone works, both in clinical care and in research, will be useful to you. Most of all, I hope that my ten plus personal years of misery in perimenopause, while I was both doing research with and taking care of some of the most symptomatic midlife women in my region, will provide insights that are helpful for you. It was disorienting for me in midlife to discover that my estrogen levels were high, not the low, dropping, and deficient levels I had been taught to expect. My purpose in this book has been to show that a concept of women's health that puts progesterone *with estrogen* as important, that understands the true chaotic physiology of perimenopause, and that offers women progesterone for treatment of hot flushes will benefit all of us—women, physicians and researchers, alike. In fact, I feel that the travesty of focusing on estrogen and blaming progesterone is an *"estrogen misogynacle"* (combining misogyny with debacle).

This exposition is necessarily from my point of view. My concept is that adding an accurate understanding of progesterone to current concepts in women's health will improve both science and clinical care. My viewpoint is ultimately positive and constructive, although I will admit, especially in this final chapter it seems to be almost overwhelmed by what I feel is important critique. In this book we have faulted gynecology, not as individual physicians, many of whom are both wise and caring, but as members of a specialty of medicine that differs in how it, collectively, appears to view both women and science. My coauthor, despite her personal misery in perimenopause, does not necessarily agree that there is an estrogen conspiracy. My vision is unique, sometimes whimsical, and often complex. It includes, with equal weight, all three aspects of who I am: a woman living in a rather ordinary, perplexing, and sometimes unruly body; a hormone expert and scientist who is trying to understand the roles of ovulation and progesterone in health across women's life cycle; and a physician who has dedicated forty years to the concerns and health of my patients.

We have covered a lot of ground in this book. What we are saying is controversial and perhaps even heretical. However, putting our energy and essence into this effort to inform and improve understanding will not have been worth it unless you—the reader—change. For those readers who are physicians, we challenge you to read what we say, study our references, and criticize what we present. For those of you who are women, we trust that now, when you are told that you are fine, despite infertility and regular menstrual cycles, you will ask, *What about my ovulation and progesterone?* We hope that you who are in midlife will say, *No way.* when someone explains that dropping estrogen levels are causing your perimenopausal heavy bleeding, night sweats and fibroids requiring hysterectomy. Finally, for those of you who have graduated into the calm of menopause, we want you to ask, *Why don't **you**?* when physician or husband or friend pesters you to take estrogen for normal age-related changes.

In short, now it is up to you. We've done our best to show that our current concepts of women's reproduction are upside down and backwards. The time has come to put progesterone first—I believe that progesterone is the bellwether of women's well-being. It is way past time to see estrogen as the essential but dangerous siren that she is.

Appendix A

Understanding and Surviving/Thriving in Perimenopause

Jerilynn C. Prior, MD

LEARNING ISSUES

1. Perimenopause begins while women continue to have *regular* periods

2. Estradiol levels are *erratically* higher and poorly suppressible, rather than dropping

3. Ovulation may occur but is often inadequate, with low progesterone levels

4. Prospective clinical observations indicate that cyclic oral micronized progesterone (Prometrium) is effective for many symptoms, but controlled trials are needed

5. Of all perimenopausal women, 80 to 85 percent will be fine with information and reassurance; however, vocational and social support and appropriate medical therapy are needed for the 15 to 20 percent of women who have the highest estrogen levels and are very symptomatic

DEFINITIONS

Old Ideas and Concepts

We used to call "menopause" everything that was symptomatic for women from midlife on. Now the term *menopause* specifically means the time from one year after the final menstrual period for the remainder of a woman's life.

Perimenopause is a unique hormonal and experiential entity—different from menopause (or *"postmenopause,"* as it may be called)—often starting in the late thirties or early forties and, for some, lasting ten years or more.[1]

Figure A1.1
Phases of perimenopause.

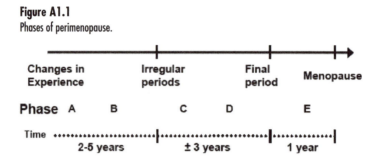

The term *menopausal transition* is not very useful—it is defined as starting many years *after* the first hormonal and experiential changes (with irregular cycles and increased FSH) and ends abruptly with the final menstrual flow (which cannot be known to be final for a further year).[2]

In this book we have used the same definition as The Centre for Menstrual Cycle and Ovulation Research, which defines perimenopause as a normal phase of every woman's life, beginning with typical experience changes and ending one year beyond the final menstrual flow. It has five variable, but helpful phases, as shown in Figure A1.1.[3]

How can you tell you are in perimenopause if you have *regular* cycles? You can tell with any three of the following:

1. New-onset heavy and/or longer menstrual flow

2. Shorter menstrual cycle lengths of less than or equal to twenty-five days

3. New, sore, swollen, and/or lumpy breasts

4. New or increased menstrual cramps

5. New mid-sleep wakening

6. Onset of night sweats, especially around flow

7. New or markedly increased migraine headaches

8. New or increased premenstrual mood swings

9. Notable weight gain without changes in exercise or food intake.[4]

Hormonal Changes in Perimenopause

1. Estrogen levels are increased and chaotic. This is the most reliable and earliest change of perimenopause that occurs in women with regular cycles.[5] The most convincing evidence that estrogen levels are higher in perimenopause is from a meta-analysis of early follicular and premenstrual serum levels comparing premenopausal and perimenopausal women.[6] Table A1.1 shows estradiol values

Table A1.1

Estrogen (estradiol) levels in women who are premenopausal compared with those who are perimenopausal showing higher levels in perimenopause.[6]

Time in cycle	Premenopausal	Perimenopausal	Fisher's F	p value
Follicular phase	$n = 292$	$n = 415$		
	175 (57) pmol/L	225 (98) pmol/L	16.12	**.041**
Premenstrual	$n = 250$	$n = 69$		
	303 (84) pmol/L	371 (97) pmol/L	15.46	**.016**

in pmol/L (SD) from cross-sectional, within-center studies of premenopausal compared with perimenopausal women with cycle-timed samples.

2. Progesterone levels are lower in perimenopause. Ovulation may persist even to the final menstrual cycle, but progesterone production is decreased or luteal phase lengths are shorter.[7]

3. Estradiol levels are poorly suppressible. Exogenous estrogen often will not suppress endogenous estrogen, probably because of aging-related changes in the normal brain–pituitary–ovarian relationships.

4. Stress hormone levels are higher, especially in women with the highest estrogen levels. Estrogen amplifies the stress responses of cortisol and norepinephrine to social stresses.[8]

Experience Changes and Concerns in Perimenopause

1. Heavy menstrual flow may occur; although it often is attributed to and occurs in women who have fibroids, the fibroids are rarely the cause for heavy flow. Instead, heavy flow is associated with higher estrogen levels and less progesterone action on the endometrium (uterine lining).[9] Heavy flow has been defined as needing more than sixteen regular-sized sanitary products per cycle and occurs in 30 percent of perimenopausal women[10] with the maximum incidence in Phases A and B. The average age at hysterectomy is the mid-forties[11] and well before the menopausal transition would be diagnosed by the onset of irregular cycles at the average age of 47.5 years.[12]

2. Hot flushes/flashes and night sweats (vasomotor symptoms) are more intense in perimenopause; they begin with cyclic night sweats near the time of flow, when cycles remain regular,[13] and peak in the year after the last flow and in the first year of menopause.[14] They are associated with increased social stress like "trouble paying for basics,"[15] smoking, paradoxically with a higher body mass index, and having had a hysterectomy.

3. Breast tenderness is a poorly recognized but common early symptom of peri-menopause that decreases closer to menopause.[16] Breast tenderness is increased premenstrually when it is associated with mood symptoms and night sweats.

Table A1.2

A Meta-analysis of percentage spinal bone density change analyzed within center for perimenopausal compared with menopausal women (in the first years of menopause) showing a greater bone loss in Phases C through E of perimenopause.[6]

Number	Perimenopausal	Number	Menopausal	Fisher's F	p value
267	−1.83 (4.49)	695	−1.22 (3.14)	34.16	**0.005**

4. Palpitations (feeling like your heart is beating strongly, irregularly, or too fast), chest pressure or pain, sleep problems, and other stress-related symptoms are very prevalent and their origin is not well understood; however, the higher stress hormones likely play a role.

5. Sleep problems—with wakening typically in mid-sleep after an hour or two of being in a sound sleep—can occur and are commonly associated with trouble falling asleep again.

6. Rapid bone loss begins during perimenopause Phase C and reaches its maximum in Phase E.[17] A meta-analysis of within-center prospective studies of spinal bone change in perimenopausal and early menopausal women showed a significantly greater rate of loss in perimenopause compared to early in menopause. This rapid bone loss occurs before estradiol levels are low, is perhaps caused by the swinging of estradiol, lower progesterone levels (which cause a decrease in bone formation), and higher stress hormone levels.[18] Increased calcium and vitamin D intake plus other lifestyle changes will help to prevent bone loss in perimenopause.* Table A1.2 shows the annual percentage changes in spine BMD by dual energy methods in perimenopausal compared with early menopausal women. Data are reported as mean % (SD).

TREATMENTS FOR PERIMENOPAUSAL SYMPTOMS

Current Controlled Trials

There is only one controlled trial (randomized, double-blind, placebo-controlled) for perimenopausal symptoms. It involved the use of a monophasic, low-dose, oral contraceptive for heavy flow or hot flushes.[19] This low dose Pill caused significantly increased mid-cycle spotting/bleeding in the first three cycles. Subsequently, flow improved; however, compared with placebo, the Pill did not significantly improve hot flushes/night sweats or quality of life. However, it did prove that placebo-controlled studies are possible in perimenopausal women.

---

*See the "ABCs of Osteoporosis Prevention (for Women in Midlife)" at http://www.cemcor.ubc.ca/ help_yourself/articles/abcs_midlife.

Cyclic Oral Micronized Progesterone (Prometrium, or Medroxyprogesterone) Therapy

Progesterone therapy cannot be expected to suppress estrogen levels in perimenopause. Its purpose is to counterbalance the tissue effects of high estrogen.

Our center previously showed that cyclic medroxyprogesterone 10 mg for ten days per month in healthy, active, normal-weight premenopausal women with abnormal menstrual cycles or amenorrhea was associated with a mean gain in bone of 2 to 3 percent a year, compared with a 2 percent loss in spinal BMD over one year in women taking the placebo ($p = .0001$).[20] This therapy was well tolerated and acceptable for premenopausal[21] and menopausal women.[22]

Cyclic progesterone in a dose of 300 mg at bedtime (or medroxyprogesterone 10 mg) on days fourteen to twenty-seven of the menstrual cycle helps with heavy flow, premenstrual night sweats, and breast tenderness.

Progesterone has the advantage that it improves sleep[23] and decreases anxiety and depression.[24] I have successfully used this therapy in my clinical practice as well as in a study of a long-distance medical consultation to family physicians (Perimenopause Experiences Project).[25]

The Daily Perimenopause Diary[26] a self-report instrument that increases women's self-knowledge and sense of control and is free for personal use on the Centre for Menstrual Cycle and Ovulation Research Web site (http://www.cemcor.ubc.ca).

INFORMATION FOR WOMEN: CYCLIC PROGESTERONE THERAPY*

Why Might I Need to Take Cyclic Progesterone Therapy?

Progesterone is one of the two important female hormones for women. (Estrogen is the one we usually hear about.) When menstrual cycles are disturbed, even in a way that is not obvious, ovulation is abnormal and progesterone levels become low or absent.

Your doctor may prescribe progesterone to control heavy periods, severe menstrual cramps (dysmenorrhea), or to help with irregular periods, acne, unwanted hair, low bone density, or sore and lumpy breasts. Cyclic progesterone therapy may help achieve fertility. It is also important therapy for night sweats, breast tenderness, or heavy flow in perimenopause.

*Reprinted from http://www.cemcor.ubc.ca. Copyright © 1997, 2002, 2003, J. C. Prior.

Figure A1.2

How cyclic progesterone therapy may be taken within the cycle days of the menstrual cycle (the first day of flow is always "cycle day 1") to treat short luteal phase or anovulatory cycles (e.g., to replace missing or low levels of endogenous progesterone) or to treat menstrual cycle problems.

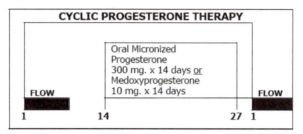

What Medications Can I Choose?

Medroxyprogesterone (previously known under the brand name Provera, a chemical form of progesterone that has been used for more than forty years) is a close cousin of natural progesterone. It is stronger, so the normal dose is 10 mg per day. Oral micronized progesterone (Prometrium) is the same as your ovaries make. Three 100-mg capsules is the normal dose. Because it causes sleepiness, take this medication on your way to bed. Either medication will have important positive effects on flow, breasts, and bones.

When Do I Take It?

If you get a period regularly and your periods are usually twenty-seven to thirty days apart, start progesterone on the fourteenth day after flow begins and take it for fourteen days, or until cycle day twenty-seven. If your cycles are regular but short (e.g., if your period starts every nineteen to twenty-six days), start cyclic medroxyprogesterone or progesterone on cycle day twelve. You would take it for fourteen days, that is, to cycle day twenty-five (see Figure A1.2).

If your period starts while you are still taking progesterone, *always continue taking it for the full fourteen days*. If this flow persists, you may need a higher dose of progesterone or to take it for a longer time. The early flow is a sign of high estrogen overstimulating the endometrium (lining of the womb).

If your period starts before you have finished the fourteen days of progesterone (e.g., on the ninth day of taking it), *finish the full fourteen days*, but start the *next* progesterone fourteen days after that new period began. This allows for "catch-up" of progesterone with your body's extra estrogen (see Figure A1.3).

If you have not started to flow after taking a cycle of progesterone, wait for fourteen days. After this fourteen-day time period, start taking progesterone again for fourteen days.

Figure A1.3
When to take cyclic progesterone therapy if your flow starts before you have finished the full fourteen days of progesterone. Each start of flow is called "cycle day 1."

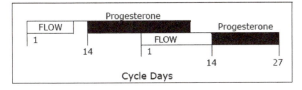

If your period is far apart or absent, take oral micronized progesterone for fourteen days and stay off of it for fourteen days. As soon as your period returns, start taking progesterone again fourteen days after the start of your flow, as shown in Figure A1.2.

Are There Any Side Effects?

There are no *serious* side effects from progesterone therapy. It does not cause blood clots or migraine headaches or increase the risk for breast cancer. It effectively prevents endometrial cancer. And its major "side effect" is a bonus—improved deep sleep. Note that medroxyprogesterone does not have this sleep enhancing effect. Pharmacy references often state that progesterone causes everything that's been shown on the Pill (high-dose estrogen and male hormone–like kinds of synthetic progesterone). In very rare instances, an allergy may occur. (Oral micronized progesterone is in peanut oil; therefore those with an allergy to peanuts *must not* take it; instead, it can be compounded in olive oil by a compounding pharmacist.)

You may notice some changes in your breasts, feelings of warmth, and other evidences of normal progesterone action. If you get moody, feel bloated, and have very sore breasts, it means that progesterone is temporarily stimulating your body to make high estrogen levels. This is rare and improves after one cycle.*

CONTINUOUS PROGESTERONE/PROGESTIN THERAPY IN PERIMENOPAUSE

There are several reasons to use progesterone/medroxyprogesterone *daily*, rather than cyclically, in perimenopause.[4] The doses continue to be 300 mg

---

*This information is made available by the Centre for Menstrual Cycle and Ovulation Research, University of British Columbia. You may make copies of handouts and tools for personal or clinical practice use. All copies must include our authorship. They may not be reproduced for profit. Further copies and guidelines for reproduction are on our Web site, http://www.cemcor.ubc.ca. Revised and reprinted from [27] J. C. Prior "Ovulatory disturbances: they do matter," *Canadian Journal of Diagnosis* February: 64–80, (1997). The article can be directly accessed here: http://www.cemcor.ubc.ca/files/uploads/Ovulatory_Disturbances_-_They_Do_Matter.pdf

at bedtime of progesterone or 10 mg of medroxyprogesterone at any convenient (but the same) time of day. Usually, the need to take daily progesterone occurs in perimenopause Phase C and later.

A woman who has had very heavy menstrual bleeding for some time, often associated with increased cramps and a low blood count (anemia), needs daily progesterone therapy to overcome the effects of prolonged high estrogen levels[28] on the lining of the uterus. Always also take 200 mg of ibuprofen about four times a day during heavy flow because it decreases flow by a different mechanism than progesterone. Usually, daily therapy for three months can be followed by cyclic therapy (as described earlier).

Sometimes flow will continue to be heavy on daily progesterone in a dose of 300 mg plus ibuprofen during heavy flow. In that case, increase the dose to 400 or 500 mg daily, and, if needed, add 10 mg of medroxyprogesterone for three months. The important thing to realize is that eventually, the flow will improve.*

If you have perimenopausal migraine headaches, because of the on–off response of those with migraines to any hormonal therapy, I would recommend *daily* progesterone.

If night sweats are continuously disturbing sleep and no longer cyclic, progesterone or medroxyprogesterone can be changed from cyclic to daily therapy. A high proportion of women will continue to have some flow.

Note that if daily progesterone/progestin therapy is adopted, because these thin the uterine lining and decrease flow, *two years* without any menstrual flow are required before a woman can be sure she is has reached menopause.

Summary

Perimenopause is a time of social and cultural status change and of ovarian chaos, during which estrogen levels overbalance progesterone and many symptoms can occur, especially in the 15 to 20 percent of women with the highest estrogen levels. Understanding of perimenopause—that these hormonal changes are natural, that the symptoms improve toward and during menopause, and that many of its unpleasant experiences result from our feelings about the negative views of aging and women in this culture—will help. Because of the high and nonsuppressible estrogen levels, therapy with oral contraceptives or estrogen should be avoided until one year has passed without flow. Cyclic or daily progesterone or medroxyprogesterone, along with emotional support and improved self-understanding (often through record keeping with the Daily Perimenopause Diary), are remarkably effective. You, too, can survive perimenopause!

---

*See "Managing Menorrhagia without Surgery" on http://www.cemcor.ubc.ca/help_yourself/articles/managing_menorrhagia.

Appendix B

Physiological, Woman-Centered Menopause Management

Jerilynn C. Prior, MD

KEY CONCEPTS

1. Menopause is normal and natural—women "get a break" from the high ovarian hormones of their reproductive lives
2. The only good reasons for menopausal "ovarian hormone therapy" follow:
   a. Early menopause starting before forty
   b. Night sweats chronically disturbing sleep plus low bone density or fracture
3. Progestin therapy is as effective for hot flushes and night sweats as estrogen—it is likely that progesterone (oral micronized progesterone, Prometrium) is even *more* effective (because it also improves sleep, and does not increase night sweats when stopped)
4. Vaginal dryness is effectively treated with information and vaginal nonhormonal therapies or very low-dose vaginal estrogen creams

PERSPECTIVES

It is not easy to accept aging in this youth-infatuated culture. In times of economic and social turmoil, women's lives always get harder, leading to a search for quick fixes. We now have good data from numerous large, randomized, double-blind, placebo-controlled trials that estrogen therapy is dangerous for healthy menopausal women. Yet those who have preached "HRT" and tried to help women are not accepting science. It is time to assert the virtue of having low ovarian hormones after the high estrogen perimenopausal stormy weather.

INFORMATION GATHERING

Much of what is written for women, unfortunately, is biased, unscientific, or motivated by profit. Therefore, you need to find Internet or print information sources that originate from reliable institutions (like the NIH, the FDA, or a university you trust) and compare multiple sources. The Centre for Menstrual Cycle and Ovulation Research (CeMCOR) Web site (http://www.cemcor.ubc.ca) contains a wealth of timely, woman-centered, accurate, and commercial-free information that is created for you.

It is natural and good to want to understand our experiences. However, those who would sell us tests of saliva or urine, blood, or other maneuvers are offering partial, at best, and questionable, at worst, answers. For example, even calm menopausal hormone levels have a pulsed pattern (dictated by brain electrical signals) and thus potentially give different answers from minute to minute.

Learn about yourself, for yourself. If you are trying to understand sleep trouble, vaginal dryness, or night sweats, record them in the context of your whole life, using the Daily Menopause Diary (you can download the diary for free from the CeMCOR Web site). If you are troubled by something not on the Diary (say, joint aches), write the troublesome symptom on an extra line and grade it on a zero to four scale.

There are many products offered to help women feel better. To see if what you try is working for you, download the Diary that includes extra lines for treatments—change one thing for a month at a time. Then you will have what is called an *experiment of one* to provide information showing what helps *you*. Show completed Diary records to your physician if herbs, soy, or over-the-counter supplements are not sufficient.

If you have had a fracture, skipped three or more periods in young adulthood, are thin or worried about weight gain, or have relatives with broken bones, it is important to get assessment and treatment. If you have no fractures but some risks, do what you can to prevent the increased bone loss in the early years of menopause. If you think your interest in sex is too low, you have incontinence, or you are wondering about thyroid balance, look for information about those also. Sign up for a two-monthly CeMCOR newsletter for the latest information.

PROGESTERONE THERAPY

The most exciting and positive aspect of women's health today, besides what should be "the death of HRT" is increasing understanding of the importance of progesterone. Progesterone that is identical to what our ovaries used to make (bioidentical and natural) is a licensed formulary drug in the United States and Canada (Prometrium) and in multiple countries from France to Argentina. Progesterone as a cream is available over the counter in the United States and by prescription in Canada where it is always compounded by a licensed pharmacist.

Sometimes women, and even physicians, are confused, thinking that progesterone should not be used alone (i.e., without estrogen). That is not true. Progesterone is safe to take alone. Estrogen is neither safe nor wise to take alone because estrogen's growth-promoting actions need progesterone to counterbalance or complement them. You ask, "What if I have had a hysterectomy?" If taking estrogen, progesterone is still needed for the breasts, brains, and bones of women who have no uterus.

As you will understand from reading this book, in women's health today, anything related to progesterone is considered "controversial and contradictory." Yet a fair assessment of all the evidence suggests that progesterone therapy is helpful for those few menopausal women who are sufficiently bothered by night sweats or sleep troubles to need a prescribed medical therapy.

Oral micronized progesterone (Prometrium) is available as cream-colored little balls, each of which contains 100 mg. The dose that is most effective and matches the levels that we had during our luteal phase (after ovulation, when progesterone is normally high) is 300 mg at bedtime. That keeps the blood level of progesterone in the luteal phase range for twenty-four hours.[1]

In using progesterone therapy orally, it is important to realize that it is quickly absorbed into the brain. Therefore, take it just before your head hits the pillow to sleep; otherwise you may feel rather dizzy and almost drunk. Its sleep effects vary with different people, but try it first on a night when you can sleep in the following morning. Those who are sleep deprived may get into such a deep sleep that they will be trying to catch up on lost sleep during the next day. The other proviso is that those who are allergic to peanuts should not use Prometrium because the progesterone is dissolved in peanut oil; instead, such women could use oral micronized progesterone compounded in olive oil.

Following are some of the potential reasons for progesterone therapy:

1. Moderate hot flushes and night sweats: progesterone cream 20 mg twice a day significantly decreases or eliminates them[2]

2. Severe night sweats chronically disturbing sleep: oral micronized progesterone (Prometrium or compounded oral micronized progesterone in olive oil) in a dose of 300 mg at bedtime daily. (The RCT that CeMCOR is doing, which will prove the extent of this clinically documented effect versus placebo, is almost complete.) Alternatively, if you do not have a family history of breast cancer, low personal risk, and breasts that are not dense, then medroxyprogesterone 10 mg daily is similarly as effective as conjugated equine estrogen (Premarin)[3]

3. Prevent the increased risk for breast cancer caused by estrogen treatment: a study from France observed more than one hundred thousand women for an average of eight years. Those on estrogen alone, or estrogen with progestins, had increased breast cancer that was not seen when estrogen therapy was combined with oral micronized progesterone[4]

4. Sleep disturbances: 300 mg at bedtime of oral micronized progesterone (Prometrium) or oral micronized progesterone compounded in olive oil by a reputable pharmacist will help falling asleep and will aid in deep and restful sleep,[5] without the side effects or addictive properties of many prescribed sleep aids

5. Prevent or treat osteoporosis: builds new bone that is especially visible when progesterone is partnered with estrogen or a bone-loss preventing medication[6]

6. Blood pressure: progesterone (300 mg at bedtime) may lower blood pressure[7]

7. Anxiety and stress: progesterone appears to increase a sense of calmness and to decrease feelings of anxiety by acting through neurotransmitters[8]

8. Help avoid obesity or diabetes: progesterone increases the number of calories burned a day (because it increases core temperature) and thus may help prevent inappropriate weight gain[9]

9. Improve blood flow: endothelial function, meaning the actions of the linings of blood vessels that increase blood flow, is a measure of the health of the whole cardiovascular system. Estrogen is known to increase flow. Progesterone is similar or even stronger in this marker of heart health.[10]

10. Help with breathing for those with sleep apnea or chronic obstructive lung disease[11]

11. Improve wrinkles: topical progesterone cream has been shown in a blinded controlled trial to decrease facial wrinkles[12]

PROGESTERONE SIDE EFFECTS

Although it is common, in fact, universal (part of "the estrogen conspiracy"), to blame progesterone for the unwanted bleeding, bloating, breast tenderness, or moodiness women may experience on ovarian hormone therapy, this is not rationally justified. If nausea, sore breasts, migraine headaches, or blood clots occur on combined therapy, it is the estrogen, and not the progesterone, that is causing them and lowering the dose of estrogen will improve the problem.

Although the combination of estrogen and medroxyprogesterone may be more likely to cause women some symptoms, two randomized, placebo-controlled trials have found no side effects related to the progestin either alone or combined with estrogen.[13]

Oral micronized progesterone has increased deep sleep as its main side effect. It will cause dizziness if taken when not in bed and ready to sleep.

One "side effect" is that oral micronized progesterone is expensive. Although there is yet no clear evidence about clots and progesterone, without estrogen, it has not been associated with clots or pulmonary embolism.

THERAPY FOR MENOPAUSAL WOMEN WHO NEED TREATMENT

Early Menopause

Women who are one year beyond their last period by age forty have early menopause. Because this means falling short of the usual thirty-five to forty years of reproductive hormones with their benefits for bones and other aspects of health, treatment with estrogen and progesterone is a healthy choice.*

Estrogen should always be a patch, gel, or cream to decrease the risk of blood clots caused by estrogen as a pill.[14] The dose should be in the low-normal range and ideally taken from the first through the twenty-fifth to twenty-eighth of the month. This gives your whole body, and especially your breasts, a healthy few days free of estrogen. The estrogen (but not the progesterone) should be gradually decreased and stopped beginning around age fifty-one (the average age at menopause in the population).† If osteoporosis is an issue for you, start a bone-loss blocking medicine, such as a bisphosphonate, before starting to taper estrogen.

Progesterone can be taken either cyclically for the last fourteen days of your monthly therapy or daily, depending on two things: if you want flow, you should take it cyclically; if you have severe hot flushes or low bone density, then progesterone should be taken daily. That will avoid flow, except, perhaps, for the first month. The dose of oral micronized progesterone is 300 mg at bedtime on day fourteen to the end of the month or daily. If using medroxyprogesterone, which is a reasonable option and less expensive, the dose is 10 mg taken on the same days as progesterone. Progesterone should be continued for at least a year after you have totally stopped estrogen to prevent and treat any hot flushes that might occur with estrogen withdrawal. If hot flushes are gone, you can stop progesterone once a year to see whether they will stay away or return. Progesterone is safe to take for many years because it does not carry the same risks as estrogen.

Severe Hot Flushes Plus Osteoporosis

Estrogen and progesterone can be taken together and daily for hot flushes waking you every night plus osteoporosis based on fractures or low bone density. Estrogen used for this purpose should be tapered gradually over at least six months and stopped after five years. Because rapid bone loss occurs when estrogen is stopped, before tapering estrogen take a medication, such as a bisphosphonate, that prevents bone loss. The estrogen should be transdermal as a patch, gel, or cream in a dose that is low-normal (50 μg patch twice a week or one pump of

---

*For more information, see "Managing Early Menopause" on the CeMCOR Web site (http://www. cemcor.ubc.ca/help_yourself/articles/oht_early_menopause).

†See "Stopping Estrogen Treatment" on the CeMCOR Web site (http://www.cemcor.ubc.ca/ help_yourself/articles/stopping_estrogen) for specific instructions on using your type of medication.

gel daily) to avoid the blood clots that pill estrogen can cause. If you develop sore breasts, then stop the estrogen for three to five days at the end of each month. If you have flow, spotting, or bloating, decrease the dose by 10 percent.

Progesterone is the mainstay for treatment of hot flushes and is needed in a dose of oral micronized progesterone of 300 mg at bedtime or medroxyprogesterone 10 mg a day. If night sweats are not effectively controlled, besides doing relaxation/meditation, exercising, and decreasing weight (which all help hot flushes), the dose of progesterone can be increased to 400 or 500 mg. If these issues are still a problem, medroxyprogesterone 5 mg can be added to the progesterone therapy. When you wish to stop progesterone, you may do so abruptly, and hot flushes will not increase beyond what they would be without treatment.

Menopause is a good time; we can go back to playing the piano, exploring our closer or wider world, enjoying grandchildren, or simply being. Enjoy!

NOTES

FOREWORD

1. N. M. Hadler, *The Last Well Person: How to Stay Well despite the Health-Care System* (McGill-Queen's University Press, Montreal, 2004), p. 201.

2. "Effects of hormone replacement therapy on endometrial histology in post-menopausal women: The Postmenopausal Estrogen/Progestin Interventions (PEPI) trial. The Writing Group for the PEPI Trial," *Journal of the American Medical Association* **275**(5), 370–375 (1996).

3. J. Groopman, *How Doctors Think* (Houghton Mifflin, Boston, 2007), p. 216.

4. Writing Group for the Women's Health Initiative Investigators, "Risks and benefits of estrogen plus progestin in healthy postmenopausal women: Principal results from the Women's Health Initiative randomized controlled trial," *Journal of the American Medical Association* **288**(3), 321–333 (2002).

5. S. Baxter, "Hormone therapy at menopause: Should you or shouldn't you?," *BC Woman*, July (1995), pp. 57–61.

6. S. Baxter and W. I. Lane, *Immune Power* (Penguin/Putnam [Avery], Garden City Park, NY, 1999), p. 188.

7. L. Payer, "United States: The virus in the machine," in *Medicine and Culture* (Henry Holt, New York, 1996), pp. 124–152.

8. W. A. Silverman, *Where's the Evidence? Debates in Modern Medicine* (Oxford University Press, Oxford, 1998).

9. M. Namenwirth, "Science seen through a feminist prism," in *Feminist Approaches to Science*, R. Bleier, ed. (Pergamon Press, New York, 1986), pp. 18–41.

10. R. Moynihan and R. Smith, "Too much medicine?," *British Medical Journal* **324**(7342), 859–860 (2002).

11. Hadler, *The Last Well Person*.

12. D. L. Sackett, "The arrogance of preventive medicine," *Canadian Medical Association Journal* **167**(4), 363–364 (2002).

13. E. Friess, H. Tagaya, L. Trachsel, F. Holsboer, and R. Rupprecht, "Progesterone-induced changes in sleep in male subjects," *American Journal of Physiology* **272**, E885–E891 (1997).

14. B. Latour, *Science in Action: How to Follow Scientists and Engineers through Society* (Harvard University Press, Cambridge, MA, 1987).

15. N. Postman, *Technopoly: The Surrender of Culture to Technology* (Vintage Books, New York, 1993).

16. C. Bartlett, J. Sterne, and M. Egger, "What is newsworthy? Longitudinal study of the reporting of medical research in two British newspapers," *British Medical Journal* **325**, 81–84 (2002).

17. S. J. Genuis, "The proliferation of clinical practice guidelines: Professional development or medicine-by-numbers?," *Journal of the American Board of Family Practice* **18**(5), 419–425 (2005).

18. R. A. Wilson, *Feminine Forever* (M. Evans, New York, 1966).

19. Hadler, *Last Well Person*.

PART 1

1. Jane Warner, *The Search for Signs of Intelligent Life in the Universe* (HarperPerennial, New York, 1990), p. 191.

CHAPTER 1

1. M. Lock, "Medicalization: Cultural concerns," in *International Encyclopedia of the Social & Behavioral Sciences*, edited by N. J. Smelser and P. B. Baltes (Pergamon, Oxford, 2001), p. 9534.

2. M. H. Whatley, "Taking feminist science to the classroom: Where do we go from here?," in *Feminist Approaches to Science*, R. Bleier, ed. (Pergamon, Oxford, 1986), p. 182.

3. J. Prior, "Perimenopause lost—reframing the end of menstruation," *Journal of Reproductive and Infant Psychology* **24**(4), 323–335 (2006).

4. M. Groves (with advice from K. Hermsmeyer, C. Reilly, J. Prior, F. Stanczyk, K. Stephenson, H. Leonetti, and D. Soholt) "Hormone therapy for mid-life and beyond: A new perspective," http://www.womeninbalance.org/pdf/ScienceAdvisor.pdf.

5. N. A. Baer, "Cardiopulmonary resuscitation on television—Exaggerations and accusations," *New England Journal of Medicine* **334**(24), 1604–1606 (1996).

6. C. Bartlett, J. Sterne, and M. Egger, "What is newsworthy? Longitudinal study of the reporting of medical research in two British newspapers," *British Medical Journal* **325**(7355), 81–84 (2002).

7. R. Bleier, *Science and Gender: A Critique of Biology and Its Theories on Women*, The Athene Series (Pergamon, New York, 1984).

8. J. D. Wilson, "The evolution of endocrinology—Plenary lecture at the 12th International Congress of Endocrinology, Lisbon, Portugal, 31 August 2004," *Clinical Endocrinology* **62**, 389–396 (2005).

9. P. A. van Keep, "The history and rationale of hormone replacement therapy," *Maturitas* **12**(3), (1990), p. 164.

10. N. Oudshoorn, "On the making of sex hormones: Research materials and the production of knowledge," *Social Studies of Science* **20**(1), (1990), p. 7.

11. R. Lewontin, *The Triple Helix—Gene, Organism, and Environment* (Harvard University Press, Cambridge, MA, 2000), p. 4.

12. Bleier, *Science and Gender*, p. 138.

13. Ibid.

14. G. Taubes, "Do we really know what makes us healthy?," *New York Times Magazine*, September 16 (2007), p. 52.

15. C. Northrup, *Women's Bodies, Women's Wisdom Creating Physical and Emotional Health and Healing*, 3rd ed. (Bantam, New York, 1998).

16. E. Pinto, "Blood pressure and ageing," *Postgraduate Medical Journal* **83**(976), 109–114 (2007).

17. Prior, "Perimenopause lost."

18. J. Prior, *Estrogen's Storm Years—Stories of Perimenopause* (Centre for Menstrual Cycle and Ovulation Research, Vancouver, 2005).

19. M. Moen, H. Kahn, K. Bjerve, and T. Halvoersen, "Menometrorrhagia in the perimenopause is associated with increased serum estradiol," *Maturitas* **47**(2), 151–155 (2004).

20. J. Prior, "Clearing confusion about perimenopause," *British Columbia Medical Journal* **47**(10), 534–538 (2005).

21. D. A. Hill, N. S. Weiss, and A. LaCroix, "Adherence to postmenopausal hormone therapy during the year after the initial prescription: A population-based study," *American Journal of Obstetrics and Gynecology* **182**(2), 270–276 (2000).

22. J. Prior, "Perimenopause: The complex endocrinology of the menopausal transition," *Endocrine Reviews* **19**, 397–428 (1998).

23. J. C. Prior, "Menopause," in *Therapeutic Choices*, J. Gray, ed. (Canadian Pharmaceutical Association, Ottawa, 1995), p. 468.

24. J. Groopman, *How Doctors Think* (Houghton Mifflin, Boston, 2007), p. 216.

25. F. Griffiths, "Women's control and choice regarding HRT," *Social Science & Medicine* **49**(4), 469–482 (1999).

26. Lock, "Medicalization," p. 9536.

27. S. Baxter, "The last word on gender differences," *Psychology Today*, March/April (1994), p. 50.

28. R. A. Wilson, *Feminine Forever* (M. Evans, New York, 1966).

29. S. M. Love, *Dr. Susan Love's Menopause & Hormone Book—Making Informed Choices*, 3rd ed. (Three Rivers Press, New York, 2003), p. 35.

30. K. H. Hall, "Reviewing intuitive decision-making and uncertainty: The implications for medical education," *Medical Education* **36**, 216–224 (2002).

31. J. C. Prior, J. D. Nielsen, C. L. Hitchcock, L. A. Williams, Y. M. Vigna, C. B. Dean, "Medroxyprogesterone and conjugated oestrogen are equivalent for hot flushes:

A 1-year randomized double-blind trial following premenopausal ovariectomy," *Clinical Science* (London) **112**(10), 517–525 (2007).

32. F. Grodstein, M. J. Stampfer, J. E. Manson, G. A. Colditz, W. C. Willett, B. Rosner, F. E. Speizer, and C. H. Hennekens, "Postmenopausal estrogen and progestin use and the risk of cardiovascular disease," *New England Journal of Medicine* **335**(7), 453–461 (1996).

33. T. Bush, E. Barrett-Connor, L. Cowan, M. Criqui, R. Wallace, C. Suchindran, H. Tyroler, and B. Rifkind, "Cardiovascular mortality and noncontraceptive use of estrogen in women: Results from the Lipid Research Clinics Program follow-up study," *Circulation* **75**(6), 1102–1109 (1987).

34. L. Voigt, T. Koepsell, and J. R. Daling, "Characteristics of telephone survey respondents according to willingness to participate," *American Journal of Epidemiology* **157**(1), 66–73 (2003).

35. D. L. Sackett, "The arrogance of preventive medicine," *Canadian Medical Association Journal* **167**(4), 363–364 (2002).

36. Taubes, "Do we really know?"

37. J. E. Manson, J. Hsia, K. C. Johnson, J. E. Rossouw, A. R. Assaf, N. L. Lasser, M. Trevisan, H. R. Black, S. R. Heckbert, R. Detrano, O. L. Strickland, N. D. Wong, J. R. Crouse, E. Stein, M. Cushman, and the Women's Health Initiative investigators, "Estrogen plus progestin and the risk of coronary heart disease," *New England Journal of Medicine* **349**(6), (2003), p. 533.

38. "Position statement: Estrogen and progestogen use in peri- and postmenopausal women: March 2007 position statement of the North American Menopause Society," *Menopause* **14**(2), 168–182 (2007).

39. J. O. Cobb, "What do midlife women expect from their gynecologists?," paper presented at the 6th annual meeting of the North American Menopause Society, San Francisco, 1995.

40. E. Friess, H. Tagaya, L. Trachsel, F. Holsboer, and R. Rupprecht, "Progesterone-induced changes in sleep in male subjects," *American Journal of Physiology* **272**, E885–E891 (1997).

41. J. Prior, Y. Vigna, B. Si, C. Rexworthy, and B. Lentle, "Cyclic medroxyprogesterone treatment increases bone density: A controlled trial in active women with menstrual cycle disturbances," *American Journal of Medicine* **96**, 521–530 (1994).

42. E. Fox-Keller, *Refiguring Life: Metaphors of Twentieth Century Biology* (Columbia University Press, New York, 1995), p. xii.

43. J. P. Vandenbroucke, "Clinical investigation in the 20th century: The ascendancy of numerical reasoning," *Lancet* **352**(Suppl. 2), 12–16 (1998).

44. R. Hubbard, *The Politics of Women's Biology* (Rutgers University Press, New Brunswick, NJ, 1990).

45. Ibid., pp. 17–18.

46. M. Lock, "Menopause: Lessons from anthropology," *Psychosomatic Medicine* **60**, 410–419 (1998).

47. G. J. Annas, "Reframing the debate on health care reform by replacing our metaphors," *New England Journal of Medicine* **332**(11), 745–748 (1995).

48. E. Martin, *The Woman in the Body: A Cultural Analysis of Reproduction* (Beacon Press, Boston, 1992).

CHAPTER 2

1. A. E. Walker, *The Menstrual Cycle* (Routledge, London, 1997), p. 13.

2. Ibid., p. 8.

3. Ibid., pp. 20–21.

4. Ibid., pp. 20–21.

5. K. Chang, T. Lee, G. Linares-Cruz, S. Fournier, and B. de Lignieres, "Influence of percutaneous administration of estradiol and progesterone on human breast epithelial cell cycle in vivo," *Fertility and Sterility* **63**, 785–791 (1995).

6. F. Tremollieres, D. Strong, D. Baylink, and S. Mohan, "Progesterone and promogestone stimulate human bone cell proliferation and insulin-like growth factor 2 production," *Acta Endocrinologica* **126**, 329–337 (1992). H. K. Nielsen, K. Brixen, R. Bouillon, and L. Mosekilde, "Changes in biochemical markers of osteoblastic activity during the menstrual cycle," *Journal of Clinical Endocrinology and Metabolism* **70**, 1431–1437 (1990).

7. K. Mather, E. Norman, J. Prior, and T. Elliott, "Preserved forearm endothelial responses with acute exposure to progesterone: A randomized cross-over trial of 17-b estradiol, progesterone, and 17-b estradiol with progesterone in healthy menopausal women," *Journal of Clinical Endocrinology and Metabolism* **85**, 4644–4649 (2000).

8. S. Berga, T. Daniels, and D. Giles, "Women with functional hypothalamic amenorrhea but not other forms of anovulation display amplified cortisol concentrations," *Fertility and Sterility* **67**, 1024–1030 (1997).

9. W. Marshall and J. Tanner, "Variations in pattern of pubertal changes in girls," *Archives of Disease in Childhood* **44**, 291–303 (1969).

10. J. Prior, Y. Vigna, and D. Watson, "Spironolactone with physiological female gonadal steroids in the presurgical therapy of male to female transsexuals: A new observation," *Archives of Sexual Behavior* **18**, 49–57 (1989).

11. N. Oudshoorn, "On the making of sex hormones: Research materials and the production of knowledge," *Social Studies of Science* **20**(1), (1990), p. 8.

12. R. Frank, *The Female Sex Hormone* (Charles C. Thomas, Springfield, IL, 1929).

13. Oudshoorn, "On the making of sex hormones," p. 8.

14. S. D. Reventlow, L. Hvas, and K. Malterud, "Making the invisible body visible: Bone scans, osteoporosis and women's bodily experiences," *Social Science and Medicine* **62**(11), 2720–2731 (2006).

15. J. Prior, S. Kirkland, L. Joseph, N. Kreiger, T. Murray, and D. Tanley, "Oral contraceptive agent use and bone mineral density in premenopausal women: Cross-sectional, population-based data from the Canadian Multicentre Osteoporosis Study," *Canadian Medical Association Journal* **165**(8), 1023–1029 (2001).

16. E. Belsey and A. P. Y Pinol, "Menstrual bleeding patterns in untreated women (from: Task Force on Long-Acting Systemic Agents for Fertility Regulation)," *Contraception* **55**, 57–65 (1997).

17. A. Treloar, R. Boyton, B. Behn, and B. Brown, "Variations of the human menstrual cycle through reproductive life," *International Journal of Fertility* **12**, 77–126 (1967).

18. G. Abraham, "The normal menstrual cycle," in *Endocrine Causes of Menstrual Disorders*, J. Givens, ed. (Year Book, Chicago, 1978), pp. 15–44.

19. K. Munster, L. Schmidt, and P. Helm, "Length and variation in the menstrual cycle—a cross-sectional study from a Danish county," *British Journal of Obstetrics and Gynaecology* **99**, 422–429 (1992).

20. C. Hitchcock and J. Prior, "Evidence about extending the duration of oral contraceptive use to suppress menstruation," *Women's Health Issues* **14**, 201–211 (2004).

21. Prior et al., "Oral contraceptive agent use."

22. M. Bracken, K. Hellenbrand, and T. Holford, "Conception delay after oral contraceptive use: The effect of estrogen dose," *Fertility and Sterility* **53**, 21–27 (1990).

23. A. Lethaby, C. Augood, and K. Duckitt, "Nonsteroidal anti-inflammatory drugs for heavy menstrual bleeding," Cochrane Database of Systematic Reviews, CD000400 (2002).

24. Walker, *Menstrual Cycle*.

25. S. Ramcharan, E. Love, G. Frick, and A. Goldfien, "The epidemiology of premenstrual symptoms in a population-based sample of 22,650 urban women: Attributable risk and risk factors," *Journal of Clinical Epidemiology* **45**, 377–392 (1992).

26. R. Frank, "The hormonal causes of premenstrual tension," *Archives of Neuropsychiatry* **26**, 1053–1057 (1931).

27. *Diagnostic and Statistical Manual of Mental Disorders*, Fourth Edition, published by the American Psychiatric Association (2005), p. 715.

28. M. L. Marvan and C. Escobedo, "Premenstrual symptomatology: Role of prior knowledge about premenstrual syndrome," *Psychosomatic Medicine* **61**(2), 163–167 (1999).

29. G. Morse, "Positive concomitants of the menstrual cycle: Nurse intervention and its effect on perimenstrual changes," *British Journal of Family Planning* **19**(Suppl.), 26–28 (1994).

30. J. Prior, Y. Vigna, N. Aojado, D. Sciaretta, and M. Schulzer, "Conditioning exercise decreases premenstrual symptoms: A prospective controlled six month trial," *Fertility and Sterility* **47**, 402–408 (1987).

31. M. Williams, R. Harris, and B. Dean, "Controlled trial of pyridoxine in the premenstrual syndrome," *Journal of International Medical Research* **13**, 174–179 (1985).

32. H. Collins and T. Pinch, "Yuppie flu, fibromyalgia and other contested diseases," in *Dr. Golem: How to Think about Medicine* (University of Chicago Press, Chicago, 2005), pp. 112–131.

33. A. E. Walker, "Premenstrual syndrome," in *The Menstrual Cycle*, p. 144.

34. A. E. Walker, "Methods in menstrual cycle research," in *The Menstrual Cycle*, pp. 59–87.

35. Ibid.

36. R. Lewontin, *Biology as Ideology: The Doctrine of DNA* (HarperPerennial, New York, 1991), p. 3.

37. R. Lewontin, "A reasonable skepticism," in *Biology as Ideology*, p. 5.

38. R. Bleier, *Science and Gender: A Critique of Biology and Its Theories on Women*, The Athene Series (Pergamon, New York, 1984), p. 71.

39. R. Bleier, "The brain and human 'nature,'" in *Science and Gender: A Critique of Biology and Its Theories on Women* (Pergamon, New York, 1984), p. 73.

40. R. Hubbard, *The Politics of Women's Biology* (Rutgers University Press, New Brunswick, NJ, 1990), pp. 26–27.

41. B. Seaman, *The Greatest Experiment Ever Performed on Women: Exploding the Estrogen Myth* (Hyperion, New York, 2003).

42. Hitchcock and Prior, "Evidence about extending the duration."

43. J. Duffin, *History of Medicine: A Scandalously Short Introduction* (University of Toronto Press, Toronto, 2000), p. 260.

44. E. Martin, *The Woman in the Body: A Cultural Analysis of Reproduction* (Beacon Press, Boston, 1992), p. 54.

45. R. Bleier, ed., *Feminist Approaches to Science* (Pergamon, New York, 1986), p. 57.

46. F. S. Greenspan and D. G. Gardner, *Basic and Clinical Endocrinology*, 7th ed. (Lange Medical Books/McGraw-Hill, New York, 2004).

47. L. Payer, "United States: The virus in the machine," in *Medicine & Culture* (Henry Holt and Company, New York, 1996), pp. 130–131.

48. J. Prior, "Perimenopause lost—reframing the end of menstruation," *Journal of Reproductive and Infant Psychology* **24**(4), 323–335 (2006).

CHAPTER 3

1. J. Prior, "Perimenopause lost—reframing the end of menstruation," *Journal of Reproductive and Infant Psychology* **24**(4), (2006), p. 323.

2. R. Atkinson, "Midlife: The crisis reconsidered," in *Encyclopaedia Britannica 1995 Medical and Health Annual*, E. Bernstein, ed. (Encyclopaedia Britannica, Chicago, 1995), pp. 61–69.

3. J. O. Cobb, "What do midlife women expect from their gynecologists?," paper presented at the 6th annual meeting of the North American Menopause Society, San Francisco, 1995.

4. B. L. Neugarten and R. J. Kraines, "'Menopausal symptoms' in women of various ages," *Psychosomatic Medicine* **27**(3), 266–273 (1965), p. 268.

5. Ibid., p. 272; J. Prior, "The ageing female reproductive axis II: Ovulatory changes with perimenopause," in *Endocrine Facets of Ageing*, D. Chadwick and J. Goode, eds. (John Wiley, Chichester, UK, 2002), pp. 172–186; G. Hale, X. Zhao, C. Hughes, H. G. Burger, D. Robertson, and I. Fraser, "Endocrine features of menstrual cycles in middle and late reproductive age and the menopausal transition classified according to the Staging of Reproductive Aging Workshop (STRAW) staging system," *Journal of Clinical Endocrinology and Metabolism* **92**, 3060–3067 (2007).

6. M. Moen, H. Kahn, K. Bjerve, and T. Halvoersen, "Menometrorrhagia in the perimenopause is associated with increased serum estradiol," *Maturitas* **47**(2), 151–155 (2004).

7. M. Wang, L. Seippel, R. Purdy, and T. Backstrom, "Relationship between symptom severity and steroid variation in women with premenstrual syndrome: Study on serum pregnenolone, prenenolone sulfat, 5a-Pregnane-3, 20-Dione, and 3a-Hydroxy-5a-Pregnan-20-one," *Journal of Clinical Endocrinology and Metabolism* **81**, 1076–1082 (1996).

8. J. Groopman, *How Doctors Think* (Houghton Mifflin, Boston, 2007), p. 5.

9. M. J. Naughton, A. S. Jones, and S. A. Shumaker, "When practices, promises, profits and policies outpace hard evidence: The post-menopausal hormone debate," *Journal of Social Issues* **61**(1), (2005), pp. 160, 163.

10. W. A. Rogers, "Evidence-based medicine in practice: Limiting or facilitating patient choice?," *Health Expectations* **5**(2), 95–103 (2002).

11. J. V. Tu, M. J. Schull, L. E. Ferris, J. E. Hux, and D. A. Redelmeier, "Problems for clinical judgement: 4. Surviving in the report card era," *Canadian Medical Association Journal* **164**(12), 1709–1712 (2001); S. J. Genuis, "The proliferation of clinical practice guidelines: Professional development or medicine-by-numbers?," *Journal of the American Board of Family Practice* **18**(5), 419–425 (2005).

12. A. R. Feinstein, "Is 'quality of care' being mislabeled or mismeasured?," *American Journal of Medicine* **112**, 472–478 (2002).

13. J. P. Vandenbroucke, "Clinical investigation in the 20th century: The ascendancy of numerical reasoning," *Lancet* **352**(Suppl. 2), 12–16 (1998).

14. Groopman, *How Doctors Think*, p. 6.

15. E. Weir, "Hot flashes . . . in January," *Canadian Medical Association Journal* **170**(1), 39–40 (2004).

16. C. Kirschbaum, N. Schommer, I. Federenko, J. Gaab, O. Neumann, and M. Oellers, "Short-term estradiol treatment enhances pituitary-adrenal axis and sympathetic responses to psychosocial stress in healthy young men," *Journal of Clinical Endocrinology and Metabolism* **81**, 3639–3643 (1996).

17. R. Hardy and D. Kuh, "Change in psychological and vasomotor symptom reporting during the menopause," *Social Science and Medicine* **55**(11), 1975–1988 (2002).

18. Neugarten and Kraines, "Menopausal symptoms," p. 272.

19. Kirschbaum et al., "Short-term estradiol treatment."

20. Hale et al., "Endocrine features of menstrual cycles."

21. J. Prior, "Premenstrual symptoms and signs," in *Conn's Current Therapy 2002*, R. Rabel and E. Bope, eds. (WB Saunders, New York, 2002), pp. 1078–1080.

22. C. P. Cannon, E. Braunwald, C. H. McCabe, D. J. Rader, J. L. Rouleau, R. Belder, S. V. Joyal, K. A. Hill, M. A. Pfeffer, A. M. Skene, and the Pravastatin or Atorvastatin Evaluation and Infection Therapy-Thrombolysis in Myocardial Infarction 22 Investigators, "Intensive versus moderate lipid lowering with statins after acute coronary syndromes," *New England Journal of Medicine* **350**(15), 1495–1504 (2004).

23. N. Freemantle, M. Calvert, J. Wood, J. Eastaugh, and C. Griffin, "Composite outcomes in randomized trials: Greater precision but with greater uncertainty?," *Journal of the American Medical Association* **289**(19), 2554–2559 (2003).

24. J. Walsh and M. Pignone, "Drug treatment of hyperlipidemia in women," *Journal of the American Medical Association* **291**, 2243–2252 (2004).

25. A. Viera, M. Bond, and S. Yates, "Diagnosing night sweats," *American Family Physician* **67**, 1019–1024 (2003).

26. L. A. Bastian, C. M. Smith, and K. Nanda, "Is this woman perimenopausal?," *Journal of the American Medical Association* **289**(7), 895–902 (2003).

27. WHO Scientific Group, *Technical Report Series: Research on the Menopause in the 1990's*, Report 866, 1–107 (World Health Organization, Geneva, Switzerland, 1996).

28. R. A. Arnowitz, *Making Sense of Illness: Science, Society and Disease* (Cambridge University Press, New York, 1998), p. 267.

29. D. Brambilla, S. McKinlay, C. Johannes, H. G. Burger, A. Green, and J. Hopper, "Defining the perimenopause for application in epidemiologic investigations," *American Journal of Epidemiology* **140**(10), 1091–1095 (1994).

30. E. Dudley, J. Hopper, J. Taffe, J. Guthrie, H. G. Burger, and L. Dennerstein, "Using longitudinal data to define the perimenopause by menstrual cycle characteristics," *Climacteric* **1**, 18–25 (1998).

31. Bastian, Smith, and Nanda, "Is this woman perimenopausal?," p. 896.

32. A. Treloar, R. Boyton, B. Behn, and B. Brown, "Variations of the human menstrual cycle through reproductive life," *International Journal of Fertility* **12**, 77–126 (1967).

33. S. McKinlay, D. Brambilla, and J. Posner, "The normal menopause transition," *Maturitas* **14**(2), 103–115 (1992).

34. M. Maresh, M. Metcalfe, K. McPherson, C. Overton, V. Hall, and J. Harbreaves, "The VALUE national hysterectomy study: Description of the patients and their surgery," *British Journal of Obstetrics and Gynaecology* **109**, 302–312 (2002).

35. A. Coulter, K. McPherson, and M. Vessey, "Do British women undergo too many or too few hysterectomies?" *Social Science and Medicine* **27**(9), (1988), p. 990.

36. R. Wallace, B. Sherman, J. Bean, A. Treloar, and L. Schlabaugh, "Probability of menopause with increasing duration of amenorrhea in middle-aged women," *American Journal of Obstetrics and Gynecology* **135**, 1021–1024 (1979).

37. Prior, "Perimenopause lost."

38. L. Dennerstein, E. Dudley, J. Hopper, J. Guthrie, and H. G. Burger, "A prospective population-based study of menopausal symptoms," *Obstetrics and Gynecology* **96**, 351–358 (2000).

39. Bastian, Smith, and Nanda, "Is this woman perimenopausal?" p. 897.

40. Cobb, "What do midlife women expect."

41. J. Prior, "Perimenopause: The complex endocrinology of the menopausal transition," *Endocrine Review* **19**, 397–428 (1998); Prior, "The ageing female reproductive axis II."

42. R. Casper, S. Dodin, and R. Reid, "The effect of 20 μg ethinyl estradiol/1 mg norethindrone acetate (MinestrinTM), a low-dose oral contraceptive, on vaginal bleeding patterns, hot flashes, and quality of life in symptomatic perimenopausal women," *Menopause* **4**(3), 138–147 (1997).

43. M. Soules, S. Sherman, E. Parrott, R. Rebar, N. Santoro, and W. Utian, "Executive summary: Stages of reproductive aging workshop (STRAW)," *Fertility and Sterility* **76**, 874–878 (2001).

44. H. G. Burger, "Diagnostic role of follicle-stimulating (FSH) measurements during the menopausal transition—an analysis of FSH, oestradiol and inhibin," *European Journal of Endocrinology* **130**, 38–42 (1994).

45. Cobb, "What do midlife women expect," p. 6.

46. D. Fischer, A. L. Stewart, D. A. Bloch, K. Lorig, D. Laurent, and H. Holman, "Capturing the patient's view of change as a clinical outcome measure," *Journal of the American Medical Association* **282**(12), 1157–1162 (1999).

47. H. G. Burger, "The endocrinology of the menopausal transition: A cross-sectional study of a population-based sample," *Journal of Clinical Endocrinology and Metabolism* **80**, 3537–3545 (1995).

48. A. J. Barsky, R. Saintfort, M. Rogers, and J. Borus, "Nonspecific medication side effects and the nocebo phenomenon," *Journal of the American Medical Association* **287**(5), 622–627 (2002).

49. Feinstein, "Is 'quality of care' being mislabeled."

50. Writing Group for the Women's Health Initiative Investigators, "Risks and benefits of estrogen plus progestin in healthy postmenopausal women: Principal results from the Women's Health Initiative randomized controlled trial," *Journal of the American Medical Association* **288**(3), 321–333 (2002).

51. G. Hale, C. Hughes, and J. Cline, "Endometrial cancer: Hormonal factors, the perimenopausal 'window of risk,' and isoflavones," *Journal of Clinical Endocrinology and Metabolism* **87**, 3–15 (2002).

52. J. Neimark, "Plastic people of the Universe: Everything you always wanted to know about the biology of plastic (but were afraid to ask)," *Discover*, May (2008), pp. 46–51.

53. G. Greer, *The Whole Woman* (Anchor, London, 2000), p. 189.

PART 2

1. G. Taubes, "Do We Really Know What Makes Us Healthy?," in *New York Times Magazine* Sept. 16 (2007), p. 52.

CHAPTER 4

1. M. J. Naughton, A. S. Jones, and S. A. Shumaker, "When Practices, Promises, Profits and Policies Outpace Hard Evidence: The Post-menopausal Hormone Debate," *Journal of Social Issues* **61**(1), 159–179 (2005).

2. M. Foucault, cited in Hardey, M, (1998) *The Social Context of Health,* Buckingham—Philadelphia: Open University Press, p. 39.

3. M. Lock, "Medicalization: Cultural Concerns," in *International Encyclopedia of the Social & Behavioral Sciences,* P. B. Baltes, ed. (Pergamon, Oxford, 2001), p. 9534–9539.

4. S. J. Williams and M. Calnan, "The 'limits' of medicalization?: Modern medicine and the lay populace in 'late' modernity," *Social Science & Medicine* **42**(12), 1609–1620 (1996).

5. Ibid.

6. C. Clements, "A Pill for Every Ill," *The Medical Post,* July 2 (2002).

7. R. A. Arnowitz, "The Social Construction of Coronary Heart Disease Risk Factors," in *Making Sense of Illness*, C. Rosenberg, ed. (Cambridge University Press, Cambridge, 1998), pp. 111–144.

8. A. R. Feinstein, "Is 'Quality of Care' Being Mislabeled or Mismeasured?," *American Journal of Medicine* **112**, 472–478 (2002).

9. F. Griffiths, "Women's control and choice regarding HRT," *Social Science & Medicine* **49**(4), 469–482 (1999).

10. See J. C. Prior, "Stopping Estrogen Treatment," http://www.cemcor.ubc.ca/help_yourself/articles/stopping_estrogen.

11. S. Blair, H. Kohl, and C. Barlow, "Physical activity, physical fitness, and all-cause mortality in women: do women need to be active?," *Journal of the American College of Nutrition* **12**, 368–371 (1993).

12. W. B. Kannel and D. L. McGee, "Diabetes and Cardiovascular Disease: The Framingham Study," *Journal of the American Medical Association* **241**(19), 2035–2038 (1979).

13. L. Payer, "United States: The Virus in the Machine," in *Medicine & Culture* (Henry Holt, New York, 1996), pp. 124–152.

14. U. Ravnskov, P. Rosch, M. Sutter, and M. Houston, "Should we lower cholesterol as much as possible?," *British Medical Journal* **332**, 1330–1332 (2006).

15. K. Harby, "Menopause: Disease State or State of Nature?," *Molecular Medicine Today* **2**(10), 414–417 (1996).

16. C. D. DeAngelis and M. A. Winker, "Women's Health—Filling the Gaps," *Journal of the American Medical Association* **285**(11), 1508–09 (2001).

17. S. A. Grover, "Estrogen replacement for women with cardiovascular disease: Why don't physicians and patients follow the guidelines?," *Canadian Medical Association Journal* **161**(1), 42–43 (1999).

18. Writing Group for the Women's Health Initiative Investigators, "Risks and Benefits of Estrogen Plus Progestin in Healthy Postmenopausal Women: Principal Results from the Women's Health Initiative Randomized Controlled Trial," *Journal of the American Medical Association* **288**(3), 321–333 (2002).

19. E. Barrett-Connor, "Hormones and Heart Disease in Women: The Timing Hypothesis," *American Journal of Epidemiology* **166**(5), 506–510 (2007).

20. N. P. Kenny, *What **Good** Is Health Care?* (CHA Press/Presse de l'ACS, Ottawa, Ontario, 2002), p. 237.

21. W. M. Hopman, T. Towheed, T. Anastassiades, A. Tenenhouse, S. Poliquin, C. Berger, L. Joseph, J. P. Brown, T. M. Murray, J. D. Adachi, D. A. Hanley, E. Papadimitropoulos, and the Canadian Multicentre Osteoporosis Study Research Group, "Canadian normative data for the SF-36 health survey," *Canadian Medical Association Journal* **163**(3), 265–271 (2000).

22. A. Sen, "Health: perception versus observation," *British Medical Journal* **324**(7342), 860–861 (2002).

23. N. M. Hadler, *The Last Well Person: How to Stay Well despite the Health-Care System* (McGill-Queen's University Press, Montreal, Quebec, 2004), p. 167.

24. S. Baxter and W. I. Lane, *Immune Power* (Penguin/Putnam [Avery], Garden City Park, New York, 1999), p. 188.

25. C. Kirschbaum, B. M. Kudielka, J. Gaab, N. C. Schommer, and D. H. Hellhammer, "Impact of Gender, Menstrual Cycle Phase, and Oral Contraceptives on the Activity of the Hypothalamus-Pituitary-Adrenal Axis," *Psychosomatic Medicine* **61**(2), 154–162 (1999).

26. A. Cassels, M. A. Hughes, C. Cole, B. Mintzes, J. Lexchin, and J. P. McCormack, "Drugs in the news: an analysis of Canadian newspaper coverage of new prescription drugs," *Canadian Medical Association Journal* **168**(9), 1133–1137 (2003).

27. P. Davis, "Health care as a risk factor," *Canadian Medical Association Journal* **170**(11), 1688–1689 (2004).

28. C. Bartlett, J. Sterne, and M. Egger, "What Is newsworthy? Longitudinal study of the reporting of medical research in two British newspapers," *British Medical Journal* **325**, 81–84 (2002).

29. Hadler, *Last Well Person,* p. 166.

30. S. E. Bell, "Changing ideas: The medicalization of menopause," *Social Science & Medicine* **24**(6), 535–542 (1987).

31. E. Tilt, *The change of life in health and disease: A practical treatise on the nervous and other afflictions incidental to women at the decline of life* (Lindsay & Blakiston, Philadelphia, 1871).

32. Bell, "Changing Ideas," p. 536.

33. N. Oudshoorn, "On the Making of Sex Hormones: Research Materials and the Production of Knowledge," *Social Studies of Science* **20**(1), 5–33 (1990).

34. J. D. Wilson, "The Evolution of Endocrinology—Plenary Lecture at the 12th International Congress of Endocrinology, Lisbon, Portugal, 31 August 2004," *Clinical Endocrinology* **62**, 389–396 (2005).

35. N. Oudshoorn, "United We Stand: The Pharmaceutical Industry, Laboratory, and Clinic in the Development of Sex Hormones into Scientific Drugs, 1920–1940," *Science, Technology & Human Values* **18**(1), 5–24 (1993).

36. Wilson, "Evolution of Endocrinology."

37. Oudshoorn, "On the Making."

38. *Female Sex Hormone Therapy, Part One, The Follicular Hormone: A Clinical Guide* (Schering Corporation, Montreal, Quebec, 1941).

39. F. B. McCrea, "The Politics of Menopause: The 'Discovery' of a Deficiency Disease," *Social Problems* **31**(1), 111–123 (1983).

40. Oudshoorn, "On the Making."

41. Bell, "Changing Ideas," p. 536.

42. McCrea, "Politics of Menopause."

43. Bell, "Changing Ideas."

44. M. L. Meldrum, "Departures from the Design: The Randomized Clinical Trial in Historical Context, 1946–1970," PhD dissertation (State University of New York at Stony Brook, 1994), p. 18.

45. Royal College of Obstetricians and Gynaecologists, "Fetal and Maternal Risks of Diethylstilboestrol Exposure in Pregnancy—RCOG Statement No. 2" (Royal College of Obstetricians and Gynaecologists, London, 2002).

46. Ibid.

47. R. Rubin, "Hidden Toll of DES, a Generation Later," *USA Today*, April 14 (2003).

48. L. Payer, *Medicine and Culture*, 2nd ed. (Henry Holt, New York, 1996).

49. Naughton et al., "When Practices."

50. McCrea, "Politics of Menopause," p. 112.

51. S. J. Genuis, "The Proliferation of Clinical Practice Guidelines: Professional Development or Medicine-by-Numbers?," *Journal of the American Board of Family Practice* **18**(5), 419–425 (2005).

52. M. J. Naughton, et al., "When Practices."

53. R. T. Hare-Mustin and J. Maracek, "The Meaning of Difference: Gender Theory, Postmodernism, and Psychology," *American Psychologist* **43**(6), 455–464 (1988).

54. McCrea, "Politics of Menopause," p. 113.

55. R. Wilson, *Feminine Forever* (M. Evans and Company Inc, New York, 1966), p. 96.

56. McCrea, "Politics of Menopause," p. 113.

57. Genius, "Proliferation of Clinical Practice," p. 419.

CHAPTER 5

1. S. B. Hulley and D. Grady, "The WHI Estrogen-Alone Trial—Do Things Look Any Better?," *Journal of the American Medical Association* **291**(14), (2004), p. 1769.

2. N. M. Hadler, "Turning Aging into a Disease," in *The Last Well Person: How to Stay Well despite the Health-Care System* (McGill-Queens University Press, Montreal, 2004), p. 155.

3. Hulley and Grady, "The WHI Estrogen-Alone Trial."

4. *Female Sex Hormone Therapy, Part Two, Corpus Luteum Hormone: A Clinical Guide* (Schering Corporation, 1941), p. 11.

5. R. A. Wilson, *Feminine Forever* (M. Evans, New York, 1966), p. 63.

6. The Writing Group for the PEPI Trial, "Effects of hormone replacement therapy on endometrial histology in postmenopausal women. The Postmenopausal Estrogen/Progestin Interventions (PEPI) Trial," *Journal of the American Medical Association* **275**(5), 370–375 (1996).

7. Hulley and Grady, "The WHI Estrogen-Alone Trial," p. 1769.

8. "Effects of hormone replacement therapy."

9. Hulley and Grady, "The WHI Estrogen-Alone Trial," p. 1769.

10. "Effects of hormone replacement therapy."

11. G. Mishra and D. Kuh, "Perceived change in quality of life during the menopause," *Social Science & Medicine* **62**(1), 93–102 (2006).

12. A. J. Welton, M. R. Vickers, J. Kim, D. Ford, B. A. Lawton, A. H. MacLennan, S. K. Meredith, J. Martin, T. W. Meade, and the WISDOM team, "Health related quality of life after combined hormone replacement therapy: randomised controlled trial," *British Medical Journal* **337**, a1190 (2008).

13. K. M. Rexrode and J. E. Manson, "Postmenopausal Hormone Therapy and Quality of Life: No Cause for Celebration," *Journal of the American Medical Association* **287**(5), (2002), p. 641.

14. Ibid.

15. D. A. Hill, N. S. Weiss, and A. LaCroix, "Adherence to postmenopausal hormone therapy during the year after the initial prescription: A population-based study," *American Journal of Obstetrics and Gynecology* **182**(2), 270–276 (2000).

16. D. T. Wade and P. W. Halligan, "Do biomedical models of illness make for good healthcare systems?," *British Medical Journal* **329**(7479), 1398 (2004).

17. Mishra and Kuh, "Perceived change in quality of life," pp. 93–94.

18. M. J. Murtagh and J. Hepworth, "Feminist ethics and menopause: Autonomy and decision-making in primary medical care," *Social Science & Medicine* **56**(8), 1643–1652 (2003).

19. J. L. Thomas and P. A. Braus, "Coronary Artery Disease in Women: A Historical Perspective," *Archives of Internal Medicine* **158**(4), (1998), p. 333.

20. Hadler, "Turning Aging into a Disease."

21. L. Mosca, "The role of hormone replacement therapy in the prevention of post-menopausal heart disease," *Archives of Internal Medicine* **160**(15), (2000), p. 2263.

22. L. Pilote, K. Dasgupta, V. Guru, K. H. Humphries, J. McGrath, C. Norris, D. Rabi, J. Tremblay, A. Alamian, T. Barnett, J. Cox, G. Wa, S. Grace, P. Hamlet, T. Ho, S. Kirkland, M. Lambert, D. Libersan, J. O'Loughlin, G. Paradis, M. Petrovich, and V. Tagalakis, "A comprehensive view of sex-specific issues related to cardiovascular disease," *Canadian Medical Association Journal* 176(6), (2007), p. S1.

23. W. A. Silverman, "Begin with 'If . . . ,'" in *Where's the Evidence? Debates in Modern Medicine* (Oxford University Press, Oxford, 1998), p. 34.

24. J. Groopman, *How Doctors Think* (Houghton Mifflin, Boston, 2007), p. 217.

25. G. Taubes, "Do we really know what makes us healthy?," *New York Times Magazine*, Sept. 16 (2007), p. 52.

26. F. Griffiths, "Women's control and choice regarding HRT," *Social Science & Medicine* 49(4), (1999), p. 470.

27. R. A. Arnowitz, "The social construction of coronary heart disease risk factors," in *Making Sense of Illness* (Cambridge University Press, Cambridge, 1998), p. 111.

28. Ibid., p. 84

29. Ibid., p. 114.

30. T. R. Fleming and D. L. DeMets, "Surrogate end points in clinical trials: Are we being misled?," *Annals of Internal Medicine* **125**(7), 605–613 (1996).

31. H. C. Bucher, G. H. Guyatt, D. J. Cook, A. Holbrook, F. A. McAlister, and the Evidence-Based Medicine Working Group, "Users' Guides to the Medical Literature: XIX. Applying Clinical Trial Results; A. How to Use an Article Measuring the Effect of an Intervention on Surrogate End Points," *Journal of the American Medical Association* **282**(8), 771–778 (1999).

32. N. M. Hadler, "Interventional Cardiology and Kindred Delusions," in *The Last Well Person*, pp. 17–34.

33. L. Payer, "United States: The Virus in the Machine," in *Medicine and Culture* (Henry Holt, New York, 1996), pp. 124–125.

34. J. Duffin, *History of Medicine: A Scandalously Short Introduction* (University of Toronto Press, Toronto, 2000).

35. D. Mechanic, "Socio-cultural implications of changing organizational technologies in the provision of care," *Social Science & Medicine* 54, 459–467 (2002).

36. W. A. Silverman, "Bradford Hill's doubts," in *Where's the Evidence?*, p. 99.

37. Ibid.

38. M. L. Meldrum, "Departures from the design: The randomized clinical trial in historical context, 1946–1970," PhD dissertation (State University of New York at Stony Brook, 1994), p. 8.

39. A. Feinstein, "Is 'Quality of Care' Being Mislabeled or Mismeasured?," *The American Journal of Medicine* **112**, 474 (2002).

40. P. Sytkowski, W. Kannel, and R. D'Agostino, "Changes in risk factors and the decline in mortality from cardiovascular disease: The Framingham Heart Study," *New England Journal of Medicine* **322**(23), 1635–1641 (1990).

41. Ibid.

42. Mosca, "The role of hormone replacement therapy."

43. T. S. Mikkola and T. B. Clarkson, "Estrogen replacement therapy, atherosclerosis, and vascular function," *Cardiovascular Research* **53**(3), 605–619 (2002).

44. Ibid., p. 605.

45. The Writing Group for the PEPI Trial, "Effects of estrogen or estrogen/progestin regimens on heart disease risk factors in postmenopausal women. The Postmenopausal Estrogen/Progestin Interventions (PEPI) Trial." *Journal of the American Medical Association* **273**(3), 199–208 (1995).

46. Ibid., p. 208.

47. Coronary Drug Project Research Group, "Coronary drug project: Initial findings leading to modifications of its research protocol," *Journal of the American Medical Association* **214**(7), 1303 (1970); Coronary Drug Project Research Group, "Coronary drug project: Findings leading to the discontinuation of the 2.5 mg/day estrogen group," *Journal of the American Medical Association* **226**, 652–657 (1973).

48. F. B. Hu, M. J. Stampfer, J. E. Manson, F. Grodstein, G. A. Colditz, F. E. Speizer, and W. C. Willett, "Trends in the incidence of coronary heart disease and changes in diet and lifestyle in women," *New England Journal of Medicine* **343**(8), 530–537 (2000).

49. Taubes, "Do we really know."

50. F. Grodstein, M. J. Stampfer, J. E. Manson, G. A. Colditz, W. C. Willett, B. Rosner, F. E. Speizer, and C. H. Hennekens, "Postmenopausal Estrogen and Progestin Use and the Risk of Cardiovascular Disease," *New England Journal of Medicine* **335**(7), (1996), p. 453.

51. N. Oudshoorn, "United We Stand: The Pharmaceutical Industry, Laboratory, and Clinic in the Development of Sex Hormones into Scientific Drugs, 1920–1940," *Science, Technology, and Human Values* **18**(1), 5–24 (1993).

52. J. P. Vandenbroucke, "Medical journals and the shaping of medical knowledge," *Lancet* **352**(9355), (1998), p. 2003.

53. Ibid., p. 2004.

54. U. Ravnskov, P. Rosch, M. Sutter, and M. Houston, "Should we lower cholesterol as much as possible?," *British Medical Journal* 332, 1330–1332 (2006); U. Ravnskov, "High cholesterol may protect against infections and atherosclerosis," *Q JM* **96**(12), 927–934 (2003).

55. T. Bush, E. Barrett-Connor, L. Cowan, M. Criqui, R. Wallace, C. Suchindran, H. Tyroler, and B. Rifkind, "Cardiovascular mortality and noncontraceptive use of estrogen in women: Results from the Lipid Research Clinics Program Follow-up Study," *Circulation* **75**(6), 1102–1109 (1987).

56. Ibid.

57. T. Bush, "*Feminine Forever* revisited: menopausal hormone therapy in the 1990's," *Journal of Women's Health* **1**(1), (1992), p. 4.

58. G. C. Bowker and S. Leigh Star, *Sorting Things Out: Classification and Its Consequences* (MIT Press, Cambridge, MA, 2000), p. 123.

59. World Health Organization, "The Accuracy and Comparability of Death Statistics," *WHO Chronicle* **21**, 7–17 (1967).

60. Hadler, "Interventional Cardiology," p. 17.

61. J. Le Fanu, "The case of the missing data," *British Medical Journal* **325**(7378), 1490–1493 (2002).

62. Feinstein, "Is 'Quality of Care' Being Mislabeled or Mismeasured?," pp. 472–478.

63. Thomas and Braus, "Coronary Artery Disease in Women," p. 335.

64. P. A. van Keep, "The history and rationale of hormone replacement therapy," *Maturitas* **12**(3), 163–170 (1990).

65. K. Matthews, E. Meilahn, L. Kuller, S. Kelsey, A. Caggiula, and R. Wing, "Menopause and risk factors for coronary heart disease," *New England Journal of Medicine* **321**(10), (1989), p. 641.

66. H. Tunstall-Pedoe, "Myth and paradox of coronary risk and the menopause," *Lancet* **351**(9113), (1998), p. 1425.

67. Ibid., p. 1425.

68. C. G. Isles and D. J. Hole, "Relation between coronary risk and coronary mortality in women of the Renfrew and Paisley survey . . . ," *Lancet* **339**(8795), 702 (1992).

69. D. J. Lerner and W. B. Kannel, "Patterns of coronary heart disease morbidity and mortality in the sexes: A 26-year follow-up of the Framingham population," *American Heart Journal* **111**(2), (1986), p. 383.

70. Tunstall-Pedoe, "Myth and paradox," p. 1425.

71. M. Moen, H. Kahn, K. Bjerve, and T. Halvoersen, "Menometrorrhagia in the perimenopause is associated with increased serum estradiol," *Maturitas* **47**(2), 151–155 (2004).

72. R. Luoto, J. Kaprio, A. Reunanen, and E. Rutanen, "Cardiovascular morbidity in relation to ovarian function after hysterectomy," *Obstetrics and Gynecology* **85**, 515–522 (1995).

73. A. Towfighi, J. Saver, R. Engelhardt, and B. Ovbiabele, "A midlife stroke surge among women in the United States," *Neurology* **69**, 1898–1904 (2007).

74. H. S. Kok, K. M. van Asselt, Y. T. van der Schouw, I. van der Tweel, P. H. M. Peeters, P. W. F. Wilson, P. L. Pearson, and D. E. Grobbee, "Heart Disease Risk Determines Menopausal Age Rather Than the Reverse," *Journal of the American College of Cardiologists* **47**(10), (2006), p. 1979.

75. M. Carr, "The emergence of the metabolic syndrome with menopause," *Journal of Clinical Endocrinology and Metabolism* **88**, 2404–2411 (2003); H. Mogul, S. Peterson, B. Weinstein, S. Zhang, and A. Southern, "Metformin and carbohydrate-modified diet: A novel obesity treatment protocol; Preliminary findings from a case series of nondiabetic women with midlife weight gain and hyperinsulinemia," *Heart Disease* **13**, 285–292 (2001); H. Mogul, B. Weinstein, D. Mogul, S. Peterson, S. Zhang, and M. Frey, "Syndrome W: a new model of hyperinsulinemia, hypertension and midlife weight

gain in healthy women with normal glucose tolerance," *Heart Disease* **4**, 78–85 (2002).

76. L. Lambert, J. Straton, M. Knuiman, and H. Barthalomew, "Health status of users of hormone replacement therapy by hysterectomy status in Western Australia," *Epidemiology and Community Health* **57**, 294–300 (2003).

77. Coronary Drug Project Research Group, "Coronary drug project: Initial findings."

78. Coronary Drug Project Research Group, "Coronary drug project; estrogens and cancer (letter)," *Journal of the American Medical Association* **239**(26), 2758–2759 (1978).

79. J. Prior, "Postmenopausal estrogen therapy and cardiovascular disease (letter)," *New England Journal of Medicine* **326**, 705–706 (1992).

80. E. Pinto, "Blood pressure and ageing," *Postgraduate Medical Journal* **83**(976), 109–114 (2007).

81. D. B. Petitti, "Hormone Replacement Therapy and Heart Disease Prevention: Experimentation Trumps Observation," *Journal of the American Medical Association* **280**(7), 650–652 (1998).

82. B. M. Rifkind and J. E. Rossouw, "Of Designer Drugs, Magic Bullets, and Gold Standards," *Journal of the American Medical Association* **279**(18), (1998), p. 1483.

83. Petitti, "Hormone Replacement Therapy and Heart Disease Prevention," p. 650.

84. E. Hemminki and K. McPherson, "Impact of postmenopausal hormone therapy on cardiovascular events and cancer: pooled data from clinical trials," *British Medical Journal* **315**(7101), (1997), p. 149.

85. S. Singleton, K. Bailey, S. Shah, L. Rhodes, V. Seagroatt, N. F. Col, J. B. Wong, S. G. Pauker, T. Sundkvist, F. Al-Azzawi, J. Thompson, A. Halligan, and R. H. Karas, "Impact of postmenopausal hormone therapy on cardiovascular events and cancer (letters)," *British Medical Journal* **315**, 676 (1997).

86. S. Hulley, D. Grady, T. Bush, C. Furberg, D. Herrington, B. Riggs, E. Vittinghoff, and the Heart and Estrogen/Replacement Study Research Group, "Randomized Trial of Estrogen Plus Progestin for Secondary Prevention of Coronary Heart Disease in Postmenopausal Women," *Journal of the American Medical Association* **280**(7), (1998), p. 605.

87. D. Grady, D. Herrington, V. Bittner, R. Blumenthal, M. Davidson, M. Hlatky, J. Hsia, S. Hulley, A. Herd, S. Khan, L. K. Newby, D. Waters, E. Vittinghoff, N. Wenger, and for the HERS Research Group, "Cardiovascular Disease Outcomes During 6.8 Years of Hormone Therapy: Heart and Estrogen/Progestin Replacement Study Follow-up (HERS II)," *Journal of the American Medical Association* **288**(1), (2002), p. 49.

88. Taubes, "Do we really know."

89. Rifkind and Rossouw, "Of Designer Drugs."

90. Writing Group for the Women's Health Initiative Investigators, "Risks and benefits of estrogen plus progestin in healthy postmenopausal women: Principal results from the Women's Health Initiative randomized controlled trial," *Journal of the American Medical Association* **288**(3), (2002), p. 321.

91. Ibid., p. 322.

92. S. Yusuf and S. Anand, "Hormone replacement therapy: a time for pause," *Canadian Medical Association Journal* **167**(4), (2002), p. 357.

93. V. M. Miller, T. B. Clarkson, S. M. Harman, E. A. Brinton, M. Cedars, R. Lobo, J. E. Manson, G. R. Merriam, F. Naftolin, and N. Santoro, "Women, hormones, and clinical trials: a beginning, not an end," *Journal of Applied Physiology* **99**(2), (2005), p. 382.

94. M. Namenwirth, "Science Seen Through A Feminist Prism," in *Feminist Approaches to Science*, R. Bleier, ed. (Pergamon, New York, 1986), p. 23.

95. Writing Group for the Women's Health Initiative Investigators, "Risks and benefits."

96. Miller et al., "Women, hormones, and clinical trials."

97. E. Barrett-Connor, "Hormones and Heart Disease in Women: The Timing Hypothesis," *American Journal of Epidemiology* **166**(5), 506–510 (2007).

98. Miller et al., "Women, hormones, and clinical trials."

99. L. Payer, "Great Britain: Keeping the Upper Lip Stiff," in *Medicine and Culture*, p. 109.

100. W. A. Silverman, "Humane limits," in *Where's the Evidence?*, pp. 20–22.

101. I. J. Kerber, R. J. Turner, V. M. Miller, T. B. Clarkson, S. M. Harman, E. A. Brinton, M. Cedars, R. Lobo, J. E. Manson, G. R. Merriam, F. Naftolin, and N. Santoro, "Euestrogenemia," *Journal of Applied Physiology* **99**(6), (2005), p. 2471.

CHAPTER 6

1. R. Moynihan, "Claims by charity exaggerate dangers of osteoporosis," *British Medical Journal* **327**(7411), 358-a (2003).

2. N. M. Hadler, "Turning aging into a disease," in *The Last Well Person: How to Stay Well despite the Health-Care System* (McGill-Queens University Press, Montreal, 2004), p. 147.

3. F. Albright, E. Bloomberg, and P. Smith, "Postmenopausal osteoporosis," *Transactions of the Association of American Physicians* **55**, 298–305 (1940).

4. P. M. Barr, Y. M. Vigna, and J. C. Prior, "Eating attitudes and habitual calcium intake in peripubertal girls are associated with initial bone mineral content and its change over 2 years," *Journal of Bone and Mineral Research* **16**(5), 940–947 (2001).

5. J. Prior, Y. Vigna, M. Schechter, and A. Burgess, "Spinal bone loss and ovulatory disturbances," *New England Journal of Medicine* **323**, 1221–1227 (1990); M. Sowers, J. Randolph, M. Crutchfield, M. Jannausch, B. Shapiro, B. Zhang, and M. La Pietra, "Urinary ovarian and gonadotropin hormone levels in premenopausal women with low bone mass," *Journal of Bone and Mineral Research* **13**(7), 1191–1202 (1998); E. Waugh, J. Polivy, R. Ridout, and G. Hawker, "A prospective investigation of the relations among cognitive dietary restraint, subclinical ovulatory disturbances, physical activity, and bone mass in healthy young women," *American Journal of Clinical Nutrition* **86**(6), 1791–1801 (2007).

6. J. C. Prior, "Perimenopause—The complex endocrinology of the menopausal transition," *Endocrine Reviews* **19**, 397–428 (1998).

7. P. A. van Keep, "The history and rationale of hormone replacement therapy," *Maturitas* **12**(3), (1990), p. 163.

8. Hadler, "Turning aging into a disease."

9. B. Lentle, J. Brown, A. Khan, W. Leslie, J. Levesque, D. Lyons, K. Siminiski, G. Tarulli, R. Josse, and A. Hodsman, "Recognizing and reporting vertebral fractures: Reducing the risk of future osteoporotic fractures," *Canadian Association of Radiologists Journal* **58**(1), 27–36 (2007).

10. J. Adachi, G. Ionnidis, L. Pickard, C. Berger, J. Prior, L. Joseph, D. A. Hanley, W. P. Olszynski, T. M. Murray, T. Anastassiades, W. Hopman, J. P. Brown, S. Kirkland, C. Joyce, A. Papaioannou, S. Poliquin, A. Tenenhouse, and E. A. Papadimitropoulos. "The association between osteoporotic fractures and health-related quality of life as measured by the Health Utilities Index in the Canadian Multicentre Osteoporosis Study (CaMos)," *Osteoporosis International* **14**, 895–904 (2003).

11. A. Cranney, S. A. Jamal, J. F. Tsang, R. G. Josse, and W. D. Leslie, "Low bone mineral density and fracture burden in postmenopausal women," *Canadian Medical Association Journal* **177**(6), 575–580 (2007).

12. R. Lindsay, S. L. Silverman, C. Cooper, D. A. Hanley, I. Barton, S. B. Broy, A. Licata, L. Benhamou, P. Geusens, K. Flowers, H. Stracke, and E. Seeman, "Risk of new vertebral fracture in the year following a fracture," *Journal of the American Medical Association* **285**(3), 320–323 (2001).

13. J. P. Brown and R. G. Josse, For the Scientific Advisory Council of the Osteoporosis Society of Canada—"2002 clinical practice guidelines for the diagnosis and management of osteoporosis in Canada," *Canadian Medical Association Journal* **167**(Suppl. 10), 1–34 (2002).

14. J. C. Prior and J. D. Wark, "Osteoporosis after menopause: An update," *British Columbia Medical Journal* **35**(9), 653–658 (1993).

15. N. M. Resnick and E. R. Marcantonio, "How should clinical care of the aged differ?" *Lancet* **350**(9085), 1157–1158 (1997).

16. R. Dobson, "Industry sponsored studies twice as likely to have positive conclusions about costs," *British Medical Journal* **327**(7422), 1006-b (2003).

17. J. M. Chandler, S. I. Zimmerman, C. J. Girman, A. R. Martin, W. Hawkes, J. R. Hebel, P. D. Sloane, L. Holder, and J. Magaziner, "Low bone mineral density and risk of fracture in white female nursing home residents," *Journal of the American Medical Association* **284**(8), (2000), p. 972.

18. Cranney et al., "Low bone mineral density," p. 575.

19. Prior, "Perimenopause—The complex endocrinology of the menopausal transition."

20. J. Prior, "Progesterone as a bone-trophic hormone," *Endocrine Reviews* **11**(2), 396–398 (1990).

21. Prior and Wark, "Osteoporosis after menopause."

22. J. Prior, Y. Vigna, S. I. Barr, C. Rexworthy, and B. Lentle, "Cyclic medroxyprogesterone treatment increases bone density: A controlled trial in active women with menstrual cycle disturbances," *American Journal of Medicine* **96**, 521–530 (1994).

23. H. Carlsten, "Immune responses and bone loss: The estrogen connection," *Immunological Reviews* **208**(1), 194–206 (2005).

24. D. Grady and S. R. Cummings, "Postmenopausal hormone therapy for prevention of fractures: How good is the evidence?" *Journal of the American Medical Association* **285**(22), 2909–2910 (2001).

25. K. Chang, T. Lee, G. Linares-Cruz, S. Fournier, and B. de Lignieres, "Influence of percutaneous administration of estradiol and progesterone on human breast epilethial cell cycle in vivo," *Fertility and Sterility* **63**, 785–791 (1995).

26. J. Foidart, C. Collin, X. Denoo, J. Desreux, A. Belliard, and S. Fournier, "Estradiol and progesterone regulate the proliferation of human breast epithelial cells," *Fertility and Sterility* 5, 063–069 (1998); A. Fournier, F. Berrino, and F. Clavel-Chapelon, "Unequal risks for breast cancer associated with different hormone replacement therapies: Results from the E3N cohort study," *Breast Cancer Research and Treatment* **107**(1), 103–111 (2008).

27. J. Prior, S. Kirkland, L. Joseph, N. Kreiger, T. Murray, D. Hanley, and the CaMOS Research Group, "Oral contraceptive agent use and bone mineral density in premenopausal women: Cross-sectional, population-based data from the Canadian Multicentre Osteoporosis Study," *Canadian Medical Association Journal* **165**(8), 1023–1029 (2001).

28. Prior and Wark, "Osteoporosis after menopause."

29. Brown and Josse, For the Scientific Advisory Council "2002 clinical practice guidelines," p. S17.

30. G. Anderson, M. Limacher, A. Assaf, T. Bassford, S. Beresford, and H. Black, "Effects of conjugated equine estrogen in postmenopausal women with hysterectomy: The Women's Health Initiative randomized controlled trial," *Journal of the American Medical Association* **291**(14), 1701–1712 (2004).

31. A. Day, "Lessons from the Women's Health Initiative: Primary prevention and gender health," *Canadian Medical Association Journal* **167**(4), 361–362 (2002).

32. Brown and Josse, For the Scientific Advisory Council. "2002 Clinical practice guidelines in osteoporosis"

33. Prior, "Perimenopause—The complex endocrinology of the menopausal transition."

34. Prior, "Progesterone as a bone-trophic hormone."

35. M. Groves, K. Hermsmeyer, C. Reilly, J. Prior, F. Stanczyk, K. Stephenson, H. Leonetti, and D. Soholt, "Hormone therapy for mid-life and beyond: A new perspective," http://www.womeninbalance.org/pdf/ScienceAdvisor.pdf.

36. Hadler, "Turning aging into a disease," p. 148.

37. J. Prior, Y. Vigna, and M. Schechter, "Spinal bone loss and ovulatory disturbances," *New England Journal of Medicine* **323**, 1221–1227 (1990).

38. Sowers et al., "Urinary ovarian and gonadotropin hormone levels."

39. B. Lentle, "Osteoporosis and bone densitometry: Does the emperor have clothes?," *Canadian Medical Association Journal* **159**(10), 1261–1264 (1998).

40. S. Mays, "Age-related cortical bone loss in women from a 3rd-4th century AD population from England," *American Journal of Physical Anthropology* **129**, 518–528 (2006).

41. J.-A. Skolbekken, W. Østerlie, and S. Forsmo, "Brittle bones, pain and fractures—Lay constructions of osteoporosis among Norwegian women attending the Nord-Trøndelag Health Study (HUNT)," *Social Science and Medicine* **66**(12), (2008), p. 2562.

42. Lentle, "Osteoporosis and bone densitometry," p. 1261.

43. Ibid.

44. WHO Scientific Group, *Technical Report Series: Assessment of Osteoporotic Fracture Risk and Its Role in Screening for Postmenopausal Osteoporosis*, Report 843 (World Health Organization, Geneva, 1994).

45. P. Alonso-Coello, A. L. Garcia-Franco, G. Guyatt, and R. Moynihan, "Drugs for pre-osteoporosis: Prevention or disease mongering?," *British Medical Journal* **336**(7636), 126–129 (2008).

46. Ibid., p. 126.

47. G. J. Strewler, "Decimal point—Osteoporosis therapy at the 10-year mark," *New England Journal of Medicine* **350**(12), (2004), p. 1172.

48. J. Rifkin, "Worlds apart on the vision thing (August 17)," *Toronto Globe and Mail*, August 17 (2004), p. A13.

49. G. Gigerenzer, *Calculated Risks*, (Simon and Schuster, NY, 2002).

50. Hadler, *Last Well Person*.

51. H. G. Bone, D. Hosking, J.-P. Devogelaer, J. R. Tucci, R. D. Emkey, R. P. Tonino, J. A. Rodriguez-Portales, R. W. Downs, J. Gupta, A. C. Santora, U. A. Liberman, and the Alendronate Phase III Osteoporosis Treatment Study Group, "Ten years' experience with alendronate for osteoporosis in postmenopausal women," *New England Journal of Medicine* **350**(12), 1189–1199 (2004).

52. Alonso-Coello et al., "Drugs for pre-osteoporosis," p. 126.

53. Day, "Lessons from the Women's Health Initiative."

54. S. R. Cummings, "A 55-year-old woman with osteopenia," *Journal of the American Medical Association* **296**(21), (2006), pp. 2602, 2603.

55. D. Marshall, O. Johnell, and H. Wedel, "Meta-analysis of how well measures of bone mineral density predict occurrence of osteoporotic fractures," *British Medical Journal* **312**(7041), (1996), p. 1258.

56. F. Griffiths, "Women's control and choice regarding HRT," *Social Science and Medicine* **49**(4), (1999), p. 470.

57. S. D. Reventlow, L. Hvas, and K. Malterud, "Making the invisible body visible: Bone scans, osteoporosis and women's bodily experiences," *Social Science and Medicine* **62**(11), (2006), pp. 2720, 2721–2723.

58. Ibid., p. 2721.

59. J. Groopman, "The eye of the beholder," in *How Doctors Think* (Houghton Mifflin, Boston, 2007), p. 178.

60. D. M. Eddy, *Clinical Decision Making: From Theory to Practice: A Collection of Essays from the Journal of the American Medical Association* (Jones and Bartlett, Sudbury, MA, 1996).

61. Hadler, *Last Well Person*.

62. D. M. Eddy, "Anatomy of a decision," in *Clinical Decision Making*, pp. 10–17.

63. Hadler, "Turning aging into a disease."

64. Alonso-Coello et al., "Drugs for pre-osteoporosis," p. 128.

65. T. L. N. Jarvinen, H. Sievanen, K. M. Khan, A. Heinonen, and P. Kannus, "Shifting the focus in fracture prevention from osteoporosis to falls," *British Medical Journal* **336**(7636), (2008), p. 125.

66. L. H. Curtis, T. Ostbye, V. Sendersky, S. Hutchison, P. E. Dans, A. Wright, R. L. Woosley, and K. A. Schulman, "Inappropriate prescribing for elderly Americans in a large outpatient population," *Archives of Internal Medicine* **164**(15), (2004), p. 1621.

67. van Keep, "The history and rationale of hormone replacement therapy."

68. M. Elwood, *Critical Appraisal of Epidemiological Studies and Clinical Trials*, 2nd ed. (Oxford Medical, Oxford University Press, Oxford, 1998).

69. K.-A. Phillips, G. Glendon, and J. Knight, "Putting the risk of breast cancer in perspective," *New England Journal of Medicine* **340**, 141–144 (1999).

70. Skolbekken et al., "Brittle bones, pain and fractures."

CHAPTER 7

1. W. Kondro, "Decline in breast cancer since HRT study," *Canadian Medical Association Journal* **176**(2), (2007), p. 160.

2. N. M. Hadler, "Breast Cancer and How the Women's Movement Got it Wrong," in *The Last Well Person: How to Stay Well Despite the Health-Care System* (McGill-Queen's University Press, Montreal, 2004), p. 77.

3. J. Prior, "Ovulatory disturbances: they do matter," *Canadian Journal of Diagnosis* February, 64–80 (1997).

4. P. A. Wingo, P. M. Layde, N. C. Lee, G. Rubin, and H. W. Ory, "The risk of breast cancer in postmenopausal women who have used estrogen replacement therapy," *Journal of the American Medical Association* **257**(2), 209–215 (1987); Writing Group for the Women's Health Initiative Investigators, "Risks and Benefits of Estrogen Plus Progestin in Healthy Postmenopausal Women: Principal Results From the Women's Health Initiative Randomized Controlled Trial," *Journal of the American Medical Association* **288**(3), 321–333 (2002); S. Yusuf and S. Anand, "Hormone replacement therapy: a time for pause," *Canadian Medical Association Journal* **167**(4), 357–359 (2002).

5. C.-L. Chen, N. S. Weiss, P. Newcomb, W. Barlow, and E. White, "Hormone Replacement Therapy in Relation to Breast Cancer," *Journal of the American Medical Association* **287**(6), 734–741 (2002).

6. P. H. Gann and M. Morrow, "Combined Hormone Therapy and Breast Cancer: A Single-Edged Sword," *Journal of the American Medical Association* **289**(24), (2003), p. 3304.

7. J. Cheek, J. Lacy, S. Toth-Fejel, K. Morris, K. Calhoun, and R. F. Pommier, "The Impact of Hormone Replacement Therapy on the Detection and Stage of Breast Cancer," *Archives of Surgery* **137**(9), (2002), p. 1015.

8. Writing Group for the Women's Health Initiative Investigators, "Risks and benefits of estrogen plus progestin."

9. C. I. Li, J. L. Stanford, and J. R. Daling, "Anthropometric variables in relation to risk of breast cancer in middle-aged women," *International Journal of Epidemiology* **29**(2), 208–213 (2000).

10. S. M. Gapstur, M. Morrow, and T. A. Sellers, "Hormone Replacement Therapy and Risk of Breast Cancer with a Favorable Histology: Results of the Iowa Women's Health Study," *Journal of the American Medical Association* **281**(22), 2091–2097 (1999).

11. Chen et al., "Hormone replacement therapy," p. 738.

12. Collaborative Group on Hormonal Factors in Breast Cancer. "Breast cancer and hormone replacement therapy: collaborative reanalysis of data from 51 epidemiological studies of 52,705 women with breast cancer and 108,411 without breast cancer," *Lancet* **350**(9084), 1047–1059 (1997).

13. V. Beral, "Breast cancer and hormone-replacement therapy in the Million Women Study," *Lancet* **362**(9382), 419–427 (2003).

14. G. Anderson, M. Limacher, A. Assaf, T. Bassford, S. Beresford, and H. Black, "Effects of conjugated equine estrogen in postmenopausal women with hysterectomy: The Women's Health Initiative randomized controlled trial," *Journal of the American Medical Association* **291**(14), 1701–1712 (2004).

15. K. L. Noller, "Estrogen Replacement Therapy and Risk of Ovarian Cancer," *Journal of the American Medical Association* **288**(3), 368–369 (2002).

16. N. Kreiger, M. Sloane, M. Cotterchio, and V. Kirsch, "The risk of breast cancer following reproductive surgery," *European Journal of Cancer* **35**, 97–101 (1999).

17. A. Fournier, F. Berrino, and F. Clavel-Chapelon, "Unequal risks for breast cancer associated with different hormone replacement therapies: results from the E3N cohort study," *Breast Cancer Research and Treatment* **107**(1), 103–111 (2008).

18. L. Payer, "United States: The Virus in the Machine," in *Medicine & Culture* (Henry Holt, New York, 1996), pp. 124–152.

19. "Systemic treatment of early breast cancer by hormonal, cytotoxic, or immune therapy. (Early Breast Cancer Trialists' Collaborative Group)," *Lancet* **339**(8784), two articles in series 1–15, 71–85 (1992).

20. S. R. Cummings, S. Eckert, K. A. Krueger, D. Grady, T. J. Powles, J. A. Cauley, L. Norton, T. Nickelsen, N. H. Bjarnason, M. Morrow, M. E. Lippman, D. Black, J. E. Glusman, A. Costa, and V. C. Jordan, "The Effect of Raloxifene on Risk of Breast Cancer in Postmenopausal Women: Results From the MORE Randomized Trial," *Journal of the American Medical Association* **281**(23), 2189–2197 (1999).

21. J. Cauley, F. Lucas, L. Kuller, K. Stone, W. Broner, and S. R. Cummings, "Elevated serum estradiol and testosterone concentrations are associated with a high risk for breast cancer: Study of Osteoporotic Fractures Research Group," *Annals of Internal Medicine* **130**(4 Pt. 1), 270–277 (1999).

22. C. Coulam, J. Annegers, and J. Kranz, "Chronic anovulation syndrome and associated neoplasia," *Obstetrics and Gynecology* **61**, 403–407 (1983); L. Cowan, L. Gordis, J. Tonascia, and G. Jones, "Breast cancer incidence in women with a history of progesterone deficiency," *American Journal of Epidemiology* **114**(2), 209–217 (1981).

23. D. Ferguson and T. Anderson, "Morphological evaluation of all turnover in relation to the menstrual cycle in the 'resting' human breast," *British Journal of Cancer* **44**, 177–181 (1981).

24. K. Chang, T. Lee, G. Linares-Cruz, S. Fournier, and B. de Lignieres, "Influence of percutaneous administration of estradiol and progesterone on human breast epilethial cell cycle in vivo," *Fertility and Sterility* **63**, 785–791 (1995).

25. Cowan et al., "Breast cancer incidence in women."

26. Coulam et al., "Chronic anovulation syndrome."

27. D. L. Sackett, "The arrogance of preventive medicine," *Canadian Medical Association Journal* **167**(4), 363–364 (2002).

28. K.-A. Phillips, G. Glendon, and J. Knight, "Putting the risk of breast cancer in perspective," *New England Journal of Medicine* **340**, 141–144 (1999).

29. H. G. Welch, *Should I Be Tested for Cancer? Maybe Not and Here's Why* (University of California Press, Berkeley, 2004).

30. H. G. Welch, "Your pathologist may say it's cancer, while others say it's not," in *Should I Be Tested for Cancer?*, pp. 90–105.

31. J. Elmore, C. Wells, and C. Lee, "Variability in radiologists' interpretations of mammograms," *New England Journal of Medicine* **331**, 1493–1499 (1994).

32. M. Retsky, R. Demicheli, and W. J. M Hrushesky, "Does surgery induce angiogenesis in breast cancer? Indirect evidence from relapse pattern and mammography paradox," *International Journal of Surgery* **3**(3), 179–187 (2005).

33. P-H. Zahl, J. Maehlen, H. G. Welch, "The Natural History of Invasive Breast Cancers Detected by Screening Mammography," *Archives of Internal Medicine* **168**(21), 2311–2316 (2008).

34. Hadler, "Breast cancer and how the women's movement got it wrong," p. 79.

35. H. G. Welch, "You may rather not know," in *Should I Be Tested for Cancer?*, pp. 66–89.

36. J. Elmore, M. Barton, and V. Moceri, "Ten-year risk of false positive screening mammograms and clinical breast examinations," *New England Journal of Medicine* **338**, 1089–1096 (1998).

37. Welch, "You may rather not know."

38. J. Prior, "Letter from Dr. Kailey Madrona to Dr. Mark Aster," in *Estrogen's Storm Season: Stories of Perimenopause* (CeMCOR, Vancouver, 2005), pp. 214–220.

39. "Breast cancer drug backfires in rare cases," *New Scientist Magazine*, http://www.newscientist.com/.

40. "The controlling interests of research (Editorial)," *Canadian Medical Association Journal* **167**(11), 1221 (2002).

41. R. Moynihan and R. Smith, "Too much medicine?," *British Medical Journal* **324**(7342), 859–860 (2002).

42. A. Miller, C. Baines, T. To, and C. Wall, "Canadian National Breast Screening Study 1. Breast cancer detection and death rates among women aged 40 to 49 years," *Canadian Medical Association Journal* **147**, 1459–1476 (1992); A. Miller, C. Baines, T. To, and C. Wall, "Canadian National Breast Screening Study 2. Breast cancer detection and death rates among women aged 50 to 59 years," *Canadian Medical Association Journal* **147**, 1477–1488 (1992).

43. Hadler, "Breast cancer and how the women's movement got it wrong."

44. Ibid.

45. Ibid.

46. C. J. McDonald, "Medical Heuristics: The Silent Adjudicators of Clinical Practice," *Annals of Internal Medicine* **124**(1 Pt. 1), 56–62 (1996).

47. Hadler, "Breast cancer and how the women's movement got it wrong."

48. K. Malterud, "The art and science of clinical knowledge: evidence beyond measures and numbers," *Lancet* **358**(9279), (2001), p. 398.

49. S. Baxter, "The last word on gender differences," *Psychology Today,* **27**(2), (1994), p. 50.

50. R. Hubbard, *The Politics of Women's Biology* (Rutgers University Press, New Brunswick, NJ, 1990), p. 98.

51. F. S. Greenspan and D. G. Gardner, *Basic and Clinical Endocrinology,* 7th ed. (Lange Medical Books/McGraw-Hill, New York, 2004).

52. E. Martin, *The Woman in the Body: A Cultural Analysis of Reproduction* (Beacon Press, Boston, 1992).

53. G. Irvine, M. Campbell-Brown, M. Lumsden, A. Heikkila, J. Walker, and I. Cameron, "Randomised comparative trial of the levonorgestrel intrauterine system and norethisterone for treatment of idiopathic menorrhagia," *British Journal of Obstetrics and Gynaecology* **105**, 592–598 (1998).

54. E. Friess, H. Tagaya, L. Trachsel, F. Holsboer, and R. Rupprecht, "Progesterone-induced changes in sleep in male subjects," *American Journal of Physiology* **272**, E885–E891 (1997).

55. L. Dennerstein, C. Spencer-Gardner, B. Gotts, J. Brown, and M. Smith, "Progesterone and the premenstrual syndrome: A double blind crossover trial," *British Medical Journal* **290**, 1617–1621 (1985).

56. J. Prior, "Perimenopause: The complex endocrinology of the menopausal transition," *Endocrine Review* **19**, 397–428 (1998).

57. J. Prior, J. Nielsen, C. Hitchcock, L. Williams, Y. Vigna, and C. Dean, "Medroxyprogesterone and conjugated oestrogen are equivalent for hot flushes: A 1-year randomized double-blind trial following premenopausal ovariectomy," *Clinical Science (London)* **112**(10), 517–525 (2007).

58. Fournier et al., "Unequal risks for breast cancer."

59. Collaborative Group on Hormonal Factors and Breast Cancer, "Breast cancer and hormone replacement therapy: Collaborative reanalysis of data from 51 epidemiological studies with 52,705 women with breast cancer and 109,411 without breast cancer," *Lancet* **350**(9084), 1047–1059 (1997).

60. J. L. Thomas and P. A. Braus, "Coronary Artery Disease in Women: A Historical Perspective," *Archives of Internal Medicine* **158**(4), 333–337 (1998).

61. Ibid.

62. A. Knottnerus and G. J. Dinant, "Medicine based evidence, a prerequisite for evidence based," *British Medical Journal* **315**(7116), 1109–1110 (1997).

63. W. A. Silverman, "Hawthorne effects," in *Where's the Evidence? Debates in Modern Medicine* (Oxford University Press, Oxford, 1998), pp. 58–61.

64. Ibid., p. 59.

AFTERWORD

1. G. Greer, *The Whole Woman* (Anchor, London, 1999), p. 134.

2. A. Rich, *The Dream of a Common Language: Poems 1974–77* (W. W. Norton, New York, 1978).

3. J. C. Prior, J. D. Nielsen, C. L. Hitchcock, L. A. Williams, Y. M. Vigna, and C. B. Dean, "Medroxyprogesterone and conjugated oestrogen are equivalent for hot flushes: a 1-year randomized double-blind trial following premenopausal ovariectomy," *Clinical Science (London)* **112**, 517–525 (2007).

4. Ibid.

5. S. Hulley, T. Bush, C. Furberg, D. Herrington, B. Riggs, and E. Vittinghoff, "Randomized trial of estrogen plus progestin for secondary prevention of coronary heart disease in postmenopausal women," *Journal of the American Medical Association* **280**, 605–613 (1998); Writing Group for the Women's Health Initiative Investigators, "Risks and benefits of estrogen plus progestin in health postmenopausal women: Principal results from the Women's Health Initiative randomized control trial," *Journal of the American Medical Association* **288**, 321–333 (2002); G. L. Anderson, M. Limacher, A. R. Assaf, T. Bassford, S. A. Beresford, H. Black, D. Bonds, R. Brunner, R Bruzyski, B. Caan, R. Cheblowski, D. Curb, M. Gass, J. Hayes, G. Heiss, S. Hendrix, R. Jackson, K. C. Johnson, M. J. O'Sullivan, L. Philips, R. L. Prentice, C. Ritenbaugh, J. Robbins, J. E. Rossouw, G. Sarto, M. L. Stefanick, L. Van Horn, J. Wactawski-Wende, R. Wallace, S. Wassertheil-Smoller., "Effects of conjugated equine estrogen in postmenopausal women with hysterectomy: The Women's Health Initiative randomized controlled trial," *Journal of the American Medical Association* **291**, 1701–1712 (2004).

6. D. Grady, "A 60-year-old woman trying to discontinue hormone replacement therapy," *Journal of the American Medical Association* **287**, 2130–2137 (2002).

7. J. C. Prior, "Postmenopausal estrogen therapy and cardiovascular disease (letter)," *New England Journal of Medicine* **326**, 705–706 (1992).

8. A. MacLennan, S. Lester, and V. Moore, "Oral estrogen replacement therapy versus placebo for hot flushes: A systematic review," *Climacteric* **4**, 58–74 (2001).

9. M. C. Klein, J. Kaczorowski, J. M. Robbins, R. J. Gauthier, S. H. Jorgensen, and A. K. Joshi, "Physicians' beliefs and behaviour during a randomized controlled trial of episiotomy: Consequences for women in their care," *Canadian Medical Association Journal* **153**, 769–779 (1995).

10. M. L. Power, J. Baron, and J. Schulkin, "Factors associated with obstetrician-gynecologists' response to the Women's Health Initiative trial of combined hormone therapy," *Medical Decision Making* **28**, 411–418 (2008).

11. P. Y. Scarabin, E. Oger, and Plu-Bureau, "Differential association of oral and transdermal oestrogen-replacement therapy with venous thromboembolism risk," *Lancet* **362**, 428–432 (2003).

12. J. A. Simon, M. M. Shangold, M. C. Andrews, J. C. Buster, and G. D. Hodgen, "Micronized progesterone therapy: The importance of route of administration and pharmacokinetics on clinical outcome," *Journal of Contraception Fertility and Sex* **20**, 13–18 (1992).

13. C. Kirkham, P. M. Hahn, D. A. Van Vugt, J. A. Carmichael, and R. L. Reid, "A randomized, double-blind, placebo-controlled, cross-over trial to assess the side effects of medroxyprogesterone acetate in hormone replacement therapy," *Obstetrics and Gynecology* **78**, 93–97 (1991); J. C. Prior, N. Alojado, D. W. McKay, and Y. M. Vigna, "No adverse effects of medroxyprogesterone treatment without estrogen in postmenopausal women:

Double-blind, placebo-controlled, cross-over trial," *Obstetrics and Gynecology* **83**, 24–28 (1994).

14. J. C. Prior, Y. M. Vigna, S. I. Barr, C. Rexworthy, and B. C. Lentle, "Cyclic medroxyprogesterone treatment increases bone density: A controlled trial in active women with menstrual cycle disturbances," *American Journal of Medicine* **96**, 521–530 (1994).

15. R. Eisler, *The Chalice and the Blade* (HarperCollins, New York, 1987).

16. J. C. Prior, K. Cameron, Y. B. Ho, and J. Thomas, "Menstrual cycle changes with marathon training: Anovulation and short luteal phase," *Canadian Journal of Applied Sport Science* **7**, 173–177 (1982).

17. S. I. Barr, K. C. Janelle, and J. C. Prior, "Vegetarian versus nonvegetarian diets, dietary restraint, and subclinical ovulatory disturbances: Prospective six month study," *American Journal of Clinical Nutrition* **60**, 887–894 (1994).

18. J. C. Prior, "Endocrine 'conditioning' with endurance training: A preliminary review," *Canadian Journal of Applied Sport Science* **7**, 149–157 (1982).

19. J. C. Prior, Y. M. Vigna, N. Alojado, D. Sciarretta, and M. Schulzer, "Conditioning exercise decreases premenstrual symptoms: A prospective controlled six month trial," *Fertility and Sterility* **47**, 402–408 (1987).

20. J. C. Prior, "Progesterone as a bone-trophic hormone," *Endocrine Reviews* **11**, 386–398 (1990).

21. J. C. Prior, Y. M. Vigna, M. T. Schechter, and A. E. Burgess, "Spinal bone loss and ovulatory disturbances," *New England Journal of Medicine* **323**, 1221–1227 (1990).

22. N. Kreiger, A. Tenenhouse, L. Joseph, M. D. Mackenzie, S. Poliquin, J. P. Brown, J. C. Prior, R. S. Rittmaster. "The Canadian Multicentre Osteoporosis Study (CaMos): Background, rationale, methods," *Canadian Journal of Aging* **18**, 376–387 (1999).

23. Prior et al., "Cyclic medroxyprogesterone treatment."

24. R. F. Casper, S. Dodin, R. L. Reid, and study investigators, "The effect of 20 μg ethinyl estradiol/1 mg norethindrone acetate (Minestrin™), a low-dose oral contraceptive, on vaginal bleeding patterns, hot flashes, and quality of life in symptomatic perimenopausal women," *Menopause* **4**, 139–147 (1997).

25. M. Sowers, J. F. Randolph, M. Crutchfield, M. L. Jannausch, B. Shapiro, B. Zhang, M. La Pietra, "Urinary ovarian and gonadotropin hormone levels in premenopausal women with low bone mass," *Journal of Bone and Mineral Research* **13**, 1191–1202 (1998).

26. Ibid.

27. Coronary Drug Project Research Group, "Coronary drug project: initial findings leading to modifications of its research protocol," *Journal of the American Medical Association* **214**, 1303–1313 (1970); Coronary Drug Project Research Group, "Coronary drug project: findings leading to the discontinuation of the 2.5 mg/day estrogen group." *Journal of the American Medical Association* **226**, 652–657 (1973).

28. Prior, "Progesterone as a bone-trophic hormone."

29. Prior et al., "Spinal bone loss and ovulatory disturbances"; Sowers et al., "Urinary ovarian and gonadotropin hormone levels"; E. J. Waugh, J. Polivy, R. Ridout, and G. A. Hawker, "A prospective investigation of the relations among cognitive dietary restraint, subclinical ovulatory disturbances, physical activity, and bone mass in healthy young women," *American Journal of Clinical Nutrition* **86**, 1791–1801 (2007).

30. Prior et al., "Cyclic medroxyprogesterone treatment"; R. Lindsay, J. C. Gallagher, M. Kleerekoper, and J. H. Pickar, "Effect of lower doses of conjugated equine estrogens with and without medroxyprogesterone acetate on bone in early postmenopausal women," *Journal of the American Medical Association* **287**, 2668–2676 (2002).

APPENDIX A

1. J. C. Prior, "Perimenopause: The complex endocrinology of the menopausal transition," *Endocrine Reviews* **19**, 397–428 (1998).

2. M. R. Soules, S. Sherman, E. Parrott, R. Rebar, N. Santoro, W. Utian, and N. Woods, "Executive summary: stages of reproductive aging workshop (STRAW)" *Fertility and Sterility* **76**, 874–878 (2001).

3. J. C. Prior, "The ageing female reproductive axis II: Ovulatory changes with perimenopause," in *Endocrine Facets of Ageing*, D. J. Chadwick and J. A. Goode, eds. (John Wiley, Chichester, UK, 2002), pp. 172–186.

4. J. C. Prior, "Clearing confusion about perimenopause," *British Columbia Medical Journal* **47**, 534–538 (2005).

5. N. Santoro, J. Rosenberg, T. Adel, and J. H. Skurnick, "Characterization of reproductive hormonal dynamics in the perimenopause," *Journal of Clinical Endocrinology and Metabolism* **81**, 1495–1501 (1996); G. E. Hale, X. Zhao, C. L. Hughes, H. G. Burger, D. M. Robertson, and I. S. Fraser, "Endocrine features of menstrual cycles in middle and late reproductive age and the menopausal transition classified according to the Staging of Reproductive Aging Workshop (STRAW) staging system," *Journal of Clinical Endocrinology and Metabolism* **92**, 3060–3067 (2007).

6. Prior, "Perimenopause: The complex endocrinology of the menopausal transition."

7. Santoro et al., "Characterization of reproductive hormonal dynamics"; Prior, "The ageing female reproductive axis II"; Hale et al., "Endocrine features of menstrual cycles."

8. C. Kirschbaum, N. Schommer, I. Federenko, J. Gaab, O. Neumann, M. Oellers, N. Rohleder, A. Untiedt, J. Hanker, "Short-term estradiol treatment enhances pituitary-adrenal axis and sympathetic responses to psychosocial stress in healthy young men," *Journal of Clinical Endocrinology and Metabolism* **81**, 3639–3643 (1996).

9. M. H. Moen, H. Kahn, K. S. Bjerve, and T. B. Halvorsen, "Menometrorrhagia in the perimenopause is associated with increased serum estradiol," *Maturitas* **47**(2), 151–155 (2004).

10. P. A. Kaufert, "The perimenopausal woman and her use of health services," *Maturitas* **2**, 191–205 (1980).

11. A. E. Weel, A. G. Uitterlinden, I. C. Westendorp, H. Burger, S. C. Schuit, A. Hofman, T. J. Helmerhorst, J. P. van Leeuwen, H. A. Pols, "Estrogen receptor polymorphism predicts the onset of natural and surgical menopause," *Journal of Clinical Endocrinology and Metabolism* **84**(9), 3146–3150 (1999); M. Tuppurainen, H. Kroger, S. Saarikoski, R. Honkanen, and E. Alhava, "The effect of gynecological risk factors on lumbar and femoral bone mineral density in peri- and postmenopausal women," *Maturitas* **21**(2), 137–145 (1995).

12. D. J. Brambilla, S. M. McKinlay, C. B. Johannes, H. G. Burger, A. Green, J. Hopper, M. Ryan, "Defining the perimenopause for application in epidemiologic investigations," *American Journal of Epidemiology* **140**(10), 1091–1095 (1994).

13. G. E. Hale, C. L. Hitchcock, L. A. Williams, Y. M. Vigna, and J. C. Prior, "Cyclicity of breast tenderness and night-time vasomotor symptoms in mid-life women: Information collected using the Daily Perimenopause Diary," *Climacteric* **6**(2), 128–139 (2003).

14. L. Dennerstein, E. C. Dudley, J. L. Hopper, J. R. Guthrie, and H. G. Burger, "A prospective population-based study of menopausal symptoms," *Obstetrics and Gynecology* **96**, 351–358 (2000).

15. E. B. Gold, B. Sternfeld, J. L. Kelsey, C. Brown, C. Mouton, N. Reame, L. Salamone, and R. Stellato, "Relation of demographic and lifestyle factors to symptoms in a multi-racial/ethnic population of women 40–55 years of age," *American Journal of Epidemiology* **152**, 463–473 (2000).

16. Dennerstein et al., "A prospective population-based study."

17. Prior, "Perimenopause: The complex endocrinology of the menopausal transition."

18. Ibid.

19. R. F. Casper, S. Dodin, R. L. Reid, and Study Investigators, "The effect of 20 ug ethinyl estradiol/1 mg norethindrone acetate (Minestrin™), a low-dose oral contraceptive, on vaginal bleeding patterns, hot flashes, and quality of life in symptomatic perimenopausal women," *Menopause* **4**, 139–147 (1997).

20. J. C. Prior, Y. M. Vigna, S. I. Barr, C. Rexworthy, and B. C. Lentle, "Cyclic medroxyprogesterone treatment increases bone density: A controlled trial in active women with menstrual cycle disturbances," *American Journal of Medicine* **96**, 521–530 (1994).

21. Ibid.

22. C. Kirkham, P. M. Hahn, D. A. Van Vugt, J. A. Carmichael, and R. L. Reid, "A randomized, double-blind, placebo-controlled, cross-over trial to assess the side effects of medroxyprogesterone acetate in hormone replacement therapy," *Obstetrics and Gynecology* **78**, 93–97 (1991).

23. E. Friess, H. Tagaya, L. Trachsel, F. Holsboer, and R. Rupprecht, "Progesterone-induced changes in sleep in male subjects," *American Journal of Physiology* **272**, E885–E891 (1997).

24. L. Dennerstein, C. Spencer-Gardner, G. Gotts, J. B. Brown, and M. A. Smith, "Progesterone and the premenstrual syndrome: A double blind crossover trial," *British Medical Journal* **290**, 1617–1621 (1985).

25. J. C. Prior, C. Hitchcock, P. Sathi, and M. Tighe, "Walking the talk: Doing science with perimenopausal women and their health care providers," *Journal of Interdisciplinary Feminist Thought* **2**(1), 43–57 (2007).

26. Hale et al., "Cyclicity of breast tenderness and night-time vasomotor symptoms."

27. J. C. Prior, "Ovulatory disturbances: they do matter" *Canadian Journal of Diagnosis*, **February**, 64–80 (1997).

28. Moen et al., "Menometrorrhagia in the perimenopause."

APPENDIX B

1. J. A. Simon, M. M. Shangold, M. C. Andrews, J. C. Buster, and G. D. Hodgen, "Micronized progesterone therapy: The importance of route of administration and pharmacokinetics on clinical outcome," *Journal of Contraception, Fertility and Sex* **20**, 13–18 (1992).

2. H. B. Leonetti, S. Longo, and J. N. Anasti, "Transdermal progesterone cream for vasomotor symptoms and postmenopausal bone loss," *Obstetrics and Gynecology* **94**, 225–228 (1999).

3. J. C. Prior, J. D. Nielsen, C. L. Hitchcock, L. A. Williams, Y. M. Vigna, and C. B. Dean, "Medroxyprogesterone and conjugated oestrogen are equivalent for hot flushes: A 1-year randomized double-blind trial following premenopausal ovariectomy," *Clinical Science (London)* **112**(10), 517–525 (2007).

4. A. Fournier, F. Berrino, and F. Clavel-Chapelon, "Unequal risks for breast cancer associated with different hormone replacement therapies: Results from the E3N cohort study," *Breast Cancer Research and Treatment* **107**(1), 103–111 (2008).

5. E. Friess, H. Tagaya, L. Trachsel, F. Holsboer, and R. Rupprecht, "Progesterone-induced changes in sleep in male subjects," *American Journal of Physiology* **272**, E885–E891 (1997).

6. R. Lindsay, J. C. Gallagher, M. Kleerekoper, and J. H. Pickar, "Effect of lower doses of conjugated equine estrogens with and without medroxyprogesterone acetate on bone in early postmenopausal women," *Journal of the American Medical Association* **287**, 2668–2676 (2002).

7. P. B. Rylance, M. Brincat, K. Lafferty, J. C. De Trafford, S. Brincat, V. Parsons, and J. W. Studd, "Natural progesterone and antihypertensive action," *British Medical Journal* **290**, 13–14 (1985).

8. L. Dennerstein, C. Spencer-Gardner, G. Gotts, J. B. Brown, and M. A. Smith, "Progesterone and the premenstrual syndrome: A double blind crossover trial," *British Medical Journal* **290**, 1617–1621 (1985); B. de Lignieres and M. Vincens, "Differential effects of exogenous oestradiol and progesterone on mood in post-menopausal women: Individual dose/effect relationship," *Maturitas* **4**(1), 67–72 (1982).

9. S. I. Barr, K. C. Janelle, and J. C. Prior, "Energy intakes are higher during the luteal phase of ovulatory menstrual cycles," *American Journal of Clinical Nutrition* **61**, 39–43 (1995).

10. K. J. Mather, E. G. Norman, J. C. Prior, and T. G. Elliott, "Preserved forearm endothelial responses with acute exposure to progesterone: A randomized cross-over trial of 17-b estradiol, progesterone, and 17-b estradiol with progesterone in healthy menopausal women," *Journal of Clinical Endocrinology and Metabolism* **85**, 4644–4649 (2000).

11. N. A. Collop, "Medroxyprogesterone acetate and ethanol-induced exacerbation of obstructive sleep apnea," *Chest* **106**, 792–799 (1994).

12. G. Holzer, E. Riegler, H. Honigsmann, S. Farokhnia, and J. B. Schmidt, "Effects and side-effects of 2% progesterone cream on the skin of peri- and postmenopausal women: Results from a double-blind, vehicle-controlled, randomized study," *British Journal of Dermatology* **153**(3), 626–634 (2005).

13. C. Kirkham, P. M. Hahn, D. A. Van Vugt, J. A. Carmichael, and R. L. Reid, "A randomized, double-blind, placebo-controlled, cross-over trial to assess the side effects of medroxyprogesterone acetate in hormone replacement therapy," *Obstetrics and Gynecology* **78**, 93–97 (1991); J. C. Prior, N. Alojado, D. W. McKay, and Y. M. Vigna, "No adverse effects of medroxyprogesterone treatment without estrogen in postmenopausal women: Double-blind, placebo-controlled, cross-over trial," *Obstetrics and Gynecology* **83**, 24–28 (1994).

14. P. Y. Scarabin, E. Oger, and J. Plu-Bureau, "Differential association of oral and transdermal oestrogen-replacement therapy with venous thromboembolism risk" *Lancet* **362**, 428–432 (2003).

CHAPTER REFERENCES

1. L. Hallberg, A. Hogdahl, L. Nillson, and G. Rybo, "Menstrual blood loss—a population study," *Acta Obstetricia et Gynecologica Scandinavica* **45**, 320–351 (1966).

2. I. Fraser, H. Critchley, M. Munro, and M. Broder, "Can we achieve international agreement on terminologies and definitions used to describe abnormalities of menstrual bleeding?," *Human Reproduction* **22**(3), 635–643 (2007), p. 635.

3. K. Munster, L. Schmidt, and P. Helm, "Length and variation in the menstrual cycle—a cross-sectional study from a Danish county," *British Journal of Obstetrics and Gynaecology* **99**, 422–429 (1992).

4. M. Soules, S. Sherman, E. Parrott, R. Rebar, N. Santoro, and W. Utian, "Executive summary: Stages of reproductive aging workshop (STRAW)," *Fertility and Sterility* **76**, 874–878 (2001).

5. V. Iyer, C. M. Farquhar, and R. Jepson, "Oral contraceptive pills for heavy menstrual bleeding (review)," *Cochrane Library, Oxford* **2**, 1–11 (1997).

6. A. Lethaby, C. Augood, and K. Duckitt, "Nonsteroidal anti-inflammatory drugs for heavy menstrual bleeding," *Cochrane Database of Systematic Reviews*, CD000400 (2002).

7. T. R. Fleming and D. L. DeMets, "Surrogate End Points in Clinical Trials: Are We Being Misled?," *Annals of Internal Medicine* **125**(7), 605–613 (1996).

8. H. C. Bucher, G. H. Guyatt, D. J. Cook, A. Holbrook, F. A. McAlister, and the Evidence-Based Medicine Working Group, "Users' Guides to the Medical Literature: XIX. Applying Clinical Trial Results; A. How to Use an Article Measuring the Effect of an Intervention on Surrogate End Points," *Journal of the American Medical Association* **282**(8), (1999), p. 771.

9. D. Echt, P. Liebson, L. Mitchell, R. Peters, D. Obias-Manno, A. Barker, D. Arensberg, A. Baker, L. Friedman, and H. Greene, "Mortality and morbidity in patients receiving encainide, flecainide, or placebo. The Cardiac Arrhythmia Suppression Trial," *New England Journal of Medicine* **324**(12), 781–788 (1991).

10. E. Lonn, "The use of surrogate endpoints in clinical trials: focus on clinical trials in cardiovascular disease," *Pharmacoepidemiology and Drug Safety* **10**(6), (2001), p. 507.

11. Ibid., p. 498.

12. W. A. Rogers, "Evidence-based medicine in practice: limiting or facilitating patient choice?," *Health Expectations* **5**(2), (2002), p. 97.

13. Fleming and DeMets, "Surrogate end points in clinical trials."

14. K. J. Rothman, *Epidemiology: An Introduction* (Oxford University Press, New York, 2002); M. C. Sutter, "Assigning Causation in Disease: Beyond Koch's Postulates," in *Perspectives in Biology and Medicine* (University of Chicago Press, Chicago, 1996), pp. 581–592.

CHAPTER REFERENCES

CHAPTER 2: CIRCADIAN RHYTHMS, MENSTRUAL CYCLES, AND CULTURE

What amount of menstrual flow is normal? On this score, we have very good data from a 1960s population-based Scandinavian study.[1] Hallberg and colleagues randomly sampled women of different ages in the population, meticulously checking for anemia (meaning a low red blood cell count). He also measured the amount of blood loss during menstruation by analyzing all the used menstrual products from one cycle. He determined, roughly, that one soaked regular-sized tampon or pad holds about 5 mL, or one teaspoon, of blood. The range for normal was enormous, but Hallberg concluded that flow greater than 80 mL (sixteen soaked regular-sized pads or tampons) in any one cycle was too much. He based this decision on the fact that 80 percent of the women whose flow was that heavy had anemia. Therefore, in one menstrual cycle, more than sixteen soaked pads or tampons are too much—that will become very relevant when we talk about perimenopause.

The newest attempt to define normal and what to call the infinite variations within and across menstrual cycles occurred recently and involved "35 clinicians (mostly gynecologists) and scientists" from "relevant international and national organizations, journal editors and individuals" who met in the United States in 2005.[2] This august panel of experts, less than half of whom were women, decided to do away with the old Latin and Greek roots like *poly* and *oligo* for frequency, *rrhagia* for flow, and *metro* for timing. They recommend considering the fifth to the ninety-fifth percentiles of something as the gold standard (but they do *not* define this related to a broad, population-based sample, and in fact, they ignore data from the one modern population-based study of menstrual cycles).[3] Further more, their purpose was to describe cycles in terms of how frequent they are, how regular they are over one year, how long flow lasts, and how these differences are related to the volume of flow. This latest version of normal for menstrual cycles, for example, simply calls it heavy flow and no longer *menorrhagia*. Menstruation can be "frequent" if cycles are shorter than twenty-four days; normal if twenty-four to thirty-eight days; and infrequent (no longer oligomenorrhea) if more than thirty-eight days apart. But the evidence that determines that a cycle may now be as long as thirty-eight days and be normal is not described. In the same vein, a prolonged menstrual flow (period) lasts more than eight days, a normal flow is four and a half to eight days, and a shortened flow is less than four and a half days (in what country and says who?). What is most interesting is that acceptable or normal menstrual cycle variability within one year may change by plus or minus two to plus or minus twenty days. That means that cycles could be forty days different in length in one year in one woman and still be considered normal. On what data is that based? I wonder what these gynecology experts will do about the current guidelines that specify that the "menopausal transition" begins when FSH is high (undefined) and cycles become irregular (meaning variable by more than plus or minus seven days in length)?[4] Experts believe that they, with these definition changes, can answer this question—do various birth control methods change cycle length, flow, and cycle regularity? Amazing.

Women with intrauterine devices tend to have heavier periods and more cramps. And although the Pill is firmly believed to reduce blood loss, the evidence that it is effective in doing this is sparse at best—only one study shows a reduction in flow, and that is a minimal reduction. There is no evidence that the Pill reduces heavy flow in teenagers.[5] However, the Pill is the usual, and often the only, recommendation for women who are flooding every month to the point of anemia. In reality, the over-the-counter pain pill ibuprofen, which does not impose hormones on a woman's menstrual cycles, works just as well at controlling heavy flow.[6]

For menstrual cramps (called *dysmenorrhea* by gynecology), although the Pill does help, if ibuprofen is taken, not every four hours, but to stay ahead of the pain of menstrual cramps,* it is highly effective for more than 95 percent of women. It also decreases the heavy menstrual bleeding by 25 to 40 percent. How does a pain pill help flow? It corrects an imbalance of two fatty acid molecules called *prostaglandins* that work in the endometrium, causing a new constriction of blood vessels. For cramps, ibuprofen literally blocks the *production* of the prostaglandin that makes the muscle of the uterus go into spasm. But because prostaglandins are being produced all of the time within the uterine lining, ibuprofen must be taken *ahead of severe pain* to prevent formation of the prostaglandins, and hence stop the misery.

---

*See "Painful Periods" at http://www.cemcor.ubc.ca/help_yourself/articles/painful_periods.

CHAPTER 5: HEARTS AND MINDS

Surrogate End Points

Conducting research that genuinely answers the broad questions of health and disease is immensely complicated, presents enormous logistical difficulties, and requires time, resources, and infinite creativity—and there are methodological problems as well as issues with long-term patient follow-up, large sample sizes, and diverse and varied patient populations. A common solution, therefore, has been to substitute *surrogate end points* for the targeted benefit: in other words, cardiac or AIDS or cancer drugs are not tested over time by measuring overall morbidity and mortality; rather, biomarkers are used as proxies, substitutes, for long-term well-being. What is measured and studied (and assumed to be a reliable indicator) is blood pressure or cholesterol for heart function; bone density for skeletal strength; CD4 cell counts for HIV-AIDS, tumor shrinkage as a measure of cancer remission; and so on. It is now commonplace to take a laboratory measure and assume that it is an accurate reflection of whatever it is that is being studied.[7] Surrogate end points are assumed to be clinically meaningful end points that measure "directly how a patient feels, functions, or survives."[8]

Only occasionally, for example in the Cardiac Arrhythmia Suppression Trial, which tested drugs that suppressed ventricular arrhythmias, is the real end point—sudden death—studied. (In this case, the hypothesis was that the intervention, drugs, would prevent sudden death after a heart attack. But they did not, and in fact, patients who were on placebo did far better than those in the treatment arm.[9]) There is much debate as to the utility of surrogates, or *biomarkers*, as pharmacologists and statisticians call them; nevertheless most researchers seem to feel that, judiciously used, surrogates "have a definite and important role in the development of new therapies" and, if wisely applied, are vital to biomedical research.[10]

Many decisions about effectiveness are dictated not only by methodological requirements, but are based on various assumptions—with the estimates of a treatment effect of a new therapy under investigation being "extremely variable, with point estimates varying largely based on different assumptions" made for the experimental conditions.[11]

For patients, many of the decisions made during this process result in "a narrowing of focus or judgement" as the question that can reasonably be answered is tailored and reduced to fit the experimental parameters. Researchers, like everyone else, create experiments in which they are likely to observe what they anticipate seeing, and as a result, "both investigators and publishers" tend to enthusiastically report studies in which large treatment effects on surrogates are demonstrated.[12]

Surrogates have had a history of spectacular failures. For instance, as was mentioned earlier, agents that suppressed ventricular arrhythmias (a kind of irregular heartbeat that is associated with an increased risk of heart attack) were assumed to prevent adverse cardiac events, yet the very opposite was found: suppressing arrhythmias was found to *increase* mortality, an unexpected finding that led to many deaths.

Similarly, CD4 cell counts proved useless as a surrogate marker in predicting the development of AIDS, even though they seemed to make sense at the time. In HIV-AIDS, as the virus advances, the quantity of CD4 cells, a subset of immune system T cells, declines. Researchers, therefore, theorized that increasing CD4 cell counts would halt or slow the progression of the disease. Unfortunately, CD4 cell counts turned out to be incidental to the progression of AIDS, as the Concorde Trial in the early 1990s demonstrated. Some 1,749 asymptomatic HIV-positive patients were randomly assigned to receive immediate or deferred treatment with the drug zidovudine (AZT), which was believed to increase CD4 cell counts. One group received the drug as soon as they were diagnosed HIV-positive, the other, after full-blown AIDS had developed. During a three-year follow-up, AZT did indeed slow the decline of CD4 cell counts, as predicted, but not only did the patients' health *not* commensurately improve, but some twenty more patients died in the early treatment group.[13] It is therefore important that as patients we not always trust trials that use surrogate end points as stand-ins for genuine health, such as lipid levels for heart health or bone density measurements for osteoporosis.

CHAPTER 6: THE BASICS OF BONE

Causality

The Nobel laureate Robert Koch (1843–1910), who initially postulated a causal role in tuberculosis for the bacillus he had isolated, proposed that a number of conditions had to be met before a scientist could say that something X caused something Y. Koch's postulates—that to establish cause, several criteria must be present—still resonate. They are as follows:

- The bacilli must be isolated from people (or animals) with the disease in question.
- The bacilli must be grown in pure culture (i.e., outside the organism).
- The bacilli, reintroduced into a different organism, must produce the original disease.

Variants of Koch's postulates have been used in identifying neurotransmitters in cellular function as well as in identifying microorganisms as putative causal agents of disease.[14] Bradford Hill, the statistician who was responsible for the first RCT, proposed a variation on Koch's postulates on causation. Hill's list had nine criteria, with wider applicability than Koch's insofar as they consider more than merely infectious agents. In descending order of importance, these revised postulates follow:

- The relationship must be strong, with greater likelihood the stronger the relationship is.
- The association must show consistency.
- The association must be specific.
- The time course of the relationship must be reasonable.
- There must be a biologic gradient.
- The relationship must evince biologic plausibility.
- It must be coherent.
- There must be evidence from experimentation.
- The relationship must show analogy.

Medical Statistics

Imagine you have just found out that your blood pressure is high, which might be a risk for cardiovascular disease. There is a drug that will reduce this risk, and it has a low incidence of side effects. Consider the following three scenarios. Would you be willing to take the drug for the next five years if results from randomized, placebo-controlled trials showed that:

1. Patients taking this drug for five years have 34 percent fewer heart attacks than patients taking placebo.
2. Of the patients taking this drug for five years, 2.7 percent had a heart attack, compared with 4.1 percent taking a placebo (a difference of 1.4%).
3. If seventy-one patients took this drug for five years, the drug would prevent one from having a heart attack.

Did you make the same decision for all three scenarios? If not, you were fooled by the numbers because all three represent the same data from the same trial presented in three different ways. The first option is the Relative Risk (RR); the second is Absolute Risk (AR), and the last is Numbers Needed to Treat (NNT).

To calculate these numbers, you need the original study data: the total number of patients in the study, how many were assigned to the treatment group, how many to the placebo (control) group, and, in each group, how many "events" there were, in other words, of the total number, how many got better or worse (depending on what the study is looking at). So if a new blood pressure medication is being tested on one hundred people with the goal being to reduce their blood pressure down to 130/80 or lower, the number of events would be the number of people whose blood pressure did in fact go down to the required number.*

Absolute Risk is the number of events in the treated or control group divided by the number of people in that group. So, in the preceding example, if there were two hundred people in the study, with one hundred in the treatment group and one hundred in the control group, and in the treatment group, eighty people had improved blood pressure, the Absolute Risk for the treatment group would be 80/100. The acronyms are as follows:

ARC: the Absolute Risk of the control group

ART: the Absolute Risk of the treatment group

ARR: the Absolute Risk Reduction, which is the ARC minus the ART (ARC − ART)

RR: the Relative Risk, which is the ART divided by the ARC (ART/ARC)

Relative Risk Reduction: the ARC minus the ART divided by the ARC (ARC − ART)/ARC (or the ARR/ARC, the ARR divided by the ARC)

Relative Risk Ratio: 1 − RR (or one minus the ART/ARC; expressed as a percentage, it becomes 1 − RR × 100)

NNT: 1/ARR (one divided by the ARR or 1/ARC − ART)

---

*For more on calculating absolute and relative risk, see http://www.cmaj.ca/cgi/content/full/171/4/353

INDEX

About the Authors

SUSAN BAXTER, PhD, is a medical writer and independent scholar with more than twenty years of experience writing on controversial medical topics, and is a lecturer at Simon Fraser University. Her focus has long been on demystifying complex subjects and providing individuals with solid, useable information that helps them make sound medical decisions. She writes for medical professionals as well as the lay public. Her work has appeared in publications such as *Psychology Today*, *Family Practice*, *Medical Post*, *HealthWatch*, *Lifeline*, and *Easy Living*, among others, and she is the author of several books, including *Immune Power*.

JERILYNN C. PRIOR, MD, is professor of medicine, Division of Endocrinology, at the University of British Columbia. She is founder and scientific director of the Centre for Menstrual Cycle and Ovulation Research, and has authored research published in journals including *The New England Journal of Medicine* and the *Annals of Internal Medicine*. Dr. Prior is a diplomate of the American Board of Internal Medicine and a fellow of the Royal College of Physicians and Surgeons of Canada. As a clinician and researcher, she has treated thousands of women. Dr. Prior has been visiting professor in Canada, Norway, Austria, Australia, and Germany (to name a few), as well as in the United States including at the New York Academy of Sciences, Harvard School of Public Health, and Albert Einstein Medical School. Dr. Prior has long lent her energies to protecting people and the planet and, in 1985, won a Nobel Peace Prize for her work with Physicians for the Prevention of Nuclear War.